NANOTECHNOLOGY TOOLS FOR INFECTION CONTROL

Micro and Nano Technologies Series

NANOTECHNOLOGY TOOLS FOR INFECTION CONTROL

Scanning New Horizons on Next-Generation Therapies to Eradicate Pathogens and Fight Drug Resistance

Edited by

ALESSANDRO POMA
Division of Biomaterials and Tissue Engineering, Eastman Dental Institute, University College London, United Kingdom

LORIS RIZZELLO
University of Milan, Department of Pharmaceutical Sciences (DISFARM), Milan, MI, Italy; The National Institute of Molecular Genetics (INGM), Milan, MI, Italy

ELSEVIER

Elsevier
Radarweg 29, PO Box 211, 1000 AE Amsterdam, Netherlands
125 London Wall, London EC2Y 5AS, United Kingdom
50 Hampshire Street, 5th Floor, Cambridge, MA 02139, United States

ISBN: 978-0-12-823994-0

For information on all Elsevier publications visit our website at
https://www.elsevier.com/books-and-journals

Publisher: Matthew Deans
Acquisitions Editor: Sabrina Webber
Editorial Project Manager: Fernanda Oliveira
Production Project Manager: Sharmila Kirouchenadassou
Cover Designer: Greg Harris

Typeset by TNQ Technologies

Contents

Contributors

Saed Abassi
Center for Nanomedicine at the Wilmer Eye Institute, The Johns Hopkins University School of Medicine, Baltimore, MD, United States

Diana Marcela Castillo
Unidad de Investigación Básica Oral-UIBO, Vicerrectoría de Investigaciones, Facultad de Odontología, Universidad El Bosque, Bogotá, Colombia

Pavani Cherukupally
Schlumberger-Doll Research, One Hampshire St, Cambridge, MA, United States; Department of Mechanical Engineering, Massachusetts Institute of Technology, Cambridge, MA, United States

Charles A. Clifford
Chemical and Biological Sciences Department, National Physical Laboratory, Teddington, United Kingdom

Anjaneyulu Dirisala
Innovation Center of NanoMedicine, Kawasaki Institute of Industrial Promotion, Kawasaki, Japan

Cher Farrugia
Bristol Dental School, University of Bristol, Bristol, United Kingdom; Bristol Dental Hospital, University Hospitals Bristol and Weston, Bristol, United Kingdom

Federico Fenaroli
University of Stavanger, Stavanger, Norway

Jens Gaitzsch
Institute for Macromolecular Chemistry, Leibniz-Institut für Polymerforschung Dresden e.V., Dresden, Germany

Daniel Gonzalez-Carter
Institute for Bioengineering of Catalonia (IBEC), Barcelona Institute for Science and Technology (BIST), Barcelona, Spain

Anna Griego
Department of Pharmaceutical Science, University of Milan, Milan, Italy; National Institute of Molecular Genetic (INGM), Milan, Italy

Junjie Li
Institute for Materials Chemistry and Engineering, Kyushu University, Fukuoka, Japan

Claudio Lourenco
Department of Chemistry, University College London (UCL), London, United Kingdom

Xiaohan Ma
Division of Biomaterials and Tissue Engineering, UCL Eastman Dental Institute, Royal Free Hospital, UCL Medical School, London, United Kingdom

Alessandra M. Martorana
Department of Pharmacological and Biomolecular Sciences, University of Milano, Milano, Italy

Caterina Minelli
Chemical and Biological Sciences Department, National Physical Laboratory, Teddington, United Kingdom

Silvia Moreno
Department of Organic and Inorganic Chemistry, University of Alcalá, Madrid, Spain

Franziska Obst
Institute of Semiconductors and Microsystems, Technische Universität Dresden, Dresden, Germany

S.A. Papadimitriou
Prolepsis Institute of Preventive Medicine Environmental and Occupational Health, Arhens, Greece; Technical Institute of Professional Practice Volos, Volos, Greece; Pharmacy School Aston University, Birmingham, United Kingdom

West Kristian Paraiso
Department of Basic Sciences, Faculty of Medicine and Health Sciences, Universitat Internacional de Catalunya, Barcelona, Spain

Yiwen Pei
Chemical and Biological Sciences Department, National Physical Laboratory, Teddington, United Kingdom

Alessandra Polissi
Department of Pharmacological and Biomolecular Sciences, University of Milano, Milano, Italy

Alessandro Poma
Division of Biomaterials and Tissue Engineering, UCL Eastman Dental Institute, Royal Free Hospital, UCL Medical School, London, United Kingdom

Loris Rizzello
Department of Pharmaceutical Sciences (DISFARM), University of Milan, Milan, MI, Italy; The National Institute of Molecular Genetics (INGM), Milan, MI, Italy

Maja Sabalic-Schoener
The ADA Forsyth Institute, Cambridge, MA, United States; Unit of Periodontology, UCL Eastman Dental Institute, London, United Kingdom

G. Saito
Formerly at GSK R&D, Stevenage, United Kingdom

Paola Sperandeo
Department of Pharmacological and Biomolecular Sciences, University of Milano, Milano, Italy

Theofilus A. Tockary
Innovation Center of NanoMedicine, Kawasaki Institute of Industrial Promotion, Kawasaki, Japan

1

Introduction

We are living a time where we believe antibiotics are the cornerstone for designing any infectious disease-based therapy. It is definitely out of question that antibiotics saved millions of people worldwide in the last century, and they still keep doing it very efficiently. Nevertheless, their extensive abuse, especially for veterinary applications, contributed to the rise of antimicrobial resistance. This latter is unanimously considered as one of the biggest threats in the current human history because it is estimated that the majority of the antibiotics, currently used in the clinics, will be completely ineffective for the eradication of infectious diseases. This has been defined as 'The New Dark Ages of Antibiotics', which is expected to start in the next decades if no actions will be taken now.

The COVID-19 outbreak, and the dramatic outcome in terms of human fatalities, further corroborated the hypothesis that new therapeutic strategies must be explored to treat infectious diseases. This is not just limited to viruses or bacteria. To provide an example, there are fungal species such as *Candida krusei* and *Candida auris* which represent a serious threat in terms of multidrug-resistant organism. An original perspective is provided by the continuously evolving pathways of nanotechnology. After no more than a few decades, when inorganic nanoparticles have seen their first dawn, we have indeed now engineered processes where nanomaterials are controlled at atomist level with unprecedented precision. New data and technologies are acquired daily, and new insight into well-studied processes come on a scale measured in weeks or months rather than years. Inevitably, this led to an exponential growth of application of the tools provided by nanotechnology to the broadest possible biomedical fields. Among these, the treatment of infectious diseases represents one of the most explored. Nanoparticles of highly controlled physicochemical properties, nanostructured substrates and responsive nano-gels are only very restricted examples of what is now tested in the perspective of finding a solution to the current and future potential pandemics, as well as for counteracting the rise in antimicrobial resistance.

Nanotechnology Tools for Infection Control. https://doi.org/10.1016/B978-0-12-823994-0.00006-2

This book is aimed at advanced students in biology, biotechnology and nanotechnology. In order to provide the most current understanding of the rapidly changing subject, we have gathered leading scientists to give a fresh and new vision to the topic, adopting their high expertise in the discipline they belong to. This book starts by 'framing' the main problem, namely what are the reasons behind the current continuous drying-up of new antibiotics released in the market. There is also a dedicated focus on the basic principles of antimicrobial resistance, the causes of it and how to potentially face the problem. Then, we provide the readers with up-to-date knowledge on the chemical strategies to assemble nanoparticles. To this respect, a whole chapter is also dedicated on the procedures adopted by international authorities to characterise nanoparticles in the most standardised way. Then, the attention is shifted towards the biological application of them, and particular attention is given to the body- and cellular distribution of nanoparticles. This is of critical importance for a clinical translation of any nanotechnology-based material. In this framework, there is also a dedicated chapter on assessing what are the best pre-clinical models to assess the safety of nanoparticles for next clinical use.

Throughout the text, we have extensively relied upon the most recent published works, without forgetting the 'back to basics' to calling back the most important milestones in the rise and development of specific subjects.

With this in mind, we truly hope that the readers will find this book informative, interesting and potentially inspiring to understand how something so small such a nanoparticle could have such a massive effect when it comes to moving towards the control of infections.

By Loris Rizzello and Alessandro Poma.

2

The significant drain in antimicrobial discovery by pharma companies

G. Saito[1] and S.A. Papadimitriou[2,3,4]

[1] *Formerly at GSK R&D, Stevenage, United Kingdom;* [2] *Prolepsis Institute of Preventive Medicine Environmental and Occupational Health, Arhens, Greece;* [3] *Technical Institute of Professional Practice Volos, Volos, Greece;* [4] *Pharmacy School Aston University, Birmingham, United Kingdom*

Summary

1. Introduction and historical background

Since the complete chemical synthesis of antimicrobials was pioneered by Paul Ehrlich more than a century ago [1], chemistry has always been crucial in the quest to find new antibacterials. Historically, discovery and development led by private pharmaceutical companies on natural, semisynthetic and synthetic molecules witnessed a 'golden period' during the 1940 to early 1960s [2].

A number of renowned holding-operating and pharmaceutical companies – Abbott, American Cyanamid (Lederle), Bristol-Myers, Eli Lilly, LEO Pharma, Merck and Pfizer amongst others – made profits as a result of large empirical screenings on natural antibiotics. As an example, up to one million antibiotic-producing strains were isolated by Abbott in 3 decades [3].

Nanotechnology Tools for Infection Control. https://doi.org/10.1016/B978-0-12-823994-0.00010-4

During World War II, the production of large quantities of penicillin became a primary need and one of the challenges pharmaceutical companies faced was to successfully bring to life some sustainable strategies for purification and scalability of antibiotics.

Pfizer succeeded in advancing the implementation of deep-tank fermentation techniques, becoming the very first supplier of this drug to the US army [4]. By 1945, 19 companies were producing penicillin in the United States [5] and prices fell from 20 dollars to 20 cents per 100,000 units during this time [6].

Boosted by the worldwide conflict, common needs and profit, scientific innovation in the field was – for the first time – driven by a joint effort of governments, pharmaceutical companies and academic scientists being part of the Penicillin Project [5,7]. Whilst chemical synthesis was not fully pursued yet [8] and American companies feared that they were wasting resources on this infant science, re-evaluation of post-war advances in synthetic approaches made a fully synthetic route accessible to penicillins only. Merck and Squibb, followed by Abbot, Hoffman-La Roche, Lilly, Parke-Davis, Pfizer, Upjohn and Wyeth were all active in this risky but profitable field [9]. Supported by Bristol company, the first non-natural fully synthetic analogue compound bearing the β-lactam or 4-membered cyclic amide function was obtained [7,10]. With such result, the synthetic race to antibiotic drugs had begun.

Synthetic programmes on penicillin salts and esters [11], p-aminosalicylic acid (PAS) derivatives [12], and sulfonamide derivatives [13] were increasing in the area. However, in the 1960s market was saturated [2]. In the 1970s, Bayer regained market shares with its three programmes on antifungals, β-lactam antibiotics and actinomycetes [14] but could not escape from the overall crisis of anti-infective drug development from the 1970s on, for which the underlying causes will be analysed in the following sections. From the 1990s, despite this half-century of success, the focus shifted on fighting antimicrobial resistance (AMR), which quickly became the primary target [15,16].

2. Challenges and role of drugmakers

Antimicrobials in general, and their extended use in particular, which creates resistance, are presently one of the most serious battles we face worldwide. The ability of microorganisms to resist antimicrobial treatments has a direct impact on the level of public health and consequently carries a heavy economic burden.

In accordance with European Centre for Disease Prevention and Control (ECDC) and a new study by World Health

Organisation (WHO) Europe and ECDC that examines variations in antibiotic consumptions in European countries, it is estimated that about 33,000 deaths are attributable to infections with antibiotic-resistant bacteria annually in the European Union/European Economic Area, and 700,000 globally. In the United States alone, an estimated 23,000 deaths each year are associated with drug-resistant bacterial infections [17].

Microbes possess by nature the ability to replicate fast and mutate rapidly, giving them by default the advantage of AMR per se at some point. Nevertheless, it is safe to state that antibiotics are not the ones to blame for AMR.

Clinicians do play a significant role. Based on the European CDC information in hospital treatment on any given day, one in three patients received at least one antimicrobial. Some of these prescriptions may be unnecessary.

The agricultural sector may have also played a role in the problem. Veterinary use of antimicrobials for promotion of animal growth with sub-therapeutic doses can foster resistance.

Inadequate treatment of the pharmaceutical effluent, with a mix of concentrated antibiotics and antibiotic resistance genes, are also responsible for the spread of AMR [18].

The challenge of AMR is indeed an enduring threat that likely will never be eliminated [19]. The internationally recognised response to AMR advocates for a 'One Health' approach, which requires policies to be developed and implemented across human, animal, and environmental health [20]. Though ensuring prudent antimicrobial use is a key priority in an effective response to AMR, alongside comes the interest of the industry for new pharmaceutically active molecules with antibiotic characteristics as well as new techniques, technologies and devices targeting AMR.

Back to the science behind antimicrobials, Richard Smith, a health economist at the University of Exeter, said that profit is basically volume multiplied by price. For antibiotics, neither element is high enough to offset the cost of development [21].

As the global scenario has changed, bottlenecks in antimicrobials development remained, therefore the role drug-makers should play nowadays needs to differ from the past. Antibiotic discovery platforms (amongst which Waksman-platform was successful for over 40 years) [22] declined as result of costs of research and development (R&D) and big financial risks irrespective of the drug candidate. As a result, the pipeline dried up and this approach was abandoned [23]. Of the >20 pharmaceutical players active in the field in 1980s, only a handful of research-focussed pharmaceutical companies remain engaged in the

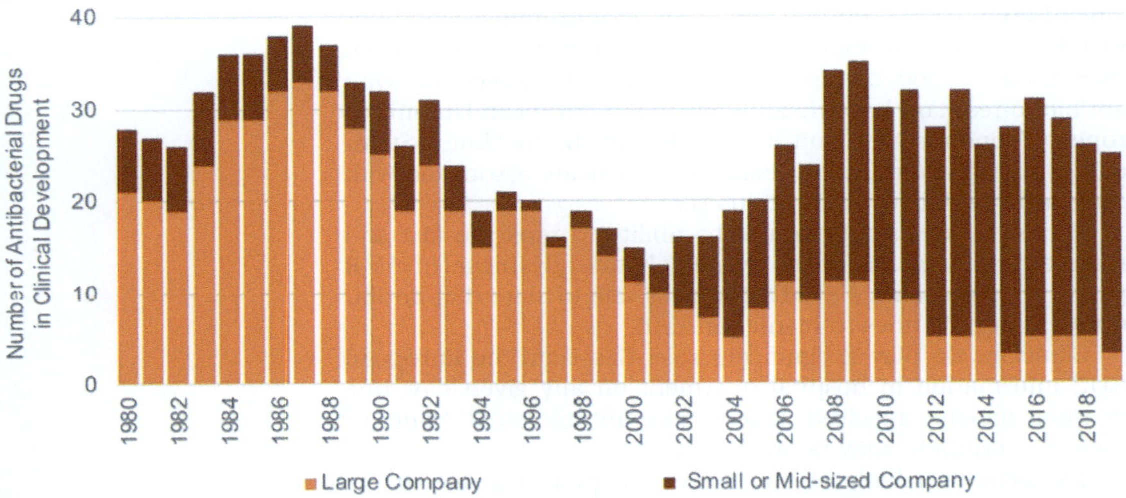

Figure 2.1 Evolution of number of antimicrobials by large and small or midsized companies. Reproduced with permission from Ref. [24].

development of antibiotics [24], and the spectrum of players engaged is continuously changing, as Fig. 2.1 shows.

With 'hightech' approaches recently explored to create new platforms and shift the 'cost result' paradigm, research groups in pharmaceutical companies focussed on alternative, innovative and promising approaches (see section 3.1) to boost a new era in antimicrobial discovery [25].

We will now revise in more details the journey through the development platforms pharmaceutical industry encountered since mid of the past century.

3. Quest for antimicrobial drug design

The transition from a factory system (i.e. screening programmes for new molecules) to industrialised research was a process that took years to complete [26], and the quest for more accessible production methods and scalability did not come without challenges.

The perceived constraints to enable a continuous development of antimicrobial drugs lied on molecular size and complexity, low toxicity profiles, specific biological targets, and scalability. Furthermore, compared to other drugs, antibiotics are effective in concentrations that are two to four magnitudes higher than other molecules affecting distinct molecular targets

[27]. Therefore, specific and highly potent molecules were the ideal candidates.

Starting with Merck focussing on the development of semisynthetic antibacterials obtained by catalytic hydrogenation of streptomycin [28], also Pfizer focussed on development of Terramycin, a derivative of six membered ring of tetracycline being among the first 'broad spectrum' antibiotics, and proved semisynthetic approach had some benefits.

Semisynthesis of β-lactams and chemical rearrangements were obtained by Eli Lilly on cephalosporins in the 1960s, followed by positive pharmacological outcomes [29]. The same approach led to the improved stability and bioavailability of erythromycin (azalide structure), amongst the most prescribed drugs in United States a decade ago.

Despite having opened a number of interesting possibilities to access improved molecules within the major families of natural antibiotics, this was not enough – except for a few cases – to deploy successful clinical candidates. Hence, in parallel, a fully synthetic approach was explored to cut costs and incorporate processes for scale ups.

Along with the non trivial mission, the thalidomide scandal that occurred in 1961 triggered new and stricter regulations including proof of efficacy, purity and safety.

Thalidomide, a drug developed by the German company Grünenthal and taken by pregnant women to alleviate morning sickness, was marketed in the 1950 and 1960s.

By the time it was belatedly pulled from the market because it was causing serious malformations and miscarriages, the drug had been distributed in 50 countries under 40 trade names.

It is widely believed that as many as 100,000 babies were affected by the drug in total. It is generally estimated that some 20,000 babies – the majority of them European – were born worldwide with seriously malformed limbs and today fewer than 3000 survive [30].

All of this translated in massive increase in costs of research and development and clinical testing, putting additional constraint [31].

Medicinal chemists restlessly worked to identify full synthetic routes aiming to access novel antimicrobials. In their hands was the ability to incorporate new chemical elements in the key structures of the active molecules known at the time. This investigative effort opened up to the possibility for enterprises to screen the potency and safety of an increased number of chemical entities and eventually finely tune their physicochemical properties. If we considered the 'List of Essential Medicine', some of the most widely used drugs – chloramphenicol, trimethoprim, fosfomycin, and some quinolones – were then manufactured using this fully synthetic approach.

New classes of antibiotics, such as a synthetic oxazolidinone, emerged from research led by DuPont. More recently, Merck succeeded in the fully synthetic modification of tetracycline – the structure of which was firstly elucidated back in 1953 – to yield 6-thiotetracycline. Investments in the development of this candidate however ceased at a clinical stage due to adverse effects on the liver.

Regardless the class of antibiotics, access to bulk production at large scale allowed for reducing costs and achieving a higher level of access to medicines.

As an example, β-lactams catalysed the attention in 1980s and 1990s due to elucidation of the full chemical synthesis (condensation) of their ring. In the early 2000s, at a time when AMR was not as impactful as nowadays, the annual market for this class of antibiotics was approximately $15 billion of USD (~$9.9 bn for cephalosporin alone), which accounted for up to 65% of the total antibiotics market [32,33].

Whereas the effort of multinational drug developers was hitting a 'hard spot', smaller pharmaceutical and biotechnology companies, which differentiated the knowledge and contributed to the development of some promising candidates, were rising [34].

As per earlier development, the almost infinite possibilities offered by synthetic manufacturing capability eventually collided with the saturation of effective molecules and suitability of known targets. But, with AMR on the rise, only few groups of antibacterial agents (i.e. oxazolidinones, pleuromutilins, tiacumicins, diarylquinolines, lipopeptides and streptogramins) have been marketed in the last 4 decades and most of them are specific for treatment of Gram-positive bacterial infections [35]. Fig. 2.2 shows the chemical structures of the main antimicrobials discussed in this chapter.

3.1 Few weapons against a bigger challenge: AMR

The large majority of marketed antibacterials have been targeted against the bacterial cell wall or macromolecular biosynthesis (DNA, RNA or protein). As mentioned, pathogens resistant to currently available treatments – as a result of use and abuse of antibiotics – claim human lives and are expected

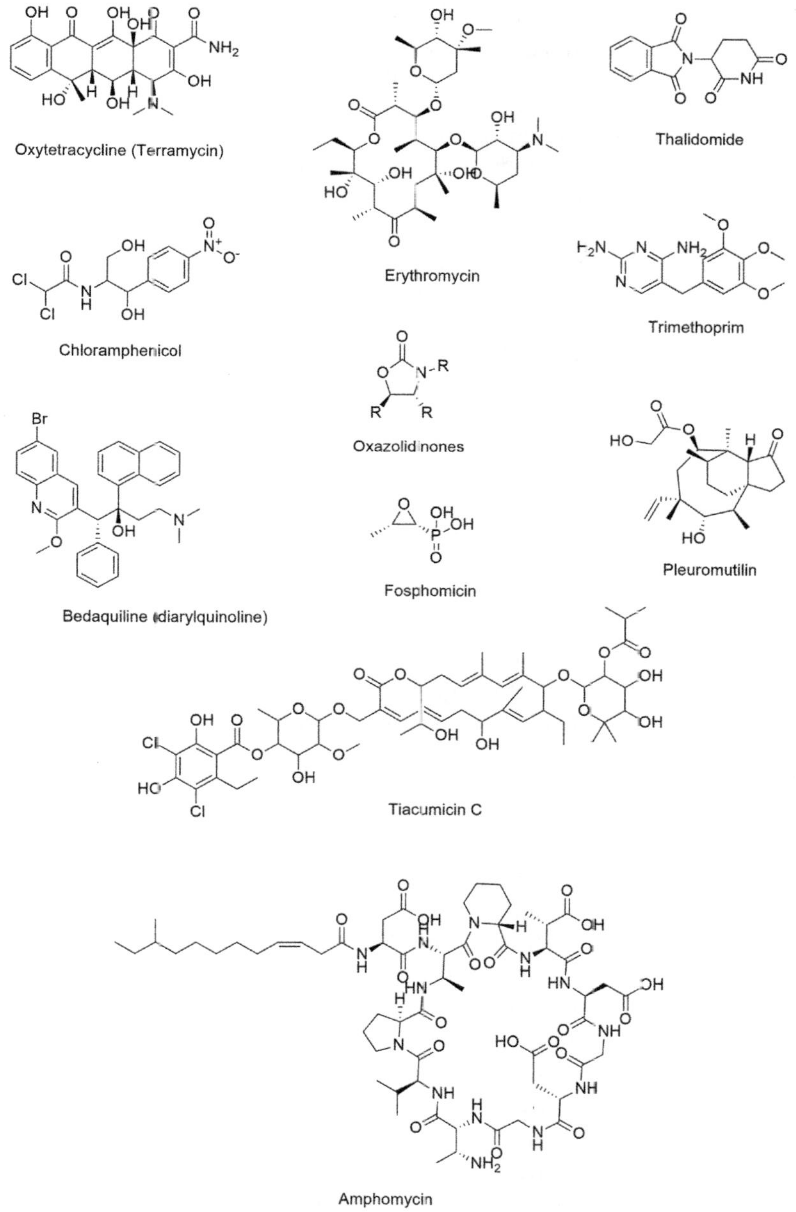

Figure 2.2 Chemical structures of the main antimicrobials.

to cost 100 billion USD by 2050 [36]. Conventional strategies – semisynthesis, chemical modification of known antimicrobials, potentiation of activity of known compounds, hybrid agents – were eventually considered not adequate anymore. Structural modifications did not fundamentally change molecular interaction with their target, which resulted in not having a direct and effective antimicrobial therapy. Moreover, this reflected in poor management of the rising AMR tide, being these drugs not suitable to stem it.

With the sequencing of the first complete bacterial genome (1995), emerging technologies in the 1990s were indicated as perhaps the only way to stop the derailing course of events, and big pharmaceutical players explored this potential since their inception.

Moving away from the earlier antibiotic producing cultures/strains screening approach, the introduction of high throughput screening (HTS) methods, followed by both combinatorial chemistry approaches based on generation of chemical libraries, rational drug design (RDD) and artificial intelligence (AI), altogether pushed the field into a new and promising development phase.

We briefly dive into the benefits these strategies brought to the market through industry.

- **High throughput screening:** with HTS, assay speed far outpaced the rate of compound supply and, for the first time, it enabled the creation of high affinity low molecular weight ligands of the therapeutically significant molecular targets of human cells.

  In a review dated 2007 by a group of scientists at GSK, Payne et al. highlighted that 63 target based and 3 whole cell based HTS R&D campaigns were performed internally (1995–2001) involving thousands of molecules screened. However, the poor outcome was of only five leads delivered [37]. A total of 34 other companies active in the field performed in excess of 125 screens (1996–2004) on 60 targets, with no molecules hitting the pipeline [38]. Despite the lack of fortune alone, HTS fuelled the birth of combinatorial chemistry.
- **Combinatorial chemistry:** diverse synthetic compound libraries and HTS were not enough. As much as rational this approach was, serendipity could not stem the need to search for quality drugs as preference to vast quantity of possible candidates. Chemical reactions on immobilised resins were already being developed. The purpose was straightforward, and industry liked it: to create new molecular entities that

can be patented, proven in trials, and developed into marketable therapies. This innovation might have had and still may imply cutting costs for development, having in turn better candidates and leads. It was a strategic decision and highlights the reasons as to why natural products came back into fashion. A more logical and focussed screening process aimed at replacing the above libraries with smaller, targeted libraries. Pfizer, for instance, was operating 'under clear marching orders to accelerate leads' – for different drug families – 'into pipelines more efficiently' according to Bryan Koontz (cofounder of Optive Research and Tripos' vice president of corporate development) [39].

The preparation and screening of combinatorial libraries, biased (class of molecular target known) and unbiased (target unknown), became a hot topic in drug research at that time. GlaxoWellcome (now GSK), SmithKlineFrench, and Pfizer, whose product portfolio was predominantly based on synthetic drugs, eventually phased out natural product screening altogether [40]. Collections of natural products were disposed of by drug giants and made again accessible from specialist suppliers through fee or via risk and profit sharing agreements. By 1997, Eli Lilly already used combinatorial technologies in over 75% research programmes including infectious disease; Abbott, starting in 1994, covered 80% of its drug discovery programmes with combinatorial chemistry in 1998; Bayer was involved only in 1995, while SmithKline Beecham filed its first combinatorial patent with University of Pennsylvania in 1992 [41–43].

Yet, by 2000, large pharmaceutical firms could be accounted for 65.5% of all combinatorial libraries synthesised by industrial players, up to 76% if considering those obtained by acquisitions of small biotech companies specialised in the field. Very few results, however, were obtained in the development of novel broad spectrum antimicrobials, despite substantial financial and material investments were made. The fact that all the available technologies were used, as well as the use of good computational design was deployed – intended to have significant impact on the identification of the 'best' library members – was not enough [37,44].

- **Artificial intelligence:**

  In the last decade, moving away from quantitative structure to activity relationships (QSAR), researchers called for more sophisticated approaches to be pursued. Big data analysis and

AI applied to antibiotic resistance became promising allies after Stokes and colleagues at the Massachusetts Institute of Technology (MIT) set a milestone by training an AI system which flagged a structurally new molecule – called halicin – from scratch, capable to kill 35 of the world's most problematic disease causing bacteria, including multiresistant strains [45]. In the field of antimicrobial peptides (AMPs) – to which bacteria have probably been exposed to for millions of years and no widespread resistance has been reported – AI aims at detecting more effective and broad spectrum, non toxic sequences with optimal pharmacokinetics and selectivity profiles [46,47].

Away from academia, by 2020 a total of 30 pharmaceutical corporations were applying AI for drug discovery, pointing at delivering '4P' medicine (predictive, preventive, personalised and participatory) [48]. However, only five start ups (Acurx Pharmaceuticals, Arixa Pharmaceuticals, AGILbiotics, Geom Therapeutics and Clemedi) are currently focussing on AMR [49].

Both the Antimicrobial Resistance Benchmark 2020 and 2021 help understanding the progress made by pharma companies in the R&D environment, clinical pipeline and approved drugs (Figs. 2.3 and 2.4) [50,51].

Approximately 100 types of antibiotics have been discovered following to the development of microbiology, biochemistry and organic chemistry. Unfortunately, to date, the low ability of bacterial cell wall penetration did not enable access to their targets, resulting in an unsatisfactory spectrum of activity, with very few exceptions. Due to resistance, most of them have been gradually decreased in usage.

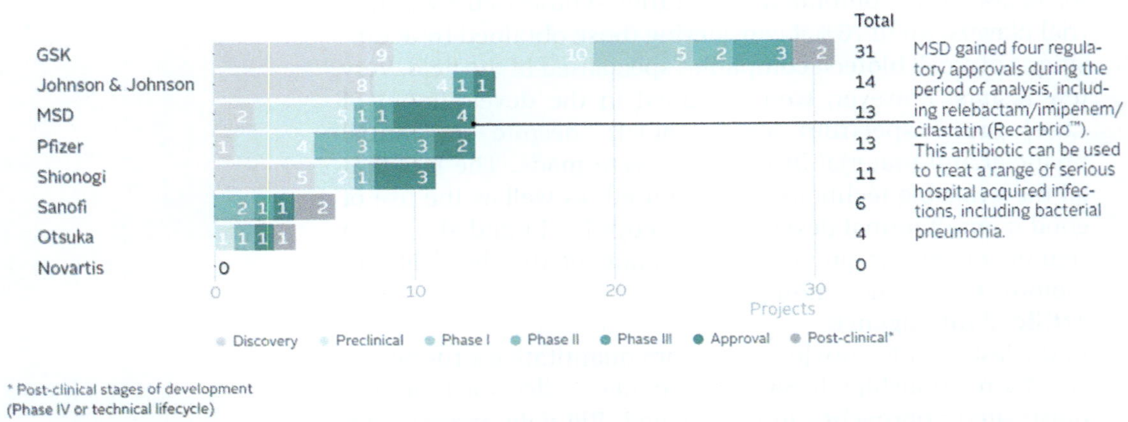

Figure 2.3 Pipelines by large antimicrobial drug developers. Reproduced with permission from Ref. [51].

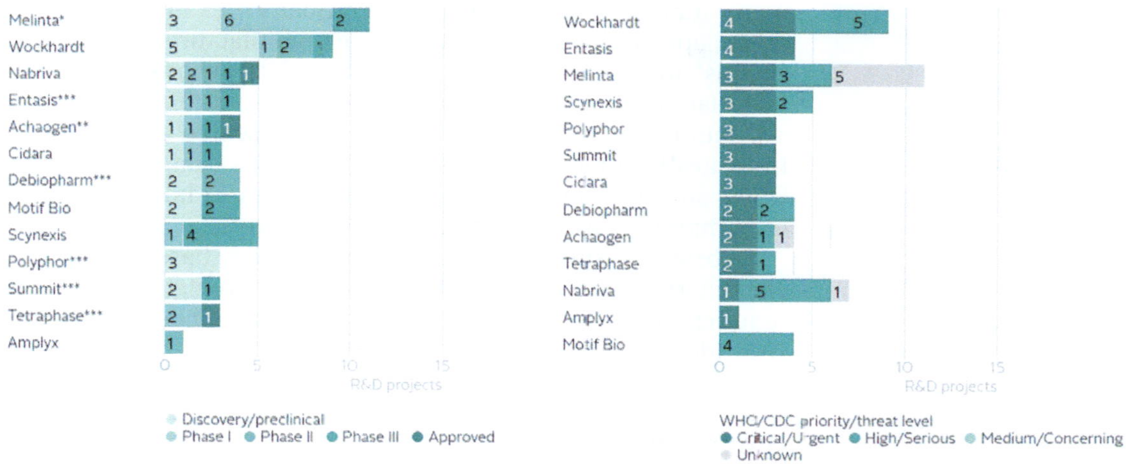

Figure 2.4 Pipelines by medium to small antimicrobial drug developer. Reproduced with permission from Ref. [50].

4. Pharmaceutical development in a 'green way'

Superbugs spread has been attributed in part to insufficient attention to management of pharmaceutical manufacturing waste. Considering that antimicrobial drugs are often prepared through synthetic chemistry with process scale up reaching tonnes amounts per year, overall process yield is known as one of the bottlenecks of the entire circus. As a consequence, the waste to product ratio has been extremely high. Calls for the incorporation of environmental considerations in International Council for Harmonisation of Technical Requirements for Pharmaceuticals for Human Use (ICH) good manufacturing practice (GMP) guidelines date back to 2007. In recent years there have been many suggestions towards the pharmaceutical industry to start introducing methods for preparation and production of 'green' pharmaceuticals [52,53].

Since 1987, there have been no new classes of antibiotics discovered for industrial production and the main industrial production techniques remain fermentation, semisynthesis and synthesis. In recent years, there has been a drive in the pharmaceutical industry to produce an active pharmaceutical ingredient (API) with a minimum amount of waste, progress has been made by industry committed to guidelines by AMR Industry Alliance. The successful story of Sitagliptin, manufactured at scale via enzymatic process by Merck, has further inspired many innovative pharmaceutical companies to integrate enzymatic approaches in the respective manufacturing processes. GSK is an example, since it invested $60 millions in greener manufacturing at Singapore amoxicillin plant in 2015. Novartis itself shut down antibacterial and antiviral research at its Novartis Institutes for Biomedical Research campus in California in 2018, whilst shortly after it invested about €150 m to improve antibiotics manufacturing at a Novartis plant in Austria [54,55].

Substantial shifting is ongoing from batch based operation, characterised by (i) a complex process flow, (ii) high consumable requirements, and (iii) mediocre yield, towards a continuous process. Ideally, a process producing no liquid waste (that had been in contact with antibiotics) would significantly limit and potentially halt the spread of AMR in industrial and urban environments.

More stringent guidelines have been provided by regulatory agencies US Food and Drug Administration (FDA) and European Medicines Agency (EMA) regarding the need for evaluation and mitigation of environmental impact whilst developing antibiotics [56]. The development of antibiotics is no longer considered an economically sensible investment for the pharmaceutical industry as antibiotics are used for relatively short periods of time, unlike drugs used to treat chronic diseases; the development costs of the latter are, among other things, much lower than those of antibiotics.

5. New technologies, devices for diagnostics and toxicology

Nowadays more than ever, in a world which faced a recent COVID pandemic while more are expected in the years to come, the need of innovative tools in early diagnosis and treatment of AMR is becoming a prerequisite. New tools in regards with self testing or massive testing and treatment of populations are the target. These tools can be used towards two different directions. Either preventive, for surveillance and potential detection of outbreaks that will help systems in achieving a quick response. Alternatively, therapeutic, tools that can be easily used to guide or change the clinical decision making for clinical therapies to be provided (i.e. diagnostic tool can quickly distinguish between viral and bacterial aetiologies of respiratory illness). Real time PCR plays a significant role as relatively quick, since within a few hours it is possible for the strain of the microbe to be identified and a targeted therapy with a particular antimicrobial to be prescribed.

5.1 Start-ups in the field of antimicrobial synthesis

In the area of the new antimicrobials as treatments, a number of start up companies have emerged worldwide during the last years, with the aim to synthesise new molecules as antimicrobials, or repurposing of already existing molecules in different directions. To the best of our knowledge, only one company is currently targeting the creation of specific diagnostic tools for clinicians [57].

Globally, there are 289 anti bacterial drugs companies, and here is the list of the 15 most interesting and most promising ones based on advanced preclinical/clinical phase and disruptive potential of their platform. Each one of them usually focusses either on a specific antimicrobial and potential changes on the chemical structure or on a certain disease (Table 2.1).

Although the research is strong and ongoing, it seems that almost 50% of the products manufactured by the abovementioned start ups manage to move to clinical trials, confirming the high value of the platforms introduced. Though less than 7% of the visualised products manage to move to market.

5.2 Start ups active in the field of microfluidics/ organ on a chip for diagnostics in antimicrobial and AMR

As nanotechnology products are starting now to have a strong presence in the global market with the term of nanomedicine, new tools and start up companies arise based on microfluidics/ organ on a chip approach, some of which are also using nanotechnology, and aim to meet the urgent global need for precision results in AMR testing. An organ on a chip is a microfluidic cell culture device created with microchip manufacturing methods, which contains continuously perfused chamber(s) inhabited by living cells arranged to simulate tissue level or organ level physiology [58].

Three groups of start up companies are of interest in the field, which use microfluidics and lab on a chip technologies as

- Associated with AI to design or identify new pharmaceutically active molecules;
- Diagnostic tools from general public;
- To design applications for point of care situation of recognising the presence of a microbe or tackling and finding potential solutions to patients affected by resistant microbe strains [59].

Some of the most interesting start ups worth highlighting – based on innovative approach, focus on unmet needs, capability

Table 2.1 Start-ups landscape in antimicrobial field.

Company	Target project	Product	Market
Arixa Pharmaceuticals	Oral antibiotics for gram-negative infections	Compound *AV-006/ARX-1796*, a proprietary prodrug of Avibactam	Currently in clinical trials
Acurx Pharmaceuticals	Antibiotics for *C. difficile* infections (CDI)	*Ibezapolstat* For the treatment of clostridium difficile infections. The antibiotic blocks the Pol 3IIIC enzymes in streptococcal, staphylococcal, and enterococcal infections	
AGILeBiotics	Novel antibiotics for the treatment of hospital-acquired infections (ventilator pneumonia, bloodstream infections, and neonatal sepsis)	*Toframicin*	Preclinical development and is already delivering in vitro results
Geom Therapeutics	Multidrug resistant (MDR) bacterial infections	*GT-1*, a novel cephalosporin class antibiotic	
Clemedi	Diagnostics for multi drug resistance. Optimal antibiotic therapies, for sexually transmitted infections and diseases	Artificial intelligence (AI) and next-generation sequencing, this in-vitro diagnostic test detects 13 pathogens and other resistance markers from a patient's sample	
Paratek Pharmaceuticals	Discovery and development of new class of antibiotics to treat bacterial infections	Omadacycline Sarecycline Once-daily oral tetracycline-derived compound for the potential treatment of acne and rosacea	Phase 3
Locus Biosciences	Early-stage biotech that uses reprogrammed CRISPR-Cas3 to develop antimicrobials against diseases that are increasingly resistant to antibiotics	Locus Biosciences uses the CRISPR-cas3 system to create custom CRISPRs and associated type-I Cas proteins that will cause the bacteria to self-destruct	

Table 2.1 Start-ups landscape in antimicrobial field.—*continued*

Company	Target project	Product	Market
Symbiomix	Focussed on developing treatments for prevalent gynaecological infections	Solosec (secnidazole in oral granules form), a 5-nitroimidazole antibiotic, is anticipated to be the first and only single-dose oral treatment approved for bacterial vaginosis (BV)	Solosec has been designated a Qualified Infectious Disease Product (QIDP) by the FDA for the treatment of BV and has received Fast Track designation from the agency in 2015. Solosec was approved by the FDA for BV with benefits of 10-year exclusivity
Bioversys	Developer of drugs that switch off drug resistance and restore the efficacy of approved antibiotics 'TRIC' Transcriptional regulator Inhibitory compounds	One of their lead series already exhibited good characteristics in rendering multi-resistant *Mycobacterium tuberculosis* sensitive again to the classical antibiotic prodrug ethionamide	Entered into a collaboration with GlaxoSmithKline (GSK) to develop a preclinical candidate against tuberculosis (TB)
Destiny	Developer of drugs for the treatment of infectious diseases	XF-73 contains exeporfinium chloride for the prevention of post-surgical staphylococcal infections NTCD-M3 for *Clostridioides difficile* SPOR-COV for COVID-19 XF drugs biofilm for the treatment of antibiotic-resistant biofilm and bacterial aggregate associated infections	
Spero Therapeutics	Novel therapies to treat highly resistant bacterial infections	SPR994 (Oral Beta-Lactam Gram-Negative Program, for complicated urinary tract infections) SPR741 & SPR206, which is an IV Potentiator Platform, which is an adjunctive, Potentiator approach to disrupt the LipoPolysaccharide layer	

Continued

Table 2.1 Start-ups landscape in antimicrobial field.—*continued*

Company	Target project	Product	Market
Tetraphase	Developing tetracycline analogues for multidrug-resistant infections	Eravacycline, a novel, fully synthetic fluorocycline antibiotic	In phase 3 clinical development for the treatment of complicated intra-abdominal infections (cIAI) and complicated urinary tract infections (cUTI)
Oxford Drug Design	Spin off Dr. Graham Richards Novel antibiotics for multidrug resistance bacterial infections	**1.** 3D ElectroShape technology **2.** Aminoacyl tRNA Synthetase inhibitors **3.** Two compound series that have shown antibiotic activity against Gram-negative pathogens	
Entasis Therapeutics	Serious drug-resistant bacterial infections	ETX0914	Currently in phase 2 clinical trials for the treatment of uncomplicated gonorrhoea
Melinta Therapeutics	Bacterial ribosome-targeting drugs for MDR infections	Delafloxacin	In market for: 1. Skin (Staphylococcus strains, Streptococcus strains, Enterococcus strain, *E. coli*, *Enterobacter cloacae*, *Klebsiella pneumoniae* and *P. aeruginosa*) 2. Pneumonia 3. Complicated urinary tract infections

to disrupt the market – clearly referring to microbial presence or tackling AMR are described below:

- **Day Zero Diagnostics** developed a molecular diagnostic technique that uses high throughput sequencing and

computational analysis to identify, within hours, both the species and the antibiotic resistance profile of a pathogen.
- **Fluid-Screen** is a start up company spun out of Dr Mark Reed's lab at Yale University. Fluid-Screen integrates four core technologies into a portable device for rapid bacteria detection.
- **Karius** is a life sciences company focussed on conquering infectious diseases through the innovative use of next generation sequencing to analyse microbial cell free DNA. The company's genomics platform uses a combination of machine learning, proprietary signal processing algorithms and next generation sequencing to enable the broad and rapid detection of microbial cell free DNA through a standard blood draw.
- **LexaGene** develops a fully automated pathogen detection platform for use at the site of sample collection, which offers unprecedented ease of use, sensitivity and breadth of pathogen detection.
- **Linear Diagnostics Limited (LDL)** is a diagnostics company developing a microfluidic cartridge based platform to detect multidrug resistant bacteria in hospitals.
- **ReoLab** focusses on intelligent point of care screening to combat the antibiotics crisis.
- **SpinDiag** develops an easy to use, compact, and automated point of care system for the broad, fast and affordable screening for drug-resistant pathogens.

6. Active public and private initiatives against AMR

According to WHO's 2020 update of the global review of antibacterial products, a total of 245 antibacterial candidates are in preclinical development (179 by private companies) and clinical pipeline as of September 2020 accounted for 68 new chemical entities [60].

At the time of writing, it is clear that no single action is sufficient to tackle the problem of AMR. To succeed in addressing AMR, international public–private partnerships (PPPs) are trying to bridge the gap and this last decade's exercise counts a number of initiatives.

- Innovative Medicines Initiative (IMI) started in 2012 with the programme New Drugs for Bad Bugs (ND4BB) [61];
- Global Health Innovation Technology (GHIT) in 2013 granted support to five Japanese drug companies, with sponsorship by the Bill & Melinda Gates Foundation and the United Nations Development Programme [62];

- Centres for Excellence in Translational Research (CETRs) in 2014 granted through NIH many academic-industrial collaborations [63];
- European Gram Negative Anti-Bacterial Engine (ENABLE) project (2014–21), as part of IMI [64];
- Combating Antibiotic Resistant Bacteria Biopharmaceutical Accelerator (CARB-X), started by Boston University in 2016, funded research for $24 m to 11 companies in 2021 [65];
- The Global Antibiotic Research and Development Partnership (GARDP) was established by the WHO and the Drugs for Neglected Disease initiative (DNDi) in 2016 [66].

The AMR Industry Alliance, established in 2017, is one of the largest private sector coalitions with approximately 100 companies [67]. Moreover, funding for basic research comes through grants and fellowships provided by agencies such as the Directorate General for Research and Innovation, European Commission (DG-RTD), the US National Institutes of Health (NIH) and the UK National Institute for Health Research (NIHR).

European Commission actively introduced on the research budget for 2021–27 the aim of tackling AMR, showing that this specific issue remains at the top of its agenda. Two main pillars of funding are available. The two main acts are

1. HORIZON-HLTH-2021-IND-07-02: Development, procurement and responsible management of new antimicrobials [68]. This focusses on creating the conditions for future innovation partnerships, by modelling the purchase agreements signed for COVID-19 vaccines and applying them to priority pathogens such as those identified by WHO.
2. HORIZON-HLTH-2021-DISEASE-04-05: A roadmap towards the creation of the European partnership on One Health AMR (OH AMR) [69]. This focusses on the development of a Strategic Research and Innovation Agenda (SRIA), with a focus on improving effective information exchange between scientific disciplines and sectors.

Although in contrast with commercial objectives, companies operating in the infectious diseases space have a social responsibility to support antimicrobial stewardship (AMS) [70]. The private sector is now investing in antimicrobial stewardship (education, patient engagement/advocacy, and novel reimbursement and sales incentive models) becoming more and more engaged [71]. Finally, performance and alignment of 30 major pharmaceutical companies to common goals described above are monitored and evaluated by Access to Medicines Foundation, which has recently published the 2020 AMR Benchmark (Fig. 2.5) [50].

		ACCESS						STEWARDSHIP		
	Company	Expanded Access; Managed Access; Compassionate Use Programmes	Equitable Pricing	Registration	Concrete provisions or other agreed-upon measures	Responsible IP arrangements, licensing arrangements	Supply Chain Strengthening, Donations	Avoid expansion of use in unnecessary indications	Surveillance	Concrete provisions or other agreed-upon measures
Small and medium-sized enterprises	Amplyx	●								
	Cidara					●			●	
	Entasis		●	●	●	●		●	●	●
	Melinta					●				
	Motif Bio		●	●						
	Scynexis	●								
	Summit					●		●		
	Tetraphase		●			●			●	
	Wockhardt			●						
Large research-based pharmaceutical companies	GSK		●	●	●	●			●	
	Johnson & Johnson	●	●	●	●		●		●	●
	Merck & Co, Inc			●						
	Otsuka				●	●				
	Pfizer	●	●		●		●		●	
	Sanofi		●							
	Shionogi		●	●						

● Reports component or principle

Figure 2.5 Details an overview of companies' stewardship and access strategy. With permission from Ref. [50], with a focus on benefits derived from this plan.

7. Final remarks and perspectives

AMR is posing a threat to the ability to prevent and cure severe bacterial infections. AMR can be intrinsic, acquired, or adaptive, each characterised by different genetic and epigenetic molecular pathways [72]. Differential genetic and epigenetic mechanisms can contribute to the development of bacterial resistance [73].

Since epigenetic changes can be easily reverted by small agents, known as 'epidrugs', they might provide useful drug targets to prevent and fight multidrug resistant (MDR) infections [74].

Actually, the answer to AMR phenomenon could potentially be the reprogramming of bacteria by the use of epidrugs instead of killing them through the use of antimicrobials. New era of research and potential application is now opening using epigenomics of microbes as the strategic goal for the design of new drug molecules.

It is clear today that, together with innovation, a major challenge for antibiotic development is the economic model. Policymakers, regulators, manufacturers, researchers and the community need to collaborate so that antibiotics are produced sustainably, are restricted to the practice of medicine and continue to stay effective in treating bacterial infections by exploring approaches unthinkable a decade ago.

Pharmaceutical industry as a one, despite decades of struggle and failed attempts in the field, could have now found new ways forward, which need to be pursued with better degree of maturity.

References

[1] A. Travis, O. Chernova, V. Chernov, R. Aminov, Antimicrobial drug discovery: lessons of history and future strategies, Expert Opinion on Drug Discovery 13 (2018) 983, https://doi.org/10.1080/17460441.2018.1515910.
[2] J.J. Leisner, The diverse search for synthetic, semisynthetic and natural product antibiotics from the 1940s and up to 1960 exemplified by a small pharmaceutical player, Frontiers in Microbiology 11 (2020) 976, https://doi.org/10.3389/fmicb.2020.00976.
[3] L. Katz, R.H. Baltz, Natural product discovery: past, present, and future, Journal of Industrial Microbiology and Biotechnology 43 (2016) 155, https://doi.org/10.1007/s10295-015-1723-5.
[4] American Chemical Society National Historic Chemical Landmarks. Penicillin Production through Deep-tank Fermentation. http://www.acs.org/content/acs/en/education/whatischemistry/landmarks/penicillin.html.
[5] J.P. Swann, The search for synthetic penicillin during World War II, The British Journal for the History of Science 16 (1983) 154, https://doi.org/10.1017/s0007087400026789.
[6] J.G. Lombardino, A brief history of Pfizer central research, Bulletin for the History of Chemistry 25 (2000) 10.
[7] P.M. Wright, I.B. Seiple, A.G. Myers, The evolving role of chemical synthesis in antibacterial drug discovery, Angewandte Chemie International Edition 53 (2014) 8840, https://doi.org/10.1002/anie.201310843.
[8] J.C. Sheehan, The Enchanted Ring, The Untold Story of Penicillin, MIT Press Cambridge, 1982.
[9] C. Nathan, Cooperative development of antimicrobials: looking back to look ahead, Nature Reviews Microbiology 13 (2015) 651, https://doi.org/10.1038/nrmicro3523.
[10] J.C. Sheehan, E.L. Buhle, E.J. Corey, G.D. Laubach, J.J. Ryan, The total synthesis of a 5-phenyl penicillin: methyl 5-phenyl-(2-carbomethoxyethyl)-penicillinate, Journal of the American Chemical Society 72 (1950) 3828, https://doi.org/10.1021/ja01164a534.
[11] M. Lobanovska, G. Pilla, Penicillin's discovery and antibiotic resistance: lessons for the future? Yale Journal of Biology and Medicine 90 (2017) 135.
[12] Para-aminosalicylic acid in the treatment of pulmonary tuberculosis, JAMA 141 (1949) 605, https://doi.org/10.1001/jama.1949.02910090031009.
[13] D. Greenwood, Antimicrobial Drugs: Chronicle of a Twentieth Century Medical Triumph, Oxford University Press, 2008.

[14] C. Grandmann, Re-inventing infectious disease: antibiotic resistance and drug development at the Bayer company 1945–80, Medical History 60 (2016) 155, https://doi.org/10.1017/mdh.2016.2.
[15] M.L. Cohen, Epidemiology of drug resistance: implications for a post-antimicrobial era, Science 257 (1992) 1050, https://doi.org/10.1126/science.257.5073.1050.
[16] H. Goossens, M. Ferech, S.R. Vander, M. Elseviers, ESAC Project Group, Outpatient antibiotic use in Europe and association with resistance: a cross-national database study, Lancet 365 (2005) 579, https://doi.org/10.1016/S0140-6736(05)17907-0.
[17] Centers for Disease Control and Prevention, 2013. Threat report, http://www.cdc.gov/drugresistance/threat-report-2013. (Accessed 24 January 2022).
[18] A. Kotwani, J. Joshi, D. Kaloni, Pharmaceutical effluent: a critical link in the interconnected ecosystem promoting antimicrobial resistance, Environmental Science & Pollution Research 28 (2021) 32111, https://doi.org/10.1007/s11356-021-14178-w.
[19] A.S. Fauci, L.D. Marston, The perpetual challenge of antimicrobial resistance, JAMA 311 (2014) 1853, https://doi.org/10.1001/jama.2014.2465.
[20] M. Anderson, M. Cecchini, E. Mossialos, Challenges to Tackling Antimicrobial Resistance: Economic and Policy Responses, Cambridge University Press, 2019.
[21] B. Plackett, Why big pharma has abandoned antibiotics, Nature 586 (2020) S50, https://doi.org/10.1038/d41586-020-02884-3.
[22] M. Gajdács, The concept of an ideal antibiotic: implications for drug design, Molecules 24 (2019) 892, https://doi.org/10.3390/molecules24050892.
[23] K. Lewis, Platforms for antibiotic discovery, Nature Reviews Drug Discovery 12 (2013) 371, https://doi.org/10.1038/nrd3975.
[24] N. Dheman, N. Mahoney, E.M. Cox, J.J. Farley, T. Amini, M.L. Lanthier, An analysis of antibacterial drug development trends in the United States, 1980–2019, Clinical Infectious Diseases 73 (2021) e4444, https://doi.org/10.1093/cid/ciaa859.
[25] D. Payne, M. Gwynn, D. Holmes, et al., Drugs for bad bugs: confronting the challenges of antibacterial discovery, Nature Reviews Drug Discovery 6 (2007) 29, https://doi.org/10.1038/nrd2201.
[26] M.J. Santesmases, Screening antibiotics: industrial research by CEPA and Merck in the 1950s, Dynamis 31 (2011) 407, https://doi.org/10.4321/S0211-95362011000200008.
[27] L. Brunton, B.A. Chabner, B. Knollman, Goodman and Gilman's: The Pharmacological Basis of Therapeutics, twelfth ed., The McGraw-Hill Companies, Inc., New York, 2011.
[28] R.L. Peck, C.E. Hoffhine Jr., K. Folkers, Streptomyces antibiotics. IX. Dihydrostreptomycin, Journal of the American Chemical Society 68 (1946) 1390, https://doi.org/10.1021/ja01211a513.
[29] R.R. Chauvette, E.H. Flynn, B.G. Jackson, E.R. Lavagnino, R.B. Morin, R.A. Mueller, R.P. Pioch, R.W. Roeske, C.W. Ryan, J.L. Spencer, E. Van Heyningen, Chemistry of cephalosporin antibiotics. II. Preparation of a new class of antibiotics and the relation of structure to activity, Journal of the American Chemical Society 84 (1962) 3401, https://doi.org/10.1021/ja00876a035.
[30] J.H. Kim, A.R. Scialli, Thalidomide: the tragedy of birth defects and the effective treatment of disease, Toxicological Sciences 122 (2011) 1, https://doi.org/10.1093/toxsci/kfr088.

[31] Anon, US Public Law 87-781, Statute 76, 1962, p. 781.
[32] R.P. Elander, Industrial production of beta-lactam antibiotics, Applied Microbiology and Biotechnology 61 (2003) 385, https://doi.org/10.1007/s00253-003-1274-y.
[33] B. Thakuria, K. Lahon, The beta lactam antibiotics as an empirical therapy in a developing country: an update on their current status and recommendations to counter the resistance against them, Journal of Clinical and Diagnostic Research 7 (2013) 1207, https://doi.org/10.7860/JCDR/2013/5239.3052.
[34] R.C. Moellering, Discovering new anti microbial agents, International Journal of Antimicrobial Agents 37 (2011) 2, https://doi.org/10.1016/j.ijantimicag.2010.08.018.
[35] E.D. Brown, G.D. Wright, Antibacterial drug discovery in the resistance era, Nature 529 (2016) 336, https://doi.org/10.1038/nature17042.
[36] J. O'Neill, Antimicrobial resistance: tackling a crisis for the health and wealth of nations, Review on Antimicrobial Resistance 20 (2014) 1.
[37] D.J. Payne, M.N. Gwynn, D.J. Holmes, D.L. Pompliano, Drugs for bad bugs: confronting the challenges of antibacterial discovery, Nature Reviews Drug Discovery 6 (2007) 29, https://doi.org/10.1038/nrd2201.
[38] F.P. Chan, D.J. Holmes, D.J. Payne, Finding the gems using genomic discovery: antibacterial drug discovery strategies – the successes and the challenges, Drug Discovery Today: Therapeutic Strategies 1 (2004) 519, https://doi.org/10.1016/j.ddstr.2004.11.003.
[39] J. Carroll, Will combinatorial chemistry keep its promise? Biotechnology Healthcare 2 (2005) 26–27, 31–32.
[40] J.-Y. Ortholand, A. Ganesan, Natural products and combinatorial chemistry: back to the future, Current Opinion in Chemical Biology 8 (2004) 271, https://doi.org/10.1016/j.cbpa.2004.04.011.
[41] R.F. Service, Winning combination: combinatorial chemistry, with its high-speed, automated methods, is all the rage in drug research. Can it repeat its success in the search for new materials? Technology Review 101 (1998) 34.
[42] P. Gwynne, Focus on careers: combinatorial chemists on the fast track, Science 12 (1999).
[43] G. Karet, Abbott accelerates its combichem efforts, Research and Development Magazine (November 1998) 26–28.
[44] R. Tommasi, D.G. Brown, G.K. Walkup, J.I. Manchester, A.A. Miller, ESKAPEing the labyrinth of antibacterial discovery, Nature Reviews Drug Discovery 14 (2015) 529, https://doi.org/10.1038/nrd4572.
[45] J.M. Stokes, K. Yang, K. Swanson, W. Jin, A. Cubillos-Ruiz, N.M. Donghia, C.R. MacNair, S. French, L.A. Carfrae, Z. Bloom-Ackermann, V.M. Tran, A. Chiappino-Pepe, A.H. Badran, I.W. Andrews, E.J. Chory, G.M. Church, E.D. Brown, T.S. Jaakkola, R. Barzilay, J.J. Collins, A deep learning approach to antibiotic discovery, Cell 180 (2020) 688, https://doi.org/10.1016/j.cell.2020.01.021.
[46] C.D. Fjell, J.A. Hiss, R.E.W. Hancock, G. Schneider, Designing antimicrobial peptides: form follows function, Nature Reviews Drug Discovery 11 (2012) 37, https://doi.org/10.1038/nrd3591.
[47] P. Das, T. Sercu, K. Wadhawan, et al., Accelerated antimicrobial discovery via deep generative models and molecular dynamics simulations, Nature Biomedical Engineering (2021) 613, https://doi.org/10.1038/s41551-021-00689-x.

[48] AI for Drug Discovery, Biomarker Development and Advanced R&D Landscape Overview, Deep-Pharma Intelligence, 2020, pp. 1–130. www.deep-pharma.tech.
[49] M.C.R. Melo, J.R.M.A. Maasch, C. de la Fuente-Nunez, Accelerating antibiotic discovery through artificial intelligence, Communications Biology 4 (2021) 1050, https://doi.org/10.1038/s42003-021-02586-0.
[50] The Access to Medicine Foundation. Antimicrobial Resistance Benchmark 2020. https://accesstomedicinefoundation.org/publications/2020-antimicrobial-resistance-benchmark (Accessed February 12, 2022).
[51] The Access to Medicine Foundation. Antimicrobial Resistance Benchmark 2021. https://accesstomedicinefoundation.org/publications/2021-antimicrobial-resistance-benchmark (Accessed March 20, 2022).
[52] D. Taylor, The pharmaceutical industry and the future of drug development, Pharmaceuticals in the Environment (2015), https://doi.org/10.1039/9781782622345-00001.
[53] Commission Implementing Decision (EU) 2018/840 of 5 June 2018 establishing a watch list of substances for Union-wide monitoring in the field of water policy pursuant to Directive 2008/105/EC of the European Parliament and of the Council and repealing Commission Implementing Decision (EU) 2015/495 (notified under document C (2018) 3362). https://eur-lex.europa.eu/eli/dec_impl/2018/840/oj.
[54] P. Taylor, Despite Looming Resistance Crisis, Novartis Ducks Out of Antibiotics Research, 2018. https://www.fiercebiotech.com/biotech/despite-looming-resistance-crisis-novartis-ducks-out-antibiotics-research.
[55] Sandoz Announces Plans for Joint Investment to Help Strengthen Future of Antibiotics Manufacturing in Europe, 2020. https://www.novartis.com/news/media-releases/sandoz-announces-plans-joint-investment-help-strengthen-future-antibiotics-manufacturing-europe.
[56] N. Nijsingh, C. Munthe, D.G.J. Larsson, Managing pollution from antibiotics manufacturing: charting actors, incentives and disincentives, Environmental Health 18 (2019) 95, https://doi.org/10.1186/s12940-019-0531-1.
[57] M. Miethke, M. Pieroni, T. Weber, et al., Towards the sustainable discovery and development of new antibiotics, Nature Reviews Chemistry 5 (2021) 726, https://doi.org/10.1038/s41570-021-00313-1.
[58] S. Bhatia, D. Ingber, Microfluidic organs-on-chips, Nature Biotechnology 32 (2014) 760, https://doi.org/10.1038/nbt.2989.
[59] Emerging Microfluidic Companies (Accessed November 15, 2021) https://www.ufluidix.com/circle/microfluidic-companies/.
[60] 2020 Antibacterial Agents in Clinical and Preclinical Development: An Overview and Analysis, World Health Organization, 2021, 978-92-4-002130-3.
[61] ND4BB—New Drugs for Bad Bugs. Innovative Medicines Initiative, 2021 https://www.imi.europa.eu/projects-results/project-factsheets/nd4bb.
[62] Annual Report 2020, Global Health Innovation Technology (GHIT) Fund. (Accessed November 28, 2021). https://www.ghitfund.org/assets/othermedia/annual_report_2020_eng.pdf.
[63] Centers of Excellence for Translational Research (CETR). (Accessed December 10, 2021). https://www.niaid.nih.gov/research/centers-excellence-translational-research.
[64] ENABLE—European Gram-Negative Antibacterial Engine, 2014. https://www.imi.europa.eu/projects-results/project-factsheets/enable. (Accessed 28 November 2021).
[65] 2020–2021 Annual Report. Combating Antibiotic-Resistant Bacteria Biopharmaceutical Accelerator (CARB-X) 2021. https://carb-x.org/.

[66] Global Antibiotic Research and Development Partnership (GARDP). (Accessed December 09, 2021). https://gardp.org/.
[67] AMR Industry Alliance. (Accessed December 09, 2021). https://www.amrindustryalliance.org/.
[68] Development, Procurement and Responsible Management of New Antimicrobials. https://ec.europa.eu/info/funding-tenders/opportunities/portal/screen/opportunities/topic-details/horizon-hlth-2021-ind-07-02.
[69] A Roadmap Towards the Creation of the European Partnership on One Health Antimicrobial Resistance (OH AMR). (Accessed December 09, 2021). https://ec.europa.eu/info/funding-tenders/opportunities/portal/screen/opportunities/topic-details/horizon-hlth-2021-disease-04-05.
[70] Stewardship & Access Plan (SAP) Development Guide, 2021. https://carb-x.org/about/stewardship-and-access/. (Accessed 9 December 2021).
[71] E.D. Hermsen, R.L. Sibbel, S. Holland, The role of pharmaceutical companies in antimicrobial stewardship: a case study, Clinical Infectious Diseases 71 (2020) 677, https://doi.org/10.1093/cid/ciaa053.
[72] J.M. Blair, M.A. Webber, A.J. Baylay, D.O. Ogbolu, L.J. Piddock, Molecular mechanisms of antibiotic resistance, Nature Reviews Microbiology 13 (2015) 42, https://doi.org/10.1038/nrmicro3380.
[73] J. Casadesús, D.A. Low, Programmed heterogeneity: epigenetic mechanisms in bacteria, Journal of Biological Chemistry 288 (2013) 13929, https://doi.org/10.1074/jbc.R113.472274.
[74] E. Crimi, G. Benincasa, S. Cirri, R. Mutesi, M. Faenza, C. Napoli, Clinical epigenetics and multidrug-resistant bacterial infections: host remodelling in critical illness, Epigenetics 15 (2020) 1021, https://doi.org/10.1080/15592294.2020.1748918.

3

Design and production of nanoparticles

Silvia Moreno[1], Franziska Obst[2] and Jens Gaitzsch[3]
[1]*Department of Organic and Inorganic Chemistry, University of Alcalá, Madrid, Spain;* [2]*Institute of Semiconductors and Microsystems, Technische Universität Dresden, Dresden, Germany;* [3]*Institute for Macromolecular Chemistry, Leibniz-Institut für Polymerforschung Dresden e.V., Dresden, Germany*

1. Choice of material

1.1 Inorganic materials

Inorganic nanoparticles are mainly silica nanoparticles or metals with their derivatives. **Semiconducting nanoparticles** such as CdSe, for example, are used as tracer molecules [1,2]. Metals themselves can form clusters, which are then named **metal nanoparticles**, to become catalysts mainly for oxidation reactions. Depending on the material, they can be tailored to include a paramagnetic, radioactive or temperature-responsive behaviour. Surface plasmon resonance, to name another example, is rapidly used in the case of gold nanoparticles [3,4]. Zinc oxide as metal oxide nanoparticles and gold and silver nanoparticles from pure metals are especially well known for their antibacterial, antimicrobial and antifungal properties [3,5–9]. Metal clusters and other metal nanoparticles can, for example, be used to sense heavy metal ions as they are able to catalyse reactions in an enzyme-like manner. In order to emphasise the similarity, the term **nanozymes** is frequently used in this respect [10]. Apart from clusters, metal ions themselves can catalyse almost any kind of reaction, but they then need to have a ligand in order to be suspended in a solution. If this ligand is an entire enzyme, the complexes formed are then called **metallozymes**. They can qualify as small nanoparticles due to the size of some enzymes [11,12]. However, all types of metal nanoparticles face a biocompatibility issue. The aforementioned antibacterial zinc oxide, gold and silver nanoparticles are known to have adverse side effects, for example, when entering the gastrointestinal tract [5,13–15].

Nanotechnology Tools for Infection Control. https://doi.org/10.1016/B978-0-12-823994-0.00003-7

While silica nanoparticles, metal clusters and nanozymes are mostly toxic to living tissue, metallozymes face the issue of possible decomposition from proteases once they have been administered. Consequently, all of them need a shell which prevents a contact of the active component with the outside environment. Inorganic nanoparticles are hence the active component of a possible formulation, but do require a carrier nanoparticle from a different material. Carrier nanoparticles from lipids, proteins and polymers are the main focus of this chapter.

1.2 Lipids

Lipids are hydrophobic or amphiphilic small molecules, which are in many cases soluble in organic substances. According to LIPID MAPS (Lipid Metabolites and Pathways Strategy), they are classified into eight categories based on their chemically functional backbone. Specifically, it is distinguished between fatty acyls, glycerolipids, glycerophospholipids, sphingolipids, sterol lipids, prenol lipids, saccharo lipids and polyketides [16,17].

To develop **lipid nanoparticles** for drug delivery, mainly glycerolipids, phospholipids and glycerophospholipids are used due to their amphiphilic character and ability to form micelles and membrane-enclosed nanoscale compartments [18]. Apart from that, sterol lipids such as cholesterol are applied to improve the physical stability of lipid nanoparticles.

Glycerolipids can be **isolated** from **vegetable oils**, such as palm oil, soy bean oil and sunflower oil. Thereby a great structural variety of lipids results from the presence of various fatty acids (e.g. linoleic acid, stearic acid, palmitic acid) which form glycerol esters [19]. In addition, such lipids are **synthetically accessible** by esterification of glycerol or reaction of fatty acids with other activated precursors [19,20].

The choice of natural lipids as material basis for nanoparticle design offers the **great advantage** of biocompatibility and biodegradability and thus low inherent toxicity. This aspect is explained by the natural origin of lipids with their existing metabolic pathways for conversion and degradation in living creatures. Especially for delivering hydrophobic drugs, which present about 40% of the currently marketed drugs, lipids are highly promising to achieve high-drug loading capacity [21]. Apart from that, the high structural diversity of lipids allows designing tailored materials to obtain high-drug encapsulation efficiency as well as controlled and precise drug delivery. In contrast to many polymers, organic solvents can be avoided in the synthesis.

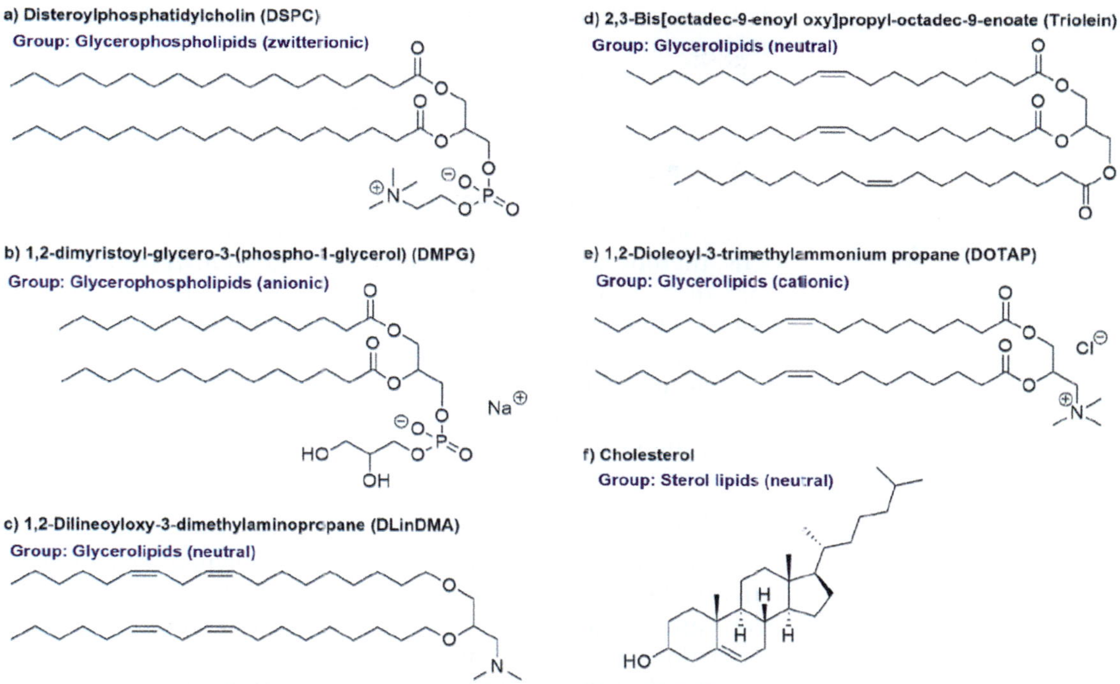

Figure 3.1 Selected lipids commonly applied for the assembly of lipid nanovesicles [23–26].

Possible disadvantages are that degradation of lipids and/or a change of the lipid modification can result in limited chemical and physical stability of lipid-based nanocarriers during sterilisation, storage and administration. Accordingly, aggregation, gelation or drug expulsion from lipid nanovesicles might occur [22].

The **structural diversity** of lipids applied for the assembly of lipid nanovesicles is illustrated in Fig. 3.1. In a lipid formulation these lipids either serve as structural compounds or are applied for the purpose of nanovesicle stabilisation, adjustment of membrane permeability, coating, e.g. with a poly ethylene glycol (PEG) shell, or control of the size and size distribution during nanovesicle synthesis [22,23]. To optimise lipid nanovesicles, e.g. regarding drug loading capacity and (controlled) drug release, various structural parameters of the lipids are considered, including the type and length of the hydrophobic chains, type and length of linker between hydrophilic headgroup and hydrophobic chains, and the acidity constant of ionisable groups. In connection with structural variations, properties such as the packing configuration, phase transition temperature, or sensitivity to enzymatic cleavage are altered, allowing an adjustment of pharmacokinetics and pharmacodynamics [24]. To treat microbial infections, fatty acids and monoglycerides with antimicrobial activity are very feasible candidates. Lauric acid and caproic acid as well as the monoglyceride of lauric acid (monolaurin) are common examples for this material group [27]. In the field of RNA delivery especially **cationic** and **ionisable lipids** (e.g. 1,2-Dioleoyl-3-trimethylammonium propane, DOTAP) are promising as they form complexes with RNA driven by electrostatic interactions, thereby shielding the negative charge of RNA [24,28]. Apart from that, also **neutral lipids** (e.g. 2,3-Bis[octadec-9-enoyl-oxy] propyl-octadec-9-enoate, Triolein) and **anionic lipids** [e.g. 1,2-dimyristoyl-sn-glycero-3-(phospho-rac-1-glycerol), DMPG] are valuable in drug delivery systems, due to their generally lower sensitivity to phagocytosis and slower clearance from the blood stream than cationic lipids [25].

1.3 Polypeptides

Amino acids are the building blocks of polypeptides and proteins in the way letters are the building blocks of words. Moreover, amino acids convey key information about structure, interactions and cells communication processes. **Natural or engineered polypeptides are particularly attractive** for multiple reasons: (1) as major structural elements in all living systems (or being able to mimic them), they are inherently biocompatible, biodegradable and water soluble; (2) they can take on multiple bio-functional roles via different compositions of residues, surface charge, ensuing conformations; (3) there is a diverse functionality considering roughly 500 natural amino acids (21 proteogenic) and their synthetic derivatives (simple synthesis, sheer limitless combinations); (4) peptide functionalisation can easily be performed by introducing additional biomolecules such as antibodies, enzymes, magnetic particles or dyes to the peptide structure; (5) they can serve as recognition and targeting moieties to mediate binding to specific disease-related markers (cell-penetrating peptides, CPPs) [29]. In contrast to conventional polymers and lipids, polypeptides form higher ordered secondary structures, such as random coils, α-helices and β-sheet associations. Therefore, not only chemical compositions but also secondary structures of polypeptides play a critical role in their properties and functions (Fig. 3.2) [30].

Additionally, antimicrobial peptides (AMPs) and CPPs have shown great potential to treat antibacterial infections by acting directly on the intracellular pathogenic bacteria (therapeutic effect per se) or performing the delivery of antibacterial cargo

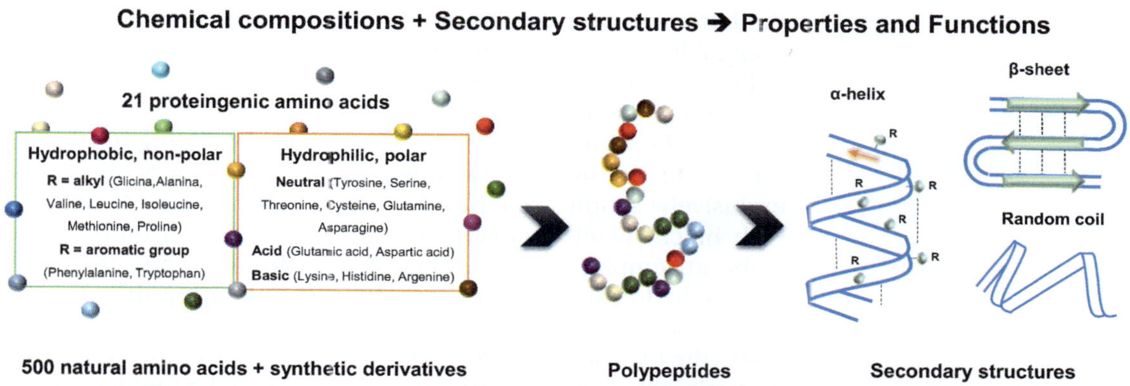

Figure 3.2 Secondary structures depending on the composition of the polypeptides and the kind of amino acids incorporated.

[29]. However, the clinical development of AMPs has shown limited success, for instance, proteolytic lability makes AMPs almost completely ineffective and difficult to apply in the clinic. **Prerequisites for modern nanocarriers** are fewer side effects, better efficacy, a prolonged circulation time in blood and release of the drug at a specific site (targeting properties). **"Smart" polypeptides** have been successfully established to achieve a better release profile at the targeted sites due to their chemical versatility [31]. The conformational transition among different secondary structures and macroscopic properties can be triggered by external stimuli (such as temperature, pH, ionic strength, light, biomolecules, etc.) [32,33]. Stimuli-responsive polypeptides can be simply synthesised with naturally occurring amino acid residues without chemical modifications. There are natural amino acids with responsive units, such as cysteine (thermo and redox), glutamic acid (pH and thermo), lysine (pH), histidine (pH and thermo sensitive) and methionine (redox). These residues possess an inherent stimuli-responsive characteristic [34]. Additionally, these stimuli-responsive natural polypeptides can be combined with a desirable functional moiety responding to another specific stimulus. The adequate designs of their chemical structures combined with appropriate stimuli-responsive groups are both responsible for their conformational transition behaviour, thus allowing to finely tune the properties.

1.4 Block-copolymers

Self-assemblies from polymeric materials are known from natural polymers (like polysaccharides) or **synthetic polymers**. Since the latter can be easier to produce, have a much larger range of accessible and useable monomers and are therefore easier to tailor towards a certain functionality, this section will focus on synthetic polymers.

Apart from macromolecules from natural building blocks like the just mentioned polypeptides, synthetic polymers are almost exclusively synthesised from synthetic monomers. A polymer with blocks of distinctively different solubility can be designed to be an amphiphile if one block is hydrophilic and the other one is hydrophobic. Such **amphiphilic blockcopolymers** can simply be AB diblock copolymers, where A is the hydrophilic and B the hydrophobic block. In their extension, either symmetric ABA triblock or asymmetric ABC triblock copolymers have been synthesised as well (where C is also hydrophilic). One of the greatest advantages of synthetic block copolymers is their chemical versatility as each of these blocks can be designed for specific purposes [35–37].

The **hydrophilic block** can be either non-ionic like PEG [38], poly(sarcosine) (PSar) [39,40], poly(vinyl alcohol) (PVA) [41] or poly(methyl oxazoline) (PMOXA) [42], anionic like in poly(acrylic acid) (PAA) [43], poly(styrene sulfonate) (PSS) [44] or be cationic as in poly(dimethylaminoethyl methacrylate) (PDMAEMA-H^+) [45]. PDMAEMA bears the additional advantage of being responsive to temperature and pH, meaning it can switch to become a hydrophobic polymer when the temperature rises above 35 °C [lower critical solution temperature (LCST)] or the pH rises above 7.5. Another well-known temperature-responsive polymer is poly(*N*-isopropyl acrylamide) (PNIPAM), which also has an LCST of 32–38°C [36].

Within the **hydrophobic block**, the pH sensitivity can be tuned by exchanging the methyl groups in PDMAEMA to ethyl (PDEA) or isopropyl (PDPA) groups. This leads to a drop in the switching pH value (pKa of the substance) to 7.0 and 6.3, respectively, while the LCST drops to 17 and 12°C in the same order. Both changes mean that the polymers are hydrophobic at ambient conditions. An LCST can also be incorporated using Oxazolines with an ethyl (PEtOz) or propyl side (PPrOz) chain, amongst others [46]. Redox-responsiveness can be included by poly(propylene sulphide) (PPS) [47,48]. The sulphur atoms in this polymer can be oxidised towards the sulfone, which renders the entire polymer hydrophilic. From the non-responsive hydrophobic polymers, poly(dimethylsiloxane) (PDMS) is important in a biomedical context since it is flexible enough to adjust the width of the membrane in order to host transmembrane proteins [49,50].

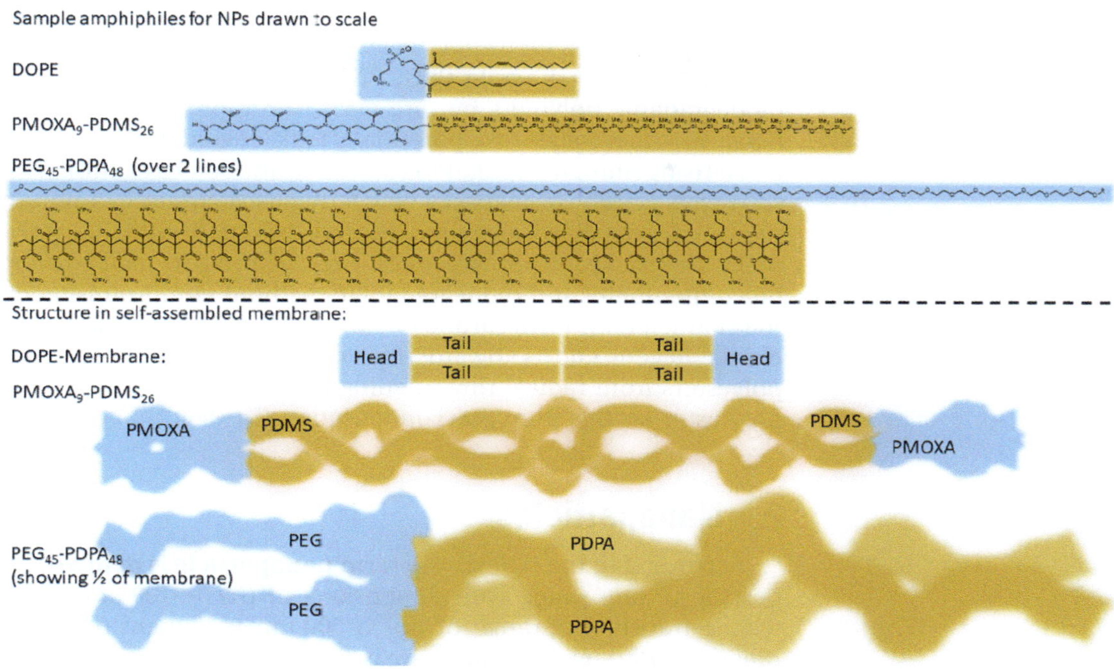

Figure 3.3 DOPE, PMOXA$_9$-PDMS$_{26}$, PEG$_{45}$-PDPA$_{48}$ all self-assemble into membranes. The upper part shows all three amphiphiles drawn to scale. Note that PEG45-PDPA48 is too long for one line in its stretched conformation. The lower part shows membranes of the amphiphiles. While the lipids do not intertwine, the polymer membranes show intertwining polymer coils, which is why they are mechanically more stable than lipid membranes (PEG$_{45}$-PDPA$_{48}$ shows only one-half of the membrane bilayer).

In addition to this chemical diversity, the higher molecular weight of polymers in comparison to lipids results in increased **physical stability**. The chains can form entanglements which increase the membrane stability significantly and thus also the stability of the nanoparticles [41]. In Fig. 3.3, a phospholipid and two block-copolymers for nanoparticles production are drawn to scale. Their corresponding membranes are shown as well to emphasise the intertwining of different copolymer chains. Additional mechanical stability can be achieved by using polymers with a high glass transition temperature like poly(styrene) (PS) [51] or semi crystalline polymers such as poly(L-lactic acid) (PLLA) or poly(caprolactone) (PCL) [52]. In PLLA, this crystallinity is commonly broken by adding glycolide to the monomer mixture. The resulting copolymer of glycolide and lactide (PGLA) is no longer semi-crystalline [53].

Besides the mentioned advantages, the enhanced **chemical stability** of polymers over peptides and lipids can result in the major disadvantage of missing biodegradability. The aforementioned polyesters P(D/L)LA, PGA and PCL are biodegradable and FDA-approved, while PEG, PNIPAM and PMOXA are non-biodegradable polymers but are also FDA-approved. With PEG, however, other issues (like potentially toxic degradation products, and a rising human population exhibiting antibodies against PEG) showcase possible drawbacks which might be common amongst non-biodegradable polymers. Hence, new biodegradable polymers, especially responsive ones, are required to facilitate the biocompatibility and biodegradability without compromising on the characteristic physical and chemical stability of polymeric materials. Recent efforts towards that direction include responsive polyesters from radical ring-opening polymerisation (RROP) and poly-ester-acetals from polycondensation [54–56].

2. Nanoparticles

According to the IUPAC, the **term nanoparticle is defined** as a particle of any shape with dimensions in the 1–100 nm range, with a transitional range of up to 500 nm in dimensions. This range already suggests that there is no sharp boundary that separates nanoparticles from non-nanoparticles. Because of their small size, they have unique material characteristics, and manufactured nanoparticles may find practical **applications in a variety of areas**, including medicine, engineering, catalysis and environmental field [57–59]. This chapter is especially focussed on the self-assembled nanoparticles with therapeutic properties [60,61].

Self-assembly is defined as the ability of a molecule, without external factors, to associate through non-covalent interactions to form highly ordered 3D structures. It is typically associated with thermodynamic equilibrium; the organised structures are characterised by a minimum in the free energy of the system. Most self-assembling molecules are **amphiphilic** with molecular amphiphilicity being the main driving force. Molecular self-assembly allows for developing a variety of thermodynamically stable and defined shapes, optimal sizes, at a quicker rate and a cheaper cost than templated nanoparticles synthesis. The molecular interactions governing the formation of such systems are predominantly **non-covalent**, such as van der Waals forces, hydrophobic interactions, electrostatic interactions, hydrogen bonding and π–π stacking (aromatic) interactions. They are weaker than covalent bonds, but strong enough to stabilise these self-assembly structures. The reversibility of these interactions

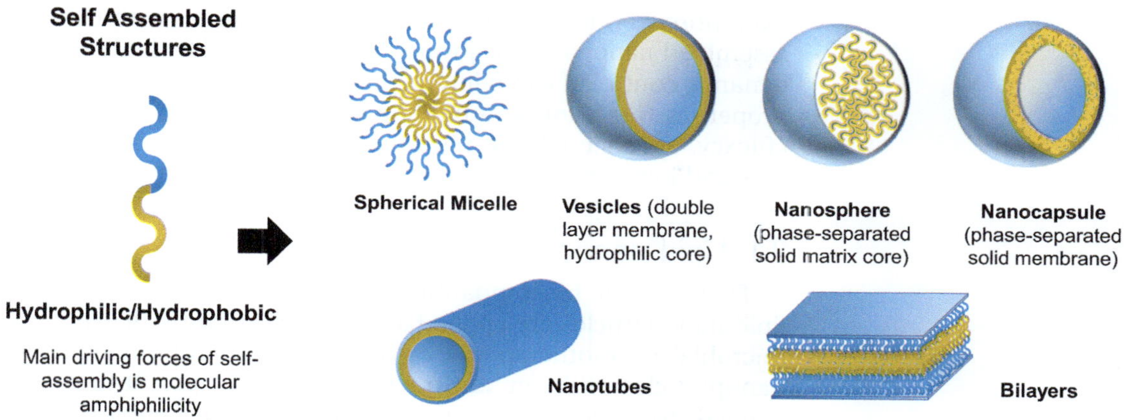

Figure 3.4 Overview of type of self-assembled nanoparticles from amphiphilic molecules, irrespective of the type of material.

implies some dynamics in the molecular architectures, therefore, their properties can be modulated to respond to external stimuli. In order to successfully exploit nanoparticle self-assembly in technological applications and to ensure efficient scale-up, a high level of control during the self-assembly process is required [60,61].

In Fig. 3.4, the most representative self-assembled structures are shown. **Different morphologies** are formed depending on the **packing parameter**. However, the following sections focus on spherical nanoparticles such as micelles, vesicles, nanocapsules and nanospheres. The main parameters of nanoparticles are their size and size distribution, shape, surface charge and porosity [58].

Nanoparticles are increasingly used to target bacteria as an alternative to antibiotics in two different ways: (i) as systems with antibacterial properties per se or (ii) as nanocarriers. Nanoparticles have been used in antibacterial coatings for implantable devices and in medicinal materials to prevent infection and promote wound healing, to treat disease, in microbial diagnostics and in antibacterial vaccines [62].

Most of the antibiotic resistance mechanisms are irrelevant for nanoparticles because their mode of action is direct contact with the bacterial cell wall, without the need to penetrate the cell, hoping less resistance in bacteria than in traditional antibiotics. Antibacterial mechanisms of nanoparticles are poorly understood, but some mechanisms are oxidative stress induction (DNA and proteins damage), metal ion release (cell wall disruption), enzyme activity inhibition and electron transport interruption

[63]. Moreover, if we compare individual materials with the self-assembled nanoparticles, properties such as multivalent binding, dynamic control of cargo interactions, cargo protection, targeting properties (precision and binding effectivity), better therapeutic efficacy, synergic effects, responsiveness to environmental triggers and long circulation times are definitely improved [62].

2.1 Lipid nanoparticles

Due to their biocompatibility and controllable disassembly, lipid nanoparticles are applied as **carrier systems** to deliver antimicrobial, chemotherapeutic or other drugs. Apart from that, lipid nanoparticles with an **antimicrobial activity** per se are also applied [64]. According to the nanoparticle's morphology, they are distinguished in lipid nanocapsules and lipid nanospheres. **Lipid nanocapsules** are formed from a lipid matrix where the cargo is incorporated, and which is mostly stabilised by emulsifiers. In case of **lipid nanospheres** (e.g. liposomes, niosomes, ethosomes), amphiphilic lipids form various membrane architectures, i.e. unilamellar and multilamellar membranes, enclosing an interior which can be loaded with the cargo [21,65]. **Further morphologies** of amphiphilic aggregates, such as micelles and worms, are formed depending on the packing parameter of the lipid, similar as for amphiphilic block copolymers (see Section 1.4) [22]. Due to the amphiphilic character of lipids, a wide range of cargo such as drugs (including hydrophobic drugs), RNA and small inorganic or lipid nanoparticles can be formulated in larger lipid nanoparticles [26].

The drug-loading capacity, release kinetics and storage stability of lipid nanoparticles largely depend on characteristics such as the crystallinity, lipid modification, particle size and shape, and zeta potential [22,66]. In that context, **solid lipid nanoparticles (SLN)**, which are obtained from solid lipids instead of lipid oils, often enable to increase drug loading capacity and to retard the drug release [22]. To prevent aggregation of SLN, emulsifiers such as sodium dodecyl sulphate (SDS) or lecithin come to use. The antimicrobial activity of glyceryl monostereate SLN filled with **anacardic acid** was recently shown by treating *Staphylococcus aureus* (*S. aureus*) biofilms. To overcome the resistance of biofilms against antibiotic therapy, SLN were coated with chitosan and the enzyme DNase to improve biofilm adhesion by electrostatic interactions and degrade enzymatic DNA, respectively [67].

For successful **drug delivery** by **nanoparticles**, a balance between chemical and physical stability during storage and administration, as well as controlled disassembly and drug release at the site of action, must be achieved. Compared to their polymer counterparts, lipid nanoparticles are often chemically and physically less stable and disassembly is induced, e.g. by shearing, changes of the solvent and/or pH value, or enzymatic cleavage [68]. This limitation can be overcome by nanoparticle stabilisation strategies such as crosslinking [69], steric stabilisation (e.g. by incorporation of PEG-lipids) [70] and the use of stabilising agents (cholesterol, other "helper" lipids, Fig. 3.1) [71]. For example, lipid nanoparticles formed from phosphatidylcholine and cholesterol were successfully applied for **the delivery of antibiotics** such as gentamicin [72], ampicillin [73], vancomycin [74] as well as nystatin and amphotericin B [75], thus resulting in improved uptake and increased antimicrobial efficiency, amongst others. To meet the challenge of increasing bacterial resistance against established antibiotics, antimicrobial peptides have been formulated in lipid nanoparticles and the antimicrobial activity of the formulations was demonstrated [76]. Furthermore, due to the ability of (mainly cationic) lipids to form complexes with RNA by electrostatic interaction, lipid nanoparticles are seen as the **leading system to deliver RNA** in vivo, e.g. small interfering RNA (siRNA). Thereby, the negative charge of RNA is shielded and the RNA is protected from degradation, improving the delivery. When developing such delivery systems, appropriate lipid design is key to realise RNA protection during circulation and at the same time release after nanoparticle uptake in the target cell. Here, advantage can be taken from the interaction of cationic lipids from the delivery system with endosome membrane-forming anionic phospholipids upon membrane disruption. Specifically, the formation of cone-shaped ion pairs results in membrane destabilisation and RNA release from endosomes [20]. Accordingly, **effective RNA delivery requires** lipids which are neutral during circulation and become positively charged in the acidic environment of endosomes (Fig. 3.5) This requirement is fulfiled by various lipids with a dimethyl amino headgroup, e.g. DLinDMA (Fig. 3.1). By structural variations in these lipids, e.g. length and degree of saturation of fatty acid chains and type of the linker, characteristics such as the sensitivity to enzymatic cleavage, phase transition temperature, and tissue accumulation can be altered to tune the effective dose (ED50 value) and thus the potency.

For example, by **systematic structural variation** of 1,2-Dilineoyloxy-3-dimethylaminopropane (DLinDMA), a lipid enabling 10-fold gene silencing potency (namely DLin-KC2-DMA, possessing a ketal linker between headgroup and tails)

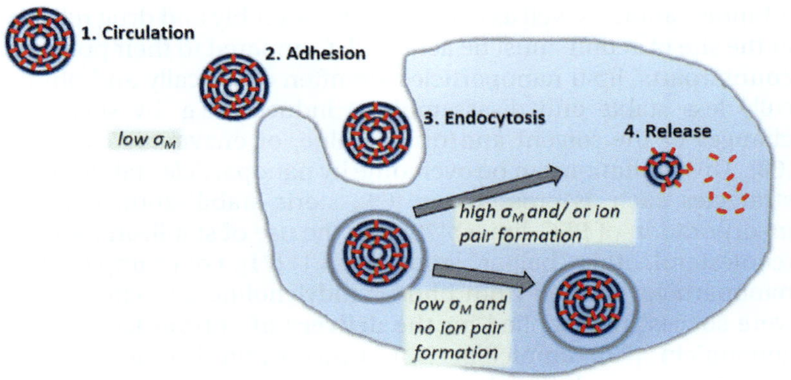

Figure 3.5 Model of the cellular uptake of a lipid —RNA complex. The dependence of the RNA release on the membrane charge density σM and the disruption of the endosome membrane is indicated. Adapted from Ref. [77].

was obtained, demonstrating the opportunities for lipid optimisation [24,78]. Thereby, lipid nanoparticles were formed from the cationic lipid together with phosphatidylcholine, cholesterol and a PEG-lipid as stabilisers. The **RNA complexation** by the lipid in the nanoparticles and thus protection from external RNases was confirmed. According to molecular simulations, the **PEG-lipid** formed a roughly homogenous coating of the nanoparticles [78].

The focussed integration of **targeting units** is enabled by the localisation of PEG-lipids on the outside of the nanoparticles. In that sense, PEG-lipids were conjugated with folate units and applied for the assembly of vancomycin loaded lipid nanoparticles. Thereby, **specific binding and uptake** by methicillin-resistant *S. aureus* (MRSA) was achieved [79,80]. As in other nanoparticulate systems, the PEG coating might interfere with the intracellular drug release, which is why cleavable, e.g. pH cleavable, linkers were developed [81]. Next to applying a PEG coating on nanoparticles, the use of **biomimetics** is a powerful strategy to improve the targeting and avoid uptake by macrophages. Similar as in naturally produced lipid nanovesicles membrane proteins can be incorporated into lipid bilayers during self-assembly of synthetic lipid nanovesicles. Prolonged circulation and improved targeting of inflamed tissue in vitro and in vivo can, for example, be achieved by integrating leucocyte membrane proteins into phosphocholine/cholesterol lipid nanovesicles [82]. To mimic a virus-like infection of bacterial cells, **surface-nanoengineered antimicrobial liposomes** (SNAL) were developed, which possess a lipid-based membrane structure and lipopeptide-enriched bilayer surface. Thereby, the SNAL combined (i) a highly efficient and selective bacteria binding, (ii) rapid fusion through the bacterial membrane, and (iii) local “burst” release were achieved i.a. in MRSA [83].

An example of **liposomes with antimicrobial activity** per se are polyunsaturated liposomes. Such liposomes targeting the endoplasmatic reticulum have been used to treat viral infections [84]. Lipid nanoparticles from antimicrobial active fatty acids such as lauric acid and caproic acid (both saturated fatty acids) as well as linoelic acid (unsaturated fatty acid) have been applied to treat i.a. *S. aureus* infections. Thereby, the antimicrobial effect is attributed to the destabilisation of the bacterial cell membrane [27].

2.2 Peptide-based nanoparticles

Synthetic peptide self-assembly has emerged as a promising research field in nanomedicine due to the following advantages [85–88]. Various peptide-based supramolecular architectures like micelles, vesicles, nanofibers, nanotubes and nanoparticles can be obtained via a rational design of the molecular building blocks [86,88–90]. Even though nature commonly uses protein sequences of up to several hundred amino acid residues as building blocks of functional materials, substantially shorter sequences (from 5 to 10 amino acids) can also exhibit highly sophisticated self-assembly behaviour. The nanostructures protect the peptide against protease degradation and preserve its functionality, improving thermal stability and peptide half-lives (from minutes to hours). Other parameters such as concentration, buffer composition (pH, ionic strength) and temperature also influence the self-assembly process [91]. **Self-assembled peptide motifs** play a large role in increasing targeting activities of drug carriers [85]. Different **classes of amphiphilic peptides** include (i) peptides that consist of both polar and nonpolar residues, giving rise to both hydrophobic and hydrophilic properties, (ii) hydrophilic peptides attached to hydrophobic lipid alkyl chains (Fig. 3.6) [70–72].

Well-defined **peptide nanoassemblies** consist of three basic components: (i) hydrophobic amino acids (e.g. leucine, alanine, valine) governing the self-assembly process through intermolecular non-covalent interactions and the subsequent formation of secondary structures; (ii) aromatic interactions, i.e. π–π stacking, contribute to the self-assembly and of secondary structures via aromatic residues (phenylalanine, tryptophan); (iii) hydrophilic amino acid residues (e.g. glutamine, asparagine) to stabilise the specific structure in a biological environment. Depending on the type of cargo delivery to be achieved, specific amino acid residues can facilitate specific interactions, e.g. in the case of

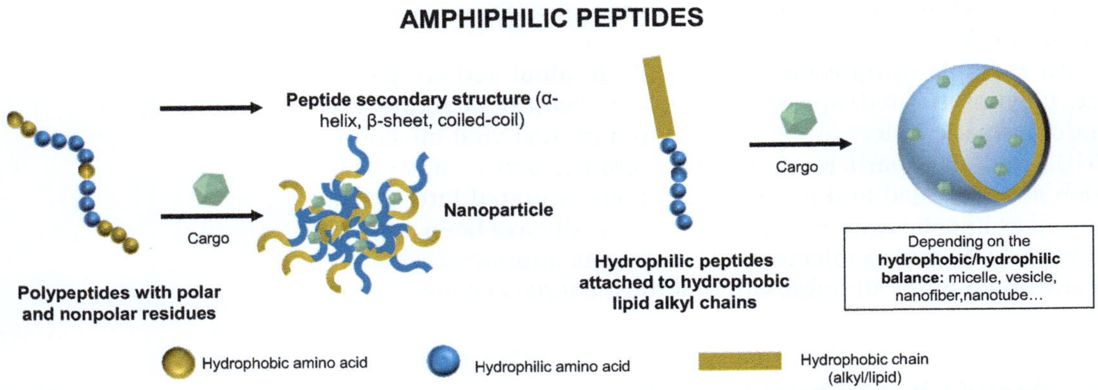

Figure 3.6 Peptide self-assembled structures based on the primary structure of the peptides and the block-length ratio in amphiphilic peptides. Adopted from Ref. [88].

negatively charged biomacromolecules such as nucleic acids, positively charged amino acid residues (lysine, arginine, and histidine) can interact electrostatically [34].

Additionally, a rational design of the building blocks is the **conjugation of hydrophobic moieties** (alkyl or lipid chain) to peptides [92]. They self-assemble into a variety of structures and sizes based upon charges (or hydrophobicity) in the peptide portion of the molecule and the nature of the hydrophobic tail [optimal hydrophilic–lipophilic balance (HLB)]. One of the **biggest advantages** of the PA-based self-assemblies is their biocompatibility and biodegradability. However, due to their amide backbone, they can be quickly degraded after systemic delivery; ongoing work has investigated limiting proteolysis in circulation. A common strategy is to synthesise peptides using D-enantiomers that are more resistant to endogenous protease degradation. Another strategy is to functionalise the surface with polymers as PEG that protect from proteolysis, increase water solubility, reduce immunogenicity and increase in vivo half-life [93]. Moreover, an amphiphilic molecule was built using hexadecanoic acid, three arginine–proline (RP) repeat peptide branches and a flexible amino acid linker. The RP repeat branches together with the hexadecanoic acid provided the peptide dendron with positive charge and hydrophobicity, respectively. Additionally, hexadecanoic acid provided the driving force for the self-assembly behaviour. The branched presentation of **AMPs as dendrons** showed a better stability towards various inhibitory factors, providing a promising potential system for addressing the antibiotic shortage without causing bacterial resistance [94].

In recent years, studies about antibacterial materials have been focussed on natural materials, such as chitosan and chitin, because of their unique biodegradable, biocompatible, non-toxic and antimicrobial nature [95]. Other natural biomacromolecules (alginate, hyaluronic acid, gelatin, heparin, etc.) can be efficiently conjugated to bioactive peptides with highly efficient coupling approaches and provide synergic properties [96].

Also, several **sequence-regulated peptides** have been identified that **exhibit stimuli-responsive structural behaviour**. For instance, elastin-like polypeptides (ELPs) exhibit a sharp temperature-reversible hydrophilic-hydrophobic phase transition (sequence of amino acids: VPGXG repeats) [97]. Another example is an acid-responsive amphiphilic peptide that contains KKGRGDS sequence in hydrophilic head. In neutral or basic medium, hydrogen bonding and hydrophobic interactions lead to the self-assembly into micelles. In an acidic environment, however, the electrostatic repulsion interaction among the ionised lysine (K) residues lead the dissociation of micelles [98]. These amphiphilic peptides are very promising as smart nanocarriers.

2.3 Polymeric nanoparticles

Polymer-based nanoparticles are colloidal systems made up of natural or synthetic polymers. They provide significant advantages such as the feasibility of scale-up and the manufacturing process under Good Manufacturing Practices (GMP). Other notable characteristics of polymeric nanoparticles are their significant physico-chemical stability in biological fluids along with the wide availability of various polymers.

2.3.1 Micelles and multi-compartment-micelles

Polymeric micelles are formed when the concentration of the amphiphilic polymer reaches a certain critical value named critical micelle concentration (CMC). At a concentration higher than the CMC, the hydrophobic segments aggregate to form a compact hydrophobic core. Polymeric micelles are then thermodynamically stabilised against disassembly. Factors such as the ratio of hydrophobic and hydrophilic chain length and the preparation process affect the formation of micelles. Depending on the polymer, they can exhibit an excellent biocompatibility, low toxicity, enhanced blood circulation time and ability to solubilise large quantities of drugs in their micellar core. The hydrophobic core serves as a reservoir in which the drug molecules can be incorporated by means of chemical, physical or electrostatic interactions [99,100].

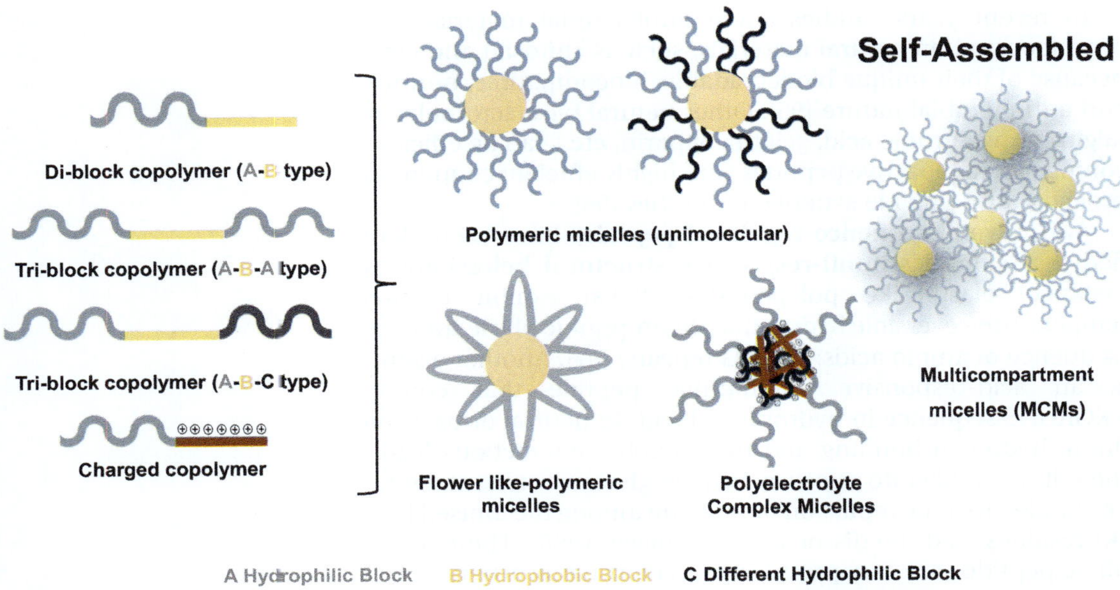

Figure 3.7 Overview of different self-assembled polymeric micelles based on the composition of the block copolymer. (A) (*blue*) and (C) (*green*) are hydrophilic, (B) (*beige*) is hydrophobic.

Amphiphilic AB diblock or ABA triblock copolymers (where A = hydrophilic and B = hydrophobic-hydrophilic) are most commonly used to prepare self-assembled polymeric micelles for drug delivery (Fig. 3.7). These block copolymers assemble into unimolecular spherical core–shell micelles of approximately 10–50 nm in diameter. Micelles always consist of a hydrophobic core for drug loading and a hydrophilic shell that acts as a main physical ("steric") barrier. The hydrophilic part prevents micelle aggregation in solution, can prevent protein binding and also stops opsonisation [i.e. the coating of non-self material with opsonins (e.g. IgG, C3b), which activates the immune response] during systemic administration. Moreover, **dendrimers or star shape molecules** are widely used as building blocks to prepare unimolecular micelles because they are highly branched, have well defined globular shape and controlled surface functionality [101]. Amphiphilic BAB triblock copolymers can generate flower like-polymeric micelles as well [102].

The ability to incorporate hydrophobic antibacterial compounds into aqueous dispersible nanocarriers allows for increased availability of the drugs at the site of the infection. The ability of triclosan-loaded micelles to penetrate into biofilms and to kill the *S. aureus* residing in the biofilms with greater efficacy than free triclosan has been recently shown [103]. In addition, the self-assembly of phosphonium-functionalised PEO-*b*-PCL copolymers into micelles (diameters less than 50 nm) shows antibacterial activity. These micelles could encapsulate and release an additional drug, providing the potential for an orthogonal mechanism of attack against bacteria during the infection process [104].

Polyelectrolyte complex micelles (PCMs), nanoparticles formed by electrostatic self-assembly of charged polymers with charged-neutral hydrophilic block copolymers, offer a potential solution to the challenging problem of delivering therapeutic nucleic acids into cells and organisms (Fig. 3.7).

Some polymeric micelles have steadily progressed through clinical trials. However, **the stability and premature disassembly** should be improved. Core-crosslinking is among the most popular methods to improve the in vivo stability and is particularly important in applications that involve changes in temperature, salt concentration, mechanical shear force, etc. Indeed, a number of core-crosslinked polymeric micelles have demonstrated enhanced stability in animal models [105].

Finally, **anisotropic nanoparticles**, such as **patchy, multicompartment and Janus** micelles, have attracted significant attention in recent years due to their novel morphologies and diverse potential applications [106,107]. They are based on the hierarchical step-wise self-assembly of a few AB diblock copolymers and most ABC triblock terpolymers (where C is also hydrophilic). The separation of incompatible compartments could enable the selective entrapment and release of various hydrophobic or hydrophilic drugs while the hydrophilic shell would permit the stabilisation of these nanostructures in physiological media [108].

2.3.2 Polymeric nanospheres

Another kind of polymeric nanoparticles that can encapsulate different types of cargo are the **polymeric nanospheres.** They are a polymeric matrix of spherical shape that ranges in size between 10 and 200 nm in diameter. The drug is encapsulated or attached uniformly to the continuous matrix of polymer. Polymeric nanospheres have demonstrated very good properties in drug delivery (they protect the drug from chemical and enzymatic degradation) and as promising theranostic platform through additional functionalities (such as inorganic nanoparticles) [109,110]. In this respect, **supramolecular polyelectrolyte complexes** based on the electrostatic interaction between anionic polymers and cationic polymers are of interest. For example, the complex between cyclodextrin-grafted chitosan derivative and carrageenan have been studied for controlled antibacterial drug release [111].

2.3.3 Polymeric vesicles

Just like lipids and peptides, amphiphilic block-copolymers can also self-assemble into vesicles with a bilayer membrane. Such vesicles are then called **polymersomes**. They can host both hydrophilic and hydrophobic substances and the bilayer is similar to the one present in natural liposomes. Following these biomimetic properties, the largest part of this segment is devoted to polymersomes.

In order to form vesicles, the hydrophilic part of an amphiphilic block-copolymer has to be about 30% (w/w) or less. The exact amount is highly dependent on the block-copolymer actually used. **AB amphiphilic diblock copolymers** are the minimum requirement to form polymersomes. Polymer block A is then present on the inner and the outer leaflet of the membrane forming the vesicle. Such symmetric membranes do not resemble natural membranes, which are usually asymmetric. However, the symmetry can be broken if polymer A bares reactive groups which can then react with molecules outside the polymersomes. The most common way to functionalise the membrane is to use responsive polymers within the hydrophobic part [36,112,113]. As soon as the responsive unit reacts with the outside environment, the entire block becomes hydrophilic, leading to a disassembly of the polymersomes and a complete release of any encapsulated cargo. A temperature-responsive block would thus lead to drug release following a temperature change in the surrounding medium. Depending on the LCST of the polymer, the cargo could be released in inflamed (i.e. warmer) tissue as the self-assemblies change when reaching the LCST. Similarly, pH-responsive units could lead to disassembly in the endosomal environment, which exhibits a lower pH value than the cytosol. Target tissues with a pronounced different redox potential (e.g. cancer) are ideal for redox responsive polymers [114].

Many polymersomes are chemically more stable than liposomes, because the underlying polymers are more difficult to degrade. This, as already discussed in Section 1.4, raises biocompatibility issues. However, it also leads to mainly impermeable membranes, making it more difficult to enable and regulate **transmembrane traffic**. Introducing cross-linking bonds in the membrane is one way to improve this aspect [115]. The cross-links prohibit a complete disassembly but result in a vesicle with a swollen membrane after the hydrophobic part has become hydrophilic. Small molecules can then diffuse through the membrane and reach the inner cavity, enabling the intended crosstalk [116]. Introducing transmembrane proteins is another way to achieve the same goal. In this approach, a transport protein is co-assembled with the block-copolymers or inserted into the membrane after it has been formed. In the simplest model, this protein is a pure channel like aquaporin, outer membrane protein F (ompF) or mellitin, enabling unregulated diffusion in and out of the vesicle [117–120]. Regulating this traffic can be achieved by putting a responsive molecular cap on the part of the protein that is supposed to end up on the outer leaflet on the membrane. For example, in case of ompF, such caps or other molecular handles lead to a directed insertion of the protein. Following sterical arguments, the spatially demanding side is then on the outside of the membrane [121,122].

If protein modification is not an option or the channel protein is a directional transporter (like proteorhodopsin or spider rhodopsin), the polymer membrane needs to be different on the inner and outer leaflet to guide the protein insertion. Such an asymmetric membrane is common in natural vesicles and can be achieved using an **ABC triblock copolymer** where one hydrophilic part (e.g. A) is on the outer leaflet and the other hydrophilic part (e.g. C) is on the inner leaflet. Following spatial arguments, the polymer for the crowded concave inner leaflet needs to be of a lower molecular weight than the one on the convex less crowded outer leaflet [35,123–126]. If the polymers A and C then have specifically different interactions with each end of the transmembrane protein, this strategy leads to a directed insertion of the protein. Proofing asymmetry of the membrane is a significant scientific challenge. In case of one charged polymer, the surface charge (zeta potential) is a very feasible indicator. In case of two neutral polymers, different reactivities of these polymers will have to be used. Reaction kits to sense the presence of amides (e.g. for oxazolines) or selective quenching of attached dyes have proven to be successful strategies in such instances [35,44].

All possible options for polymersomes discussed so far follow homogeneous surfaces on either side of the membrane, which is not close to natural membranes. **Inhomogeneous surfaces,** i.e. distinct material domains on their surfaces (Fig. 3.7), are much more common in natural membranes [127]. Following the fluidity of lipid membranes, a heterogeneous surface is much more feasible with polymeric membranes [41,127–130]. ABC block-copolymers (linear or star-shaped) can overcome this

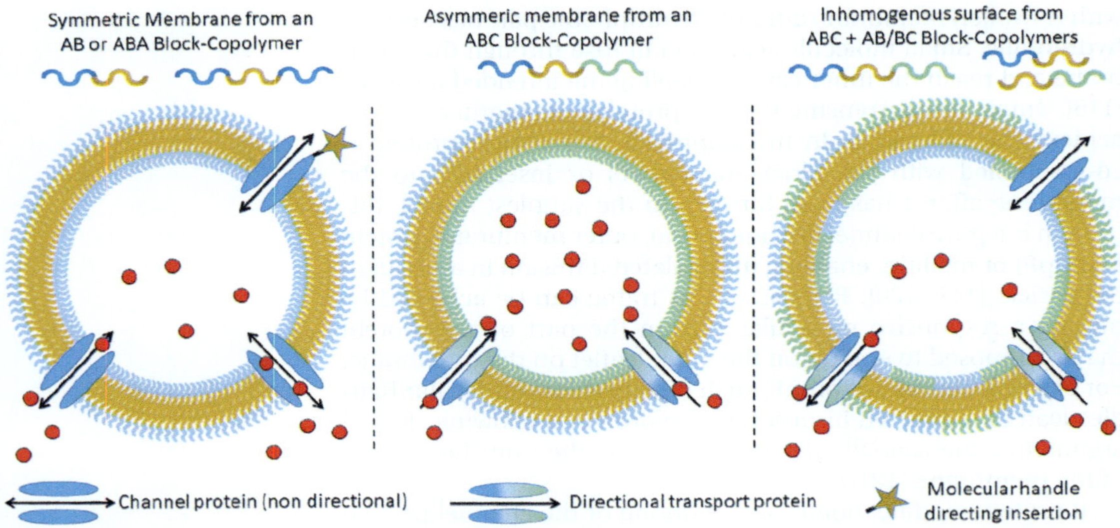

Figure 3.8 A symmetric membrane from an AB or ABA block-copolymer can host non-directional membrane proteins like OmpF or mellitin, which can be directed if they contain a molecular handle. An asymmetric membrane from an ABC triblock copolymer can host directional proteins with a preferred orientation like rhodopsins, so that gradients can evolve. Membranes with an inhomogeneous surface (both A and C on the surface) can host directional transport proteins in both directions, inducing a short circuit in transport, so that no gradient can evolve.

shortcoming of polymersomes (Fig. 3.8, right side). If the blocks A and C are similar enough in length, both of them are present on either leaflet of the membrane. Since polymers are thermodynamically stable when surrounded by similar polymers, the polymers de-mix and form domains. These domains are small for polymersomes of pure ABC triblock copolymers, since the blocks are chemically linked and thus cannot have great distances between each other. Mixing the ABC block copolymer with the corresponding AB and BC diblock-copolymers makes the separate domains grow and the ABC triblock-copolymers act as "lineactant" preventing a complete demixing of the copolymers, which occurs without this auxiliary triblock [131–133].

In addition to the linear polymers just discussed, defined branched polymers can also self-assemble effectively into vesicles. Highly defined branching refers to the combination of hydrophilic and hydrophobic dendrons onto one core to form amphiphilic dendrimers (named amphiphilic Janus Dendrimers) [134], which can self-assemble into **Dendrimersomes.** In contrast to linear polymers, they are now well defined in their molar mass with a dispersity close to 1.00. Highly defined molecules are more likely to clear the bar in a pharmaceutical approval process. In addition to the defined molecules, the final vesicles are also more uniform after their formation, which can simplify the production process considerably. However, dendrimersomes can also face the issue of lacking biodegradability if they are based on a non-degradable polymer [134,135].

3. Production of nanoparticles

All aforementioned types of nanoparticles from lipids, proteins and polymers as a drug delivery carrier via pharmaceutical encapsulation have greatly promoted the development of nanomedicine. Several approaches have been explored to **prepare nanoparticles of desired composition, size, shape and properties**. Broadly these approaches are grouped as top-down and bottom-up approaches. Both methods are widely used, however, top-down approaches (physical methods) yield imperfection of the surface structure. Such defects can have a significant impact on the physical and chemical properties. Generally spoken, bottom-up approaches yield nanoparticles with fewer defects, more homogenous chemical composition, better ordering and smaller sizes (Fig. 3.9).

3.1 Bottom-up production

The **emulsification solvent-evaporation** method was the first technique developed to prepare polymeric nanoparticles. A polar organic solvent containing the polymer and the cargo is prepared. The organic solution is emulsified in the aqueous phase containing a surfactant, and then it is processed by using high-speed homogenisation or ultrasonication, yielding a dispersion of nanodroplets. A suspension of nanoparticles is formed by

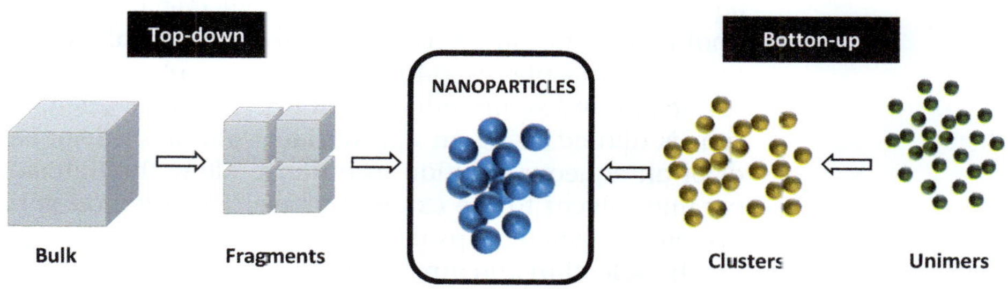

Figure 3.9 Two different approaches for polymeric nanoparticles production. They can be formed from a bulk material (*top-down, left*) or from dissolved unimers (*bottom-up, right*). Adopted from Ref. [136].

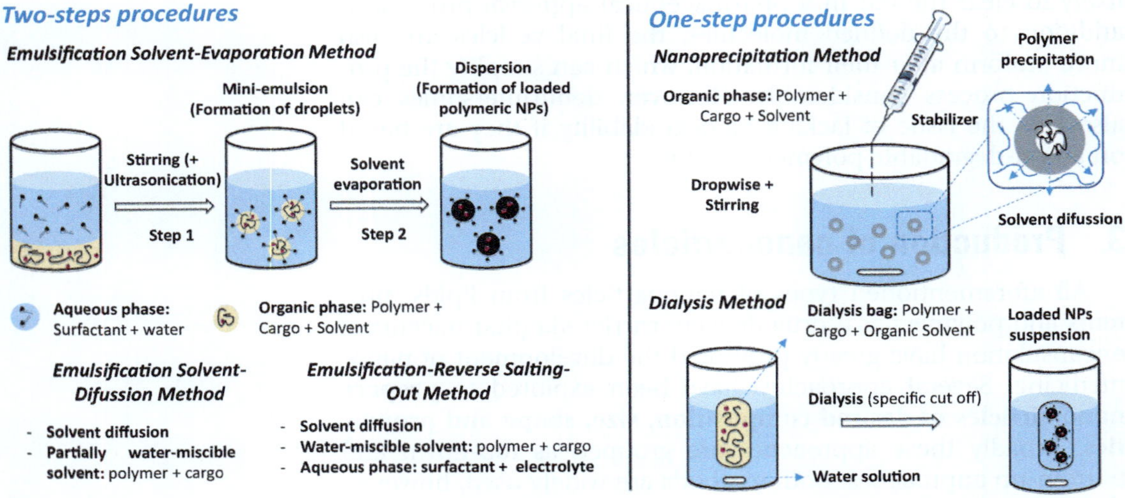

Figure 3.10 Main bottom-up production techniques based on emulsification. The names of the methods are written in a larger font size to distinguish them from different texts.

evaporation of the polymer solvent. This method leads mainly to nanospheres. The main advantages of the process are versatility with respect to the polymer, that it is easy to handle and the fast production times (Fig. 3.10) [137,138].

The **emulsification solvent-diffusion** method is a modified version to the previous one. The internal phase of this emulsion consists of a partially hydro-miscible organic solvent. By adding a large amount of water to the previously saturated water/solvent mixture, the hydrophobic part of the material becomes insoluble, resulting in the formation of colloidal particles. This method is used to produce nanospheres, but nanocapsules can also be obtained (Fig. 3.10) [139].

Emulsification-reverse salting-out is based on the separation of organic solutions which are usually water-miscible from an aqueous solution, through a salting-out effect to render hydrophobic parts insoluble. This method mainly results in the formations of nanospheres [140]. The aqueous phase consists of the surfactant and saturated solution of electrolyte. Then, the emulsion is diluted using an appropriate volume of deionised water or of an aqueous solution in order to allow the diffusion of the organic solvent to the external phase. This method is useful for protein/enzyme encapsulation (Fig. 3.10) [141].

The **selection and amount of the surfactants** is the key to successful fabrication in all previous methods. Low concentration of surfactants usually leads to a high polydispersity and particle aggregation. However, high concentration leads to a decrease of the cargo loading efficiency due to strong interactions between the cargo and surfactants.

Formation by **nanoprecipitation** requires two miscible solvents. The polymer is dissolved in a water-miscible solvent of intermediate polarity, and this solution is added stepwise into an aqueous solution under stirring. Due to the fast-spontaneous diffusion of the polymer solution into the aqueous phase, the nanoparticles form instantaneously in an attempt to avoid the water molecules, the polymer precipitates in the form of nanocapsules or nanospheres. Depending on the required nanoparticle, the organic phase is added to the aqueous solution or vice versa. The obtained nanoparticles feature a well-defined size and a narrow size distribution, but the speed of the addition can have a major impact on the shape of the nanoparticles. However, their formation is instantaneous and needs only one step (Fig. 3.10) [142,143]. Materials with stimuli-sensitive chains can also be transformed into nanoparticles by **physicochemical nanoprecipitation**. Following a change in a solvent parameter (e.g. temperature or pH), one part of the material becomes hydrophobic, inducing the self-assembly process. Some of the best known stimuli are temperature-sensitive polymers by phase inversion temperature (PIT) [144], and pH-sensitive polymers by pH switch [145,146].

The **dialysis method** is a simple and effective technique with narrow distribution. Cargo and polymers are placed inside a dialysis tube/membrane after dissolving with water miscible organic solvents with appropriate molecular weight cut-off. The organic phase diffuses through the dialysis tube/membrane into the aqueous phase which decreases the interfacial tension between them, leading to the formation of a colloidal suspension of nanoparticles. However, the large volume of counter dialysing medium could arouse a premature release of the nanoparticle payload. The morphology and particle size distribution of the obtained nanoparticles can be modulated by several experimental parameters, such as concentration of the material, solvent/non-solvent pair, dialysis molecular weight cut-off and the temperature at which the procedure is carried out [147].

Another option is **polymerisation-induced self-assembly (PISA)**. Much of the PISA literature has been based on thermally initiated RAFT-polymerisation. Formation of the nanoparticle core is initiated in situ, by a characteristic solubility change of the co-monomer, which is soluble in the initial solvent, but the corresponding polymer is not. The PISA approach can be used to prepare families of nanoparticles varying in morphology in a via a simple one-pot reaction, where polymer synthesis and assembly occur simultaneously. The most commonly observed nanoparticle morphologies obtained from PISA are spheres, worms and vesicles. Its term "PISA" is still relatively new as its first appearance in the academic literature was in 2009 [148].

A common problem statement in the pharmaceutical industry is low oral bioavailability of drug candidates with poor aqueous solubility. Many technologies exist to address issues of oral delivery and selecting the right strategy depends on the physical chemical properties of the drug and the final product. When applying the **spray drying method**, the drying of polymeric nanoparticles is used to obtain **solid amorphous dispersion** represents a promising platform to improve the physicochemical stability of formulations and/or to control the release of hydrophilic and lipophilic drugs [149].

3.2 Top-down production

For block-copolymers, one of the top-down approaches includes starting from bulk polymer in the shape of a thin film. The method is hence called **thin film rehydration**. After the polymer has been dissolved in a good solvent, this solvent gets removed slowly, leaving behind the aforementioned thin film of the used polymer. Once the polymer gets into contact with water, the hydrophilic part hydrates and begins to detach from the film. Since the hydrophobic part is moved out of the film together with the hydrophilic part, the self-assembly process gets started. If vesicles have to be produced, this method is more promising than a bottom-up approach, since it favours the thermodynamically more stable product. The underlying reason is the longer time it takes for the film to be completely rehydrated, which prevents the formation of kinetically trapped structures [150,151]. Film rehydration often leads to self-assembly structures of increased dispersity compared to bottom-up methods. **Extrusion** is thus often applied to decrease dispersity and reaching self-assemblies of dispersities equal to bottom-up methods [152,153].

With thin film rehydration, **enclosing hydrophilic** and **hydrophobic molecules** can be achieved. Any hydrophobic substance has to be pre-mixed with the polymer in the organic solvent before the film is formed and is then included in the hydrophobic part of the polymer film and thus ends up in the hydrophobic part of the final self-assembly. Any micellar core or the membrane of vesicles can be filled with hydrophobic substances that way. However, the substances need to have a common solvent with the polymer for this approach to be successful. Hydrophilic

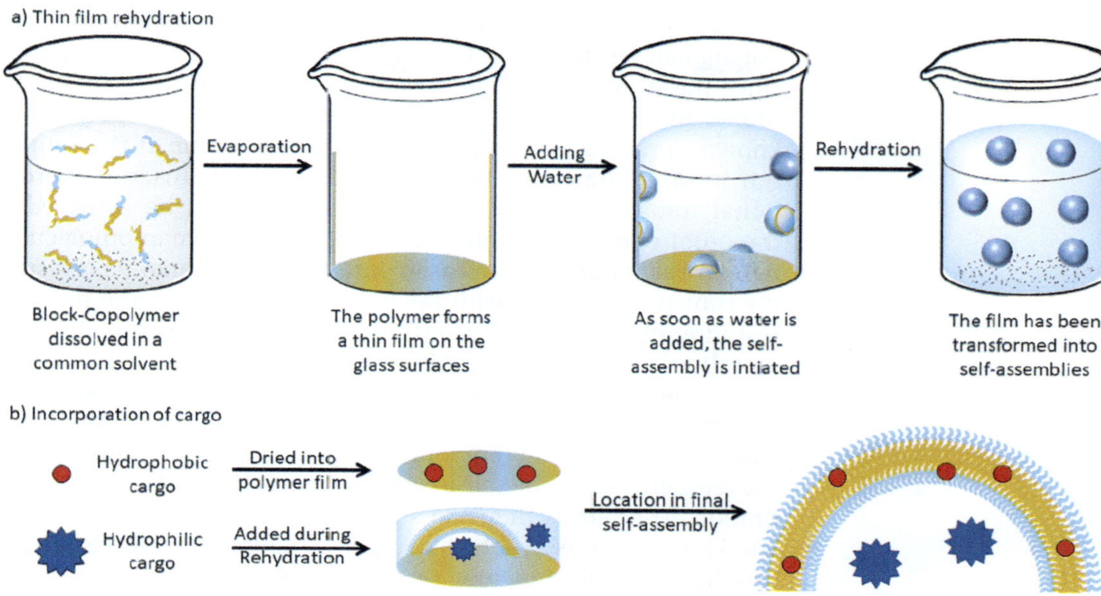

Figure 3.11 Production of nanoparticles using thin film rehydration on the example of polymersomes. (A) The polymer is dissolved in an organic solvent, which is then evaporated to leave a thin film. After adding water or an aqueous buffer, the polymer rehydrates into vesicles or other nanoparticles. (B) Hydrophobic substances are added with the polymer, while hydrophilic substances are added with the rehydration medium. If vesicles are formed, the hydrophobic substances are included in the membrane and the hydrophobic ones can be incorporated into the lumen.

substances, on the other hand, can be enclosed if they are added together with the water or buffer used to rehydrate the thin polymer film. After rehydration, they end up in the hydrophilic component of the self-assembly, i.e. the hydrophilic compartments of multi-compartment-micelles or the hydrophilic lumen of vesicles [154,155] (Fig. 3.11).

Incorporating amphiphilic components into the membrane like **transmembrane proteins** is more difficult to enclose. Especially proteins would denature if co-solved with the polymer in an organic solvent, ruling out that option in this case. However, the channels can still be included **after membrane formation**. All proteins with a hydrophobic component are stabilised by an amphiphile. Removing the amphiphile and adding it to the self-assembly structure has the effect that the hydrophobic part of the protein aligns with the hydrophobic part of the polymer. Since the hydrophilic part aligns itself with the hydrophilic part of the polymer, the protein ends up being inserted into the self-assembly [156–158]. In case of liposomes, this works well since the hydrophobic parts are designed to be surrounded by lipids. In polymersomes, however, the thicker membrane can cause issues since the protein would be too short to span through the membrane. In case of very soft polymers like PDMS, the polymer is known to rearrange and present a thin membrane at the spot of the inserted transmembrane protein [50,128]. Inserting directional transporters in a specific orientation can be achieved if the outer end of the protein is modified with a macromolecular handle that is unlikely to insert into the membrane. As a result, the transporter inserts with the non-modified end of the protein, resulting in an oriented insertion allowing for directional transmembrane transport [121,122].

Despite the many options, some materials are **not feasible for this method** or require additional energy input. Any stiff material with a glass transition temperature or melting temperature above the temperature of the self-assembly cannot be used for film rehydration. The film is then too stable and does not rehydrate into any kind of self-assembly. Strong $\pi-\pi$ interactions in PS render this hydrophobic polymer not applicable for film rehydration [37,159]. Semi-crystalline polymers (like PCL), however, have to be heated above their melting temperature for this process to work [125,160]. Any molecules that are to be included during self-assembly then have to withstand this temperature and the final self-assembly is inert to any insertion after the solution has been cooled below melting temperature due to crystallites forming in the self-assembled structure.

3.3 Microfluidics

Microfluidics is the manipulation of fluids on a small geometrical scale in miniaturised devices, which are formed by microstructuring of materials such as glass, elastomers or thermoplastics. Resulting from the small channel dimensions, the fluid flow is mostly **laminar**, thus enabling reproducible fluid mixing by diffusion. Because of these characteristics, microfluidics is a powerful method for the **bottom-up production** of **nanoparticles** achieving good size control, low polydispersity and high drug encapsulation efficiency [23]. Regarding the development of nanoparticles towards commercial application, the scalability of microfluidic synthesis is another crucial aspect [80].

In general, two approaches for can be distinguished for microfluidic nanoparticle formation, namely the production of **droplet emulsions** from **non-miscible fluids,** and the nanoparticle precipitation by mixing fluids with different polarity [161]. In the first case, oil and water phases are combined in a microfluidic device, using geometries such as the **co-flow, cross-flow** or **flow focussing** [162]. Key parameters for controlling the droplet size are (i) the channel dimensions at the junction where the fluids intersect; (ii) the flow rates of water and oil phase; (iii) the interfacial tensions; (iv) fluid viscosities; and (v) applied materials [23,163]. Repeated combination of oil and water phases, e.g. by combining a co-flow geometry and a flow-focussing geometry, allows producing double emulsions. **Nanoparticle self-assembly** of amphiphillic materials occurs at the oil-water interface, e.g. as it is described for the block copolymer PEG-*b*-PLLA [164]. However, corresponding to the channel dimensions, particles with a diameter of about 25 μm (mainly giant unilammelar vesicles, GUVs) are obtained [165], which are far too large for intravenous administration. Only in recent research, successful integration of **nanochannels** into microchannels was demonstrated, thus achieving a significant **downsizing of water-in-oil droplets** to 2.5 μm−50 nm and the assembly of protein nanogels [163]. Therefore, given sufficient reliability in production and operation despite the sensitivity to clogging, droplet nanofluidics might become a tool for controlled nanoparticle formation.

For **nanoparticle synthesis** by **precipitation**, a solution containing the nanoparticle material (e.g. polymers, peptides or lipids) and possibly further components is mixed with a nonsolvent on a microfluidic chip to induce the self-assembly process. Reproducible and complete mixing of the fluids, though, is required to obtain nanoparticles with low dispersity and adjustable size. Furthermore, to obtain diameters in the range of 1−200 nm, fast nucleation (happening in few ms, corresponding to fast mixing) is essential. Both prerequisites can be fulfiled by mixing the fluids in a microfluidic device. However, due to the laminar flow in microfluidics, efficient mixing requires the use of **mixing geometries**, such as obstacle-based mixers, split-and-recombine mixers or shearing-based mixers [166,167]. Among the obstacle-based mixers, the herringbone geometry is frequently applied as it enables reproducible and fast mixing (Fig. 3.12A) [78,168]. Correspondingly, this mixing geometry is also applied in commercial microfluidic systems for nanoparticle production, e.g. by the company PrecisionNanoSystems [82]. To realise clinically relevant production rates (L/hour), a scalable, parallelised microfluidic device with herringbone mixers was recently developed. In this context, "scalable" refers to the scaling up or scaling down of the production rate by simply adding or removing mixer channels without changing the general microfluidic design [169]. Apart from that, controlled solvent exchange (and therefore reproducible nanoparticle assembly) was

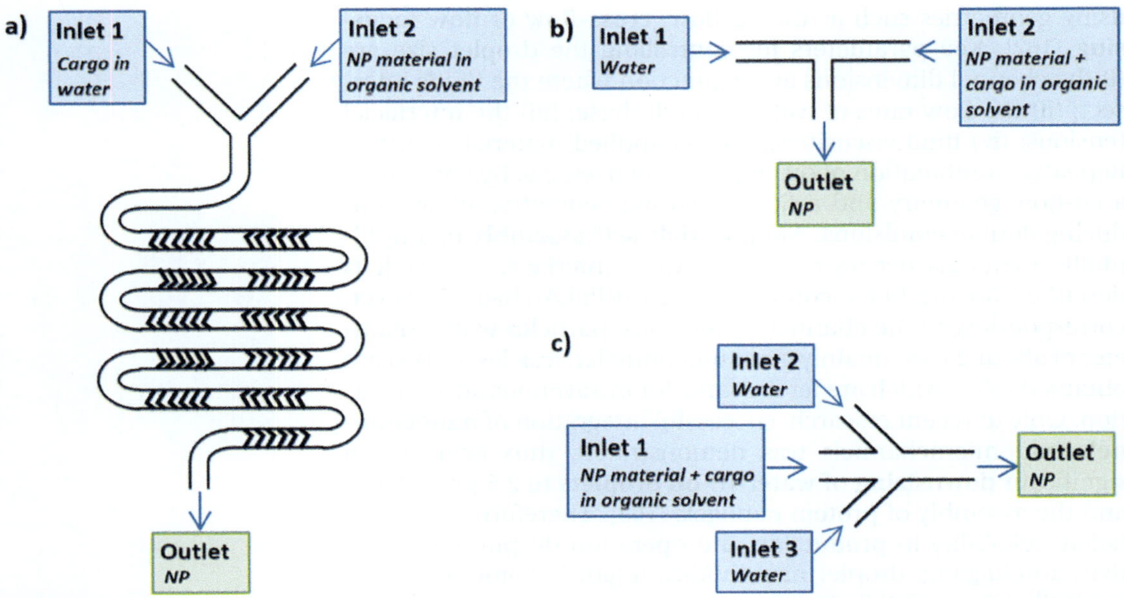

Figure 3.12 Nanoparticle production by precipitation in microfluidic devices. (A) Mixing in herringbone structure. (B) Mixing at a T-junction. (C) Solvent exchange by flow focussing. The fluids indicated at the inlets are only given as examples and are not only applicable for the respective geometry of the microfluidic device.

demonstrated with T-junction geometries (Fig. 3.12B) [26] and with flow focussing devices [80,170,171] (Fig. 3.12B and C).

4. Examples of commercialised applications

To visualise the high relevance of nanoparticulate drug delivery systems in medicine an overview of **commercialised products** is given in Table 3.1. Especially a high number of **lipid-based systems** was commercialised in the past years, to deliver various anti-cancer, anti-fungal and anti-inflammatory drugs as well as therapeutic genes [172]. In 2020, the mRNA-based COVID-19 vaccines mRNA-1273 (Moderna Therapeutics) and BNT-162 (now "Comirnaty"; BioNTech/Pfizer) received the emergency use authorisation by the FDA. Thus, the corresponding lipid nanoparticles are the first authorised formulations for the delivery of mRNA [173].

The group of **protein-based nanoparticles** contains drugs which are conjugated to protein carriers, engineered proteins (where the protein itself acts as the drug) and systems with protein motifs for targeting. Despite the challenges attached to protein

Table 3.1 Different polymers used to form polymeric nanoparticles.

Name and acronym	Molecular structure	Main use and functionality
Hydrophilic polymers		
Poly (ethylene oxide) (PEO) or poly (ethylene glycol) (PEG)	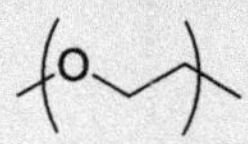	Hydrophilic, neutral
Poly([methyl/ethyl] oxazoline) (PMOXA/ PEtOz)	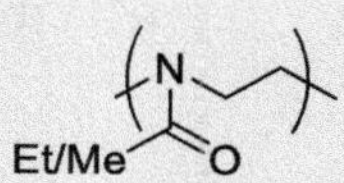	Me + Et: Hydrophilic, neutral Et: LCST 60–65°C
Poly (vinyl alcohol) (PVA)	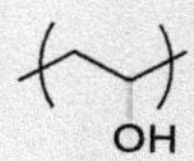	Hydrophilic, neutral
Poly(acrylic acid) (PAA)	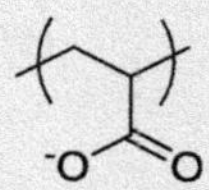 + counterion	Hydrophilic, mostly negatively charged (deprotonated)
Poly(styrene sulfonate) (PSS)	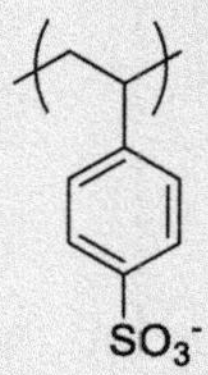 + counterion	Hydrophilic, negatively charged
Polymers for either block		
Poly(N-isopropyl acrylamide) (PNIPAM)	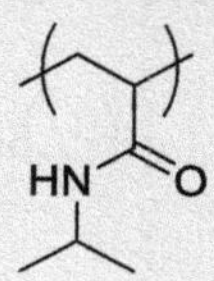	Hydrophilic, neutral LCST: 32–38°C

Continued

Table 3.1 Different polymers used to form polymeric nanoparticles.—*continued*

Name and acronym	Molecular structure	Main use and functionality
Poly(di[methyl/ethyl/iso-propyl] aminoethyl meth-acrylate) (PD[M/E/P] AEMA)	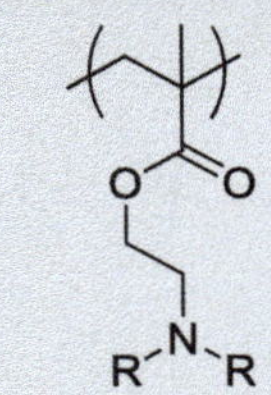	M: Hydrophilic, neutral or positively charged. LCST: 35°C, pKa: 7,5 E + P: Hydrophobic, pH + T-sensitive. pKa: 7,0 (E), 6,3 (P); LCST: 17°C (E), 12°C (P)
Poly(proylene sulphide) (PPS)	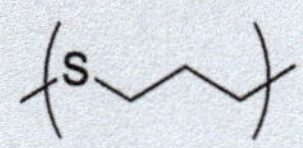	Redox responsive (possible sulphur oxidation)
Poly([L/D]lactic acid) (P[L/D]LA, R = Me) Poly(glylide) (PGA, R=H))	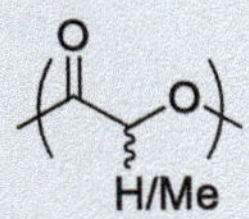	Hydrophobic PLLA: $T_m = 130°C$ PDLA: $T_m = 180°C$
Hydrophobic polymers		
Poly(ε-caprolactone) (PCL)	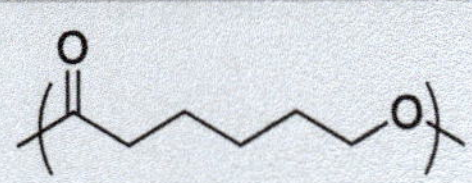	Hydrophobic $T_m = 63°C$
Poly(styrene) (PS)	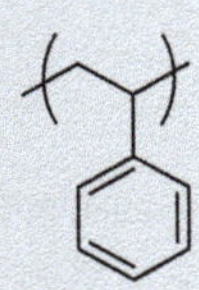	Hydrophobic $T_g = 100°C$
Poly(dimethyl siloxane) (PDMS)	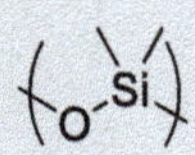	Hydrophobic, very soft

They are sorted from plain hydrophilic to hydrophilic and responsive/functional followed by hydrophobic and responsive/functional and plain hydrophobic polymers.

drug delivery, some formulations, such as albumin-bound paclitaxel nanoparticles (Abraxane), received FDA approval and others are currently in clinical studies [174].

Resulting from their often facile synthesis and wide possible range of applications, a good number of **polymer-based nanomedicines** were approved in recent years and are now in clinical use. However, a huge number of these medicines are based on hybrid materials, e.g. PEGylated drugs or random copolymers. In contrast, self-assembled nanoparticles from amphipillic block copolymers are far less represented. One of the few FDA-approved drug formulation in a polymeric micelle is the menopausal therapeutic Estrasorb. Still, several polymeric systems such as a micellar formulation of docetaxel are currently in clinical studies, demonstrating the progress in the field [174] (Table 3.2).

Table 3.2 Examples of commercial nanoparticle-based drug delivery systems.

Tradename	Active agent/ formulation	Indication	Company/year of approval	References
Lipid-based nanoparticles				
Ambisome	Mycosamine/Liposomes	Fungal infections	Astellas Pharma/1997	[172]
Doxil	Doxorubicin hydrochloride/ Liposomes	Ovarian and breast cancer, Kaposi's sarcoma	Sequus Pharmaceuticals/1995	[172]
Depocyt	Cytarabine/Liposomes	Cancer (neoplastic meningitis)	SkyPharma Inc./1999	[172]
DepoDur	Morphine sulphate/ Liposomes	Pain management	SkyPharma Inc./2004	[172]
Epaxal	Inactivated hepatitis A virus/Liposomes	Hepatitis A vaccination	Crucell, Berna Biotech/1993	[172]
Onpattro	siRNA targeting transthyretin/lipid nanoparticles	Transthyretin-induced amyloidosis (hATTR)	Alnylam Pharmaceuticals/2018	[175]
COVID-19 vaccine Moderna/ mRNA-1273	mRNA/Lipid nanoparticles	COVID-19 vaccination (immunostimulants)	Moderna Therapeutics/Phase III clinical studies; Emergency use authorisation by FDA 2020	[173]

Continued

Table 3.2 Examples of commercial nanoparticle-based drug delivery systems.—*continued*

Tradename	Active agent/ formulation	Indication	Company/year of approval	References
mRNA-1944	mRNA/Lipid nanoparticles	Chikungunya virus infection (mRNA encoding antibodies)	Moderna Therapeutics/Phase I clinical studies	[173]
BNT-162/ Comirnaty	mRNA/Lipid nanoparticles	COVID-19 vaccination (immunostimulants)	BioNTech + Pfizer/Phase III clinical studies; Emergency use authorisation by FDA 2020	[173,176]
Etomidat-Lipuro	Etomidat/Oil-in-water emulsion	Hypnotic	B. Braun Melsungen AG/1991	[22,177]
Diazepam-Lipuro	Diazepam/Oil-in-water emulsion	Sedative	B. Braun Melsungen AG/1985	[22,178]
Propofol-Lipur	Propofol/Oil-in-water emulsion	Anaesthetic	B. Braun Melsungen AG/ Emergency use authorisation by FDA 2020	[179]
Protein-based nanoparticles				
Abraxane	Paclitaxel/albumin-bound paclitaxel nanoparticles	Breast cancer/2005 Non-small cell lung cancer/2012 Pancreatic cancer/ 2013	Celgene/FDA-approved (see left column for year)	[174]
Ontak	Engineered protein combining Interleukin-2 and diphtheria toxin	Cutaneous T-cell lymphoma	Eisai Inc/1999	[174]
Polymer-based nanoparticles				
Estrasorb	Polymeric micelle	Menopausal therapy	Novavax/2003	[174]
BIND-014	Docetaxel/core-shell polymeric micelle	Prostate cancer	Bind Therapeutics/Phase II clinical studies	[174]
Adagen	PEGylated adenosine deaminase enzyme	Severe combined immunodeficiency disease	Sigma-Tau Pharmaceuticals/1990	[174]

References

[1] Y. Williams, A. Sukhanova, M. Nowostawska, A.M. Davies, S. Mitchell, V. Oleinikov, Y. Gun'ko, I. Nabiev, D. Kelleher, Y. Volkov, Probing cell-type-specific intracellular nanoscale barriers using size-tuned quantum dots, Small 5 (22) (2009) 2581–2588.

[2] V. Lesnyak, N. Gaponik, A. Eychmüller, Colloidal semiconductor nanocrystals: the aqueous approach, Chemical Society Reviews 42 (7) (2013) 2905–2929.

[3] M.J. Ndolomingo, N. Bingwa, R. Meijboom, Review of supported metal nanoparticles: synthesis methodologies, advantages and application as catalysts, Journal of Materials Science 55 (15) (2020) 6195–6241.

[4] B. Wiltschi, W. Knoll, E.K. Sinner, Binding assays with artificial tethered membranes using surface plasmon resonance, Methods 39 (2) (2006) 134–146.

[5] X. Gu, Z. Xu, L. Gu, H. Xu, F. Han, B. Chen, X. Pan, Preparation and antibacterial properties of gold nanoparticles: a review, Environmental Chemistry Letters 19 (1) (2021) 167–187.

[6] C. Marambio-Jones, E.M.V. Hoek, A review of the antibacterial effects of silver nanomaterials and potential implications for human health and the environment, Journal of Nanoparticle Research 12 (5) (2010) 1531–1551.

[7] C.G.A. Das, V.G. Kumar, T.S. Dhas, V. Karthick, K. Govindaraju, J.M. Joselin, J. Baalamurugan, Antibacterial activity of silver nanoparticles (biosynthesis): a short review on recent advances, Biocatalysis and Agricultural Biotechnology 27 (2020) 101593.

[8] R. Arvizo, R. Bhattacharya, P. Mukherjee, Gold nanoparticles: opportunities and challenges in nanomedicine, Expert Opinion on Drug Delivery 7 (6) (2010) 753–763.

[9] L.-E. Shi, Z.-H. Li, W. Zheng, Y.-F. Zhao, Y.-F. Jin, Z.-X. Tang, Synthesis, antibacterial activity, antibacterial mechanism and food applications of ZnO nanoparticles: a review, Food Additives & Contaminants: Part A 31 (2) (2014) 173–186.

[10] Y. Huang, J. Ren, X. Qu, Nanozymes: classification, catalytic mechanisms, activity regulation, and applications, Chemical Reviews 119 (6) (2019) 4357–4412.

[11] F. Schwizer, Y. Okamoto, T. Heinisch, Y. Gu, M.M. Pellizzoni, V. Lebrun, R. Reuter, V. Köhler, J.C. Lewis, T.R. Ward, Artificial metalloenzymes: reaction scope and optimization strategies, Chemical Reviews 118 (1) (2018) 142–231.

[12] J.G. Rebelein, T.R. Ward, In vivo catalyzed new-to-nature reactions, Current Opinion in Biotechnology 53 (2018) 106–114.

[13] J. Li, M. Tang, Y. Xue, Review of the effects of silver nanoparticle exposure on gut bacteria, Journal of Applied Toxicology 39 (1) (2019) 27–37.

[14] M.F. Hornos Carneiro, F. Barbosa, Gold nanoparticles: a critical review of therapeutic applications and toxicological aspects, Journal of Toxicology and Environmental Health, Part A B 19 (3–4) (2016) 129–148.

[15] B. Wang, W. Feng, M. Wang, T. Wang, Y. Gu, M. Zhu, H. Ouyang, J. Shi, F. Zhang, Y. Zhao, Z. Chai, H. Wang, J. Wang, Acute toxicological impact of nano- and submicro-scaled zinc oxide powder on healthy adult mice, Journal of Nanoparticle Research 10 (2) (2008) 263–276.

[16] E. Fahy, S. Subramaniam, H.A. Brown, C.K. Glass, J.,A.H. Merrill, R.C. Murphy, C.R.H. Raetz, D.W. Russell, Y. Seyama, W. Shaw, T. Shimizu, F. Spener, G. van Meer, M.S. VanNieuwenhze, S.H. White, J.L. Witztum,

E.A. Dennis, A comprehensive classification system for lipids, European Journal of Lipid Science and Technology 107 (5) (2005) 337–364.
[17] G. Liebisch, E. Fahy, J. Aoki, E.A. Dennis, T. Durand, C.S. Ejsing, M. Fedorova, I. Feussner, W.J. Griffiths, H. Köfeler, A.H. Merrill Jr., R.C. Murphy, V.B. O'Donnell, O. Oskolkova, S. Subramaniam, M.J.O. Wakelam, F. Spener, Update on LIPID MAPS classification, nomenclature, and shorthand notation for MS-derived lipid structures, The Journal of Lipid Research 61 (12) (2020) 1539–1555.
[18] C. Liu, Q. Feng, J. Sun, Lipid nanovesicles by microfluidics: manipulation, synthesis, and drug delivery, Advanced Materials 31 (45) (2019) 1804788.
[19] D.O. Edem, Palm oil: biochemical, physiological, nutritional, hematological and toxicological aspects: a review, Plant Foods for Human Nutrition 57 (3) (2002) 319–341.
[20] A.S. Malamas, M. Gujrati, C.M. Kummitha, R. Xu, Z.-R. Lu, Design and evaluation of new pH-sensitive amphiphilic cationic lipids for siRNA delivery, Journal of Controlled Release 171 (3) (2013) 296–307.
[21] G. Amoabediny, F. Haghiralsadat, S. Naderinezhad, M.N. Helder, E. Akhoundi Kharanaghi, J. Mohammadnejad Arough, B. Zandieh-Doulabi, Overview of preparation methods of polymeric and lipid-based (niosome, solid lipid, liposome) nanoparticles: a comprehensive review, International Journal of Polymeric Materials and Polymeric Biomaterials 67 (6) (2018) 383–400.
[22] W. Mehnert, K. Mäder, Solid lipid nanoparticles: production, characterization and applications, Advanced Drug Delivery Reviews 64 (2012) 83–101.
[23] C.B. Roces, G. Lou, N. Jain, S. Abraham, A. Thomas, G.W. Halbert, Y. Perrie, Manufacturing considerations for the development of lipid nanoparticles using microfluidics, Pharmaceutics 12 (11) (2020).
[24] S.C. Semple, A. Akinc, J. Chen, A.P. Sandhu, B.L. Mui, C.K. Cho, D.W.Y. Sah, D. Stebbing, E.J. Crosley, E. Yaworski, I.M. Hafez, J.R. Dorkin, J. Qin, K. Lam, K.G. Rajeev, K.F. Wong, L.B. Jeffs, L. Nechev, M.L. Eisenhardt, M. Jayaraman, M. Kazem, M.A. Maier, M. Srinivasulu, M.J. Weinstein, Q. Chen, R. Alvarez, S.A. Barros, S. De, S.K. Klimuk, T. Borland, V. Kosovrasti, W.L. Cantley, Y.K. Tam, M. Manoharan, M.A. Ciufolini, M.A. Tracy, A. de Fougerolles, I. MacLachlan, P.R. Cullis, T.D. Madden, M.J. Hope, Rational design of cationic lipids for siRNA delivery, Nature Biotechnology 28 (2) (2010) 172–176.
[25] L.F. Neves, J. Duan, A. Voelker, A. Khanal, L. McNally, J. Steinbach-Rankins, B.P. Ceresa, Preparation and optimisation of anionic liposomes for delivery of small peptides and cDNA to human corneal epithelial cells, Journal of Microencapsulation 33 (4) (2016) 391–399.
[26] J.A. Kulkarni, Y.Y.C. Tam, S. Chen, Y.K. Tam, J. Zaifman, P.R. Cullis, S. Biswas, Rapid synthesis of lipid nanoparticles containing hydrophobic inorganic nanoparticles, Nanoscale 9 (36) (2017) 13600–13609.
[27] C.R. Thorn, N. Thomas, B.J. Boyd, C.A. Prestidge, Nano-fats for bugs: the benefits of lipid nanoparticles for antimicrobial therapy, Drug Delivery and Translational Research 11 (4) (2021) 1598–1624.
[28] P.P.G. Guimaraes, R. Zhang, R. Spektor, M. Tan, A. Chung, M.M. Billingsley, R. El-Mayta, R.S. Riley, L. Wang, J.M. Wilson, M.J. Mitchell, Ionizable lipid nanoparticles encapsulating barcoded mRNA for accelerated in vivo delivery screening, Journal of Controlled Release 316 (2019) 404–417.

[29] D.F. Buccini, M.H. Cardoso, O.L. Franco, Antimicrobial peptides and cell-penetrating peptides for treating intracellular bacterial infections, Frontiers in Cellular and Infection Microbiology 10 (912) (2021).
[30] A. Levin, T.A. Hakala, L. Schnaider, G.J.L. Bernardes, E. Gazit, T.P.J. Knowles, Biomimetic peptide self-assembly for functional materials, Nature Reviews Chemistry 4 (11) (2020) 615–634.
[31] R. Augustine, N. Kalva, H.A. Kim, Y. Zhang, I. Kim, pH-responsive polypeptide-based smart nano-carriers for theranostic applications, Molecules 24 (16) (2019) 2961.
[32] D. Lee, N.S. Rejinold, S.D. Jeong, Y.-C. Kim, Stimuli-responsive polypeptides for biomedical applications, Polymers 10 (8) (2018) 830.
[33] Y. Shen, X. Fu, W. Fu, Z. Li, Biodegradable stimuli-responsive polypeptide materials prepared by ring opening polymerization, Chemical Society Reviews 44 (3) (2015) 612–622.
[34] K. Bauri, M. Nandi, P. De, Amino acid-derived stimuli-responsive polymers and their applications, Polymer Chemistry 9 (11) (2018) 1257–1287.
[35] E. Konishcheva, D. Daubian, J. Gaitzsch, W. Meier, Synthesis of linear ABC triblock copolymers and their self-assembly in solution, Helvetica Chimica Acta 101 (2) (2018) e1700287.
[36] J. Gaitzsch, X. Huang, B. Voit, Engineering functional polymer capsules toward smart nanoreactors, Chemical Reviews 116 (3) (2016) 1053–1093.
[37] Y. Mai, A. Eisenberg, Self-assembly of block copolymers, Chemical Society Reviews 41 (18) (2012) 5969–5985.
[38] Y. Matter, R. Enea, O. Casse, C.C. Lee, J. Baryza, W. Meier, Amphiphilic PEG-b-PMCL-b-PDMAEMA triblock copolymers: from synthesis to physico-chemistry of self-assembled structures, Macromolecular Chemistry and Physics 212 (9) (2011) 937–949.
[39] R. Luxenhofer, C. Fetsch, A. Grossmann, Polypeptoids: a perfect match for molecular definition and macromolecular engineering? Journal of Polymer Science Part A: Polymer Chemistry 51 (13) (2013) 2731–2752.
[40] C. Fetsch, J. Gaitzsch, L. Messager, G. Battaglia, R. Luxenhofer, Self-assembly of amphiphilic block copolypeptoids - micelles, worms and polymersomes, Scientific Reports 6 (2016) 33491.
[41] L. Messager, J. Gaitzsch, L. Chierico, G. Battaglia, Novel aspects of encapsulation and delivery using polymersomes, Current Opinion in Pharmacology 18 (2014) 104–111.
[42] C. Nardin, M. Winterhalter, W. Meier, Giant free-standing ABA triblock copolymer membranes, Langmuir 16 (20) (2000) 7708–7712.
[43] O. Terreau, C. Bartels, A. Eisenberg, Effect of poly(acrylic acid) block length distribution on polystyrene-b-poly(acrylic acid) block copolymer aggregates in solution. 2. A partial phase diagram, Langmuir 20 (3) (2004) 637–645.
[44] J. Gaitzsch, S. Hirschi, S. Freimann, D. Fotiadis, W. Meier, Directed insertion of light-activated proteorhodopsin into asymmetric polymersomes from an ABC block copolymer, Nano Letters 19 (4) (2019) 2503–2508.
[45] A. Car, P. Baumann, J.T. Duskey, M. Cham, N. Bruns, W. Meier, pH-responsive PDMS-b-PDMAEMA micelles for intracellular anticancer drug delivery, Biomacromolecules 15 (9) (2014) 3235–3245.
[46] M. Barz, R. Luxenhofer, R. Zentel, M.J. Vicent, Overcoming the PEG-addiction: well-defined alternatives to PEG, from structure-property

relationships to better defined therapeutics, Polymer Chemistry 2 (9) (2011) 1900–1918.
[47] A. Napoli, M. Valentini, N. Tirelli, M. Mueller, J.A. Hubbell, Oxidation-responsive polymeric vesicles, Nature Materials 3 (3) (2004) 183–189.
[48] S. Cerritelli, D. Velluto, J.A. Hubbell, PEG-SS-PPS: reduction-sensitive disulfide block copolymer vesicles for intracellular drug delivery, Biomacromolecules 8 (6) (2007) 1966–1972.
[49] C.G. Palivan, R. Goers, A. Najer, X. Zhang, A. Car, W. Meier, Bioinspired polymer vesicles and membranes for biological and medical applications, Chemical Society Reviews 45 (2) (2016) 377–411.
[50] F. Itel, A. Najer, C.G. Palivan, W. Meier, Dynamics of membrane proteins within synthetic polymer membranes with large hydrophobic mismatch, Nano Letters 15 (6) (2015) 3871–3878.
[51] General Purpose Polystyrene (GPPS). (Accessed 02 September 2019).
[52] E.V. Konishcheva, U.E. Zhumaev, M. Kratt, V. Oehri, W. Meier, Complex self-assembly behavior of bis-hydrophilic PEO-b-PCL-b-PMOXA triblock copolymers in aqueous solution, Macromolecules 50 (18) (2017) 7155–7168.
[53] H. Sah, L.A. Thoma, H.R. Desu, E. Sah, G.C. Wood, Concepts and practices used to develop functional PLGA-based nanoparticulate systems, International Journal of Nanomedicine 8 (2013) 747–765.
[54] J. Folini, C.-H. Huang, J.C. Anderson, W. Meier, J. Gaitzsch, Novel monomers in radical ring-opening polymerisation for biodegradable and pH responsive nanoparticles, Polymer Chemistry 10 (2019) 5285–5288.
[55] N. Vanparijs, L. Nuhn, B.G. De Geest, Transiently thermoresponsive polymers and their applications in biomedicine, Chemical Society Reviews 46 (4) (2017) 1193–1239.
[56] L. Bixenmann, J. Stickdorn, L. Nuhn, Amphiphilic poly(esteracetal)s as dual pH- and enzyme-responsive micellar immunodrug delivery systems, Polymer Chemistry 11 (13) (2020) 2441–2456.
[57] G. Chen, Y. Wang, R. Xie, S. Gong, A review on core-shell structured unimolecular nanoparticles for biomedical applications, Advanced Drug Delivery Reviews 130 (2018) 58–72.
[58] M.M. Modena, B. Rühle, T.P. Burg, S. Wuttke, Nanoparticle characterization: what to measure? Advanced Materials 31 (32) (2019) 1901556.
[59] R.A. Petros, J.M. DeSimone, Strategies in the design of nanoparticles for therapeutic applications, Nature Reviews Drug Discovery 9 (8) (2010) 615–627.
[60] M. Grzelczak, L.M. Liz-Marzán, R. Klajn, Stimuli-responsive self-assembly of nanoparticles, Chemical Society Reviews 48 (5) (2019) 1342–1361.
[61] M. Grzelczak, J. Vermant, E.M. Furst, L.M. Liz-Marzán, Directed self-assembly of nanoparticles, ACS Nano 4 (7) (2010) 3591–3605.
[62] L. Wang, C. Hu, L. Shao, The antimicrobial activity of nanoparticles: present situation and prospects for the future, International Journal of Nanomedicine 12 (2017) 1227–1249.
[63] V.A. Spirescu, C. Chircov, A.M. Grumezescu, E. Andronescu, Polymeric nanoparticles for antimicrobial therapies: an up-to-date overview, Polymers 13 (5) (2021) 724.
[64] R. Lakshminarayanan, E. Ye, D.J. Young, Z. Li, X.J. Loh, Recent advances in the development of antimicrobial nanoparticles for combating resistant pathogens, Advanced Healthcare Materials 7 (13) (2018) 1701400.

[65] Y. Duan, A. Dhar, C. Patel, M. Khimani, S. Neogi, P. Sharma, N. Siva Kumar, R.L. Vekariya, A brief review on solid lipid nanoparticles: part and parcel of contemporary drug delivery systems, RSC Advances 10 (45) (2020) 26777–26791.
[66] G.-H. Son, B.-J. Lee, C.-W. Cho, Mechanisms of drug release from advanced drug formulations such as polymeric-based drug-delivery systems and lipid nanoparticles, Journal of Pharmaceutical Investigation 47 (4) (2017) 287–296.
[67] M.M. Anjum, K.K. Patel, D. Dehari, N. Pandey, R. Tilak, A.K. Agrawal, S. Singh, Anacardic acid encapsulated solid lipid nanoparticles for Staphylococcus aureus biofilm therapy: chitosan and DNase coating improves antimicrobial activity, Drug Delivery and Translational Research 11 (1) (2021) 305–317.
[68] M. Grit, D.J.A. Crommelin, Chemical stability of liposomes: implications for their physical stability, Chemistry and Physics of Lipids 64 (1) (1993) 3–18.
[69] Q. Wang, L. He, D. Fan, W. Liang, J. Fang, Improving the anti-inflammatory efficacy of dexamethasone in the treatment of rheumatoid arthritis with polymerized stealth liposomes as a delivery vehicle, Journal of Materials Chemistry B 8 (9) (2020) 1841–1851.
[70] M. Silvander, Steric stabilization of liposomes — a review, in: T. Nylander, B. Lindman (Eds.), Lipid and Polymer-Lipid Systems, Springer Berlin Heidelberg, Berlin, Heidelberg, 2002, pp. 35–40.
[71] S.-C. Lee, K.-E. Lee, J.-J. Kim, S.-H. Lim, The effect of cholesterol in the liposome bilayer on the stabilization of incorporated retinol, Journal of Liposome Research 15 (3–4) (2005) 157–166.
[72] R.M. Schiffelers, G. Storm, M.T.t. Kate, I.A.J.M. Bakker-Woudenberg, Therapeutic efficacy of liposome-encapsulated gentamicin in rat *Klebsiella pneumoniae* pneumonia in relation to impaired host defense and low bacterial susceptibility to gentamicin, Antimicrobial Agents and Chemotherapy 45 (2) (2001) 464–470.
[73] I. Schumacher, R. Margalit, Liposome-encapsulated ampicillin: physicochemical and antibacterial properties, Journal of Pharmaceutical Sciences 86 (5) (1997) 635–641.
[74] L. Sande, M. Sanchez, J. Montes, A.J. Wolf, M.A. Morgan, A. Omri, G.Y. Liu, Liposomal encapsulation of vancomycin improves killing of methicillin-resistant Staphylococcus aureus in a murine infection model, Journal of Antimicrobial Chemotherapy 67 (9) (2012) 2191–2194.
[75] I.A. Yamskov, A.N. Kuskov, K.K. Babievsky, B.B. Berezin, M.A. Krayukhina, N.A. Samoylova, V.E. Tikhonov, M. Shtilman, Novel liposomal forms of antifungal antibiotics modified by amphiphilic polymers, Applied Biochemistry and Microbiology 44 (2008) 624–628.
[76] T.G. Meikle, D. Dharmadana, S.V. Hoffmann, N.C. Jones, C.J. Drummond, C.E. Conn, Analysis of the structure, loading and activity of six antimicrobial peptides encapsulated in cubic phase lipid nanoparticles, Journal of Colloid and Interface Science 587 (2021) 90–100.
[77] K.K. Ewert, A. Zidovska, A. Ahmad, N.F. Bouxsein, H.M. Evans, C.S. McAllister, C.E. Samuel, C.R. Safinya, Cationic liposome–nucleic acid complexes for gene delivery and silencing: pathways and mechanisms for plasmid DNA and siRNA, in: W. Bielke, C. Erbacher (Eds.), Nucleic Acid Transfection, Springer Berlin Heidelberg, Berlin, Heidelberg, 2010, pp. 191–226.

[78] N.M. Belliveau, J. Huft, P.J.C. Lin, S. Chen, A.K.K. Leung, T.J. Leaver, A.W. Wild, J.B. Lee, R.J. Taylor, Y.K. Tam, C.L. Hansen, P.R. Cullis, Microfluidic synthesis of highly potent limit-size lipid nanoparticles for in vivo delivery of siRNA, Molecular Therapy - Nucleic Acids 1 (2012).
[79] K. Vanamala, K. Bhise, H. Sanchez, R. Kebriaei, D. Luong, S. Sau, H. Abdelhady, M.J. Rybak, D. Andes, A.K. Iyer, Folate functionalized lipid nanoparticles for targeted therapy of methicillin-resistant Staphylococcus aureus, Pharmaceutics 13 (11) (2021) 1791.
[80] R. Krzysztoń, B. Salem, D.J. Lee, G. Schwake, E. Wagner, J.O. Rädler, Microfluidic self-assembly of folate-targeted monomolecular siRNA-lipid nanoparticles, Nanoscale 9 (22) (2017) 7442–7453.
[81] K. Maier, E. Wagner, Acid-labile traceless click linker for protein transduction, Journal of the American Chemical Society 134 (24) (2012) 10169–10173.
[82] R. Molinaro, M. Evangelopoulos, J.R. Hoffman, C. Corbo, F. Taraballi, J.O. Martinez, K.A. Hartman, D. Cosco, G. Costa, I. Romeo, M. Sherman, D. Paolino, S. Alcaro, E. Tasciotti, Design and development of biomimetic nanovesicles using a microfluidic approach, Advanced Materials 30 (15) (2018) 1702749.
[83] Y. Shi, X. Feng, L. Lin, J. Wang, J. Chi, B. Wu, G. Zhou, F. Yu, Q. Xu, D. Liu, G. Quan, C. Lu, X. Pan, J. Cai, C. Wu, Virus-inspired surface-nanoengineered antimicrobial liposome: a potential system to simultaneously achieve high activity and selectivity, Bioactive Materials 6 (10) (2021) 3207–3217.
[84] S. Pollock, N.B. Nichita, A. Böhmer, C. Radulescu, R.A. Dwek, N. Zitzmann, Polyunsaturated liposomes are antiviral against hepatitis B and C viruses and HIV by decreasing cholesterol levels in infected cells, Proceedings of the National Academy of Sciences of the United States of America 107 (40) (2010) 17176–17181.
[85] N. Habibi, N. Kamaly, A. Memic, H. Shafiee, Self-assembled peptide-based nanostructures: smart nanomaterials toward targeted drug delivery, Nano Today 11 (1) (2016) 41–60.
[86] H. Acar, S. Srivastava, E.J. Chung, M.R. Schnorenberg, J.C. Barrett, J.L. LaBelle, M. Tirrell, Self-assembling peptide-based building blocks in medical applications, Advanced Drug Delivery Reviews 110–111 (2017) 65–79.
[87] G.-B. Qi, Y.-J. Gao, L. Wang, H. Wang, Self-assembled peptide-based nanomaterials for biomedical imaging and therapy, Advanced Materials 30 (22) (2018) 1703444.
[88] S. Tarvirdipour, X. Huang, V. Mihali, C.-A. Schoenenberger, C.G. Palivan, Peptide-based nanoassemblies in gene therapy and diagnosis: paving the way for clinical application, Molecules 25 (15) (2020) 3482.
[89] J. Chen, X. Zou, Self-assemble peptide biomaterials and their biomedical applications, Bioactive Materials 4 (2019) 120–131.
[90] S. Tarvirdipour, C.-A. Schoenenberger, Y. Benenson, C.G. Palivan, A self-assembling amphiphilic peptide nanoparticle for the efficient entrapment of DNA cargoes up to 100 nucleotides in length, Soft Matter 16 (6) (2020) 1678–1691.
[91] J. Wang, K. Liu, R. Xing, X. Yan, Peptide self-assembly: thermodynamics and kinetics, Chemical Society Reviews 45 (20) (2016) 5589–5604.
[92] A. Dasgupta, D. Das, Designer peptide amphiphiles: self-assembly to applications, Langmuir 35 (33) (2019) 10704–10724.

[93] K. Knop, R. Hoogenboom, D. Fischer, U.S. Schubert, Poly(ethylene glycol) in drug delivery: pros and cons as well as potential alternatives, Angewandte Chemie International Edition 49 (36) (2010) 6288–6308.
[94] Z. Lai, Q. Jian, G. Li, C. Shao, Y. Zhu, X. Yuan, H. Chen, A. Shan, Self-assembling peptide dendron nanoparticles with high stability and a multimodal antimicrobial mechanism of action, ACS Nano 15 (10) (2021) 15824–15840.
[95] T.H.C. Petrin, V. Fadel, D.B. Martins, S.A. Dias, A. Cruz, L.M. Sergio, M. Arcisio-Miranda, M.A.R.B. Castanho, M.P. dos Santos Cabrera, Synthesis and characterization of peptide–chitosan conjugates (PepChis) with lipid bilayer affinity and antibacterial activity, Biomacromolecules 20 (7) (2019) 2743–2753.
[96] W. Tang, M.L. Becker, "Click" reactions: a versatile toolbox for the synthesis of peptide-conjugates, Chemical Society Reviews 43 (20) (2014) 7013–7039.
[97] J. Despanie, J.P. Dhandhukia, S.F. Hamm-Alvarez, J.A. MacKay, Elastin-like polypeptides: therapeutic applications for an emerging class of nanomedicines, Journal of Controlled Release 240 (2016) 93–108.
[98] J. Liang, W.-L. Wu, X.-D. Xu, R.-X. Zhuo, X.-Z. Zhang, pH Responsive micelle self-assembled from a new amphiphilic peptide as anti-tumor drug carrier, Colloids and Surfaces B: Biointerfaces 114 (2014) 398–403.
[99] C. Sousa, L.F. Gouveia, B. Kreutzer, B. Silva-Lima, R.E. Maphasa, A. Dube, M. Videira, Polymeric micellar formulation enhances antimicrobial and anticancer properties of Salinomycin, Pharmaceutical Research 36 (6) (2019) 83.
[100] C.H.N. Barros, D.W. Hiebner, S. Fulaz, S. Vitale, L. Quinn, E. Casey, Synthesis and self-assembly of curcumin-modified amphiphilic polymeric micelles with antibacterial activity, Journal of Nanobiotechnology 19 (1) (2021) 104.
[101] P. Tambe, P. Kumar, K.M. Paknikar, V. Gajbhiye, Smart triblock dendritic unimolecular micelles as pioneering nanomaterials: advancement pertaining to architecture and biomedical applications, Journal of Controlled Release 299 (2019) 64–89.
[102] M. Najafi, N. Kordalivand, M.-A. Moradi, J. van den Dikkenberg, R. Fokkink, H. Friedrich, N.A.J.M. Sommerdijk, M. Hembury, T. Vermonden, Native chemical ligation for cross-linking of flower-like micelles, Biomacromolecules 19 (9) (2018) 3766–3775.
[103] Y. Liu, H.J. Busscher, B. Zhao, Y. Li, Z. Zhang, H.C. van der Mei, Y. Ren, L. Shi, Surface-adaptive, antimicrobially loaded, micellar nanocarriers with enhanced penetration and killing efficiency in Staphylococcal biofilms, ACS Nano 10 (4) (2016) 4779–4789.
[104] B. Hisey, P.J. Ragogna, E.R. Gillies, Phosphonium-functionalized polymer micelles with intrinsic antibacterial activity, Biomacromolecules 18 (3) (2017) 914–923.
[105] M. Talelli, M. Barz, C.J.F. Rijcken, F. Kiessling, W.E. Hennink, T. Lammers, Core-crosslinked polymeric micelles: principles, preparation, biomedical applications and clinical translation, Nano Today 10 (1) (2015) 93–117.
[106] A.H. Gröschel, F.H. Schacher, H. Schmalz, O.V. Borisov, E.B. Zhulina, A. Walther, A.H.E. Müller, Precise hierarchical self-assembly of multicompartment micelles, Nature Communications 3 (1) (2012) 710.
[107] J. Du, R. O'Reilly, Anisotropic particles with patchy, multicompartment and Janus architectures: preparation and application, Chemical Society Reviews 40 (2011) 2402–2416.

[108] W. Li, H. Palis, R. Mérindol, J. Majimel, S. Ravaine, E. Duguet, Colloidal molecules and patchy particles: complementary concepts, synthesis and self-assembly, Chemical Society Reviews 49 (6) (2020) 1955–1976.

[109] S.A. Costa Lima, S. Reis, Temperature-responsive polymeric nanospheres containing methotrexate and gold nanoparticles: a multi-drug system for theranostic in rheumatoid arthritis, Colloids and Surfaces B: Biointerfaces 133 (2015) 378–387.

[110] T. Ramezanli, B.E. Kilfoyle, Z. Zhang, B.B. Michniak-Kohn, Polymeric nanospheres for topical delivery of vitamin D3, International Journal of Pharmaceutics 516 (1–2) (2017) 196–203.

[111] T.F.S. Evangelista, G.R.S. Andrade, K.N.S. Nascimento, S.B. dos Santos, M. de Fátima Costa Santos, C. Da Ros Montes D'Oca, S. dos, C. Estevam, I.F. Gimenez, L.E. Almeida, Supramolecular polyelectrolyte complexes based on cyclodextrin-grafted chitosan and carrageenan for controlled drug release, Carbohydrate Polymers 245 (2020) 116592.

[112] K. Renggli, P. Baumann, K. Langowska, O. Onaca, N. Bruns, W. Meier, Selective and responsive nanoreactors, Advanced Functional Materials 21 (7) (2011) 1241–1259.

[113] J. Nicolas, S. Mura, D. Brambilla, N. Mackiewicz, P. Couvreur, Design, functionalization strategies and biomedical applications of targeted biodegradable/biocompatible polymer-based nanocarriers for drug delivery, Chemical Society Reviews 42 (3) (2013) 1147–1235.

[114] S.J. Sigg, F. Santini, A. Najer, P.U. Richard, W.P. Meier, C.G. Palivan, Nanoparticle-based highly sensitive MRI contrast agents with enhanced relaxivity in reductive milieu, Chemical Communications 52 (64) (2016) 9937–9940.

[115] S. Moreno, B. Voit, J. Gaitzsch, The chemistry of cross-linked polymeric vesicles and their functionalization towards biocatalytic nanoreactors, Colloid and Polymer Science 299 (2021) 309–324.

[116] J. Gaitzsch, D. Appelhans, L.G. Wang, G. Battaglia, B. Voit, Synthetic bio-nanoreactor: mechanical and chemical control of polymersome membrane permeability, Angewandte Chemie, International Edition 51 (18) (2012) 4448–4451.

[117] M. Kumar, M. Grzelakowski, J. Zilles, M. Clark, W. Meier, Highly permeable polymeric membranes based on the incorporation of the functional water channel protein Aquaporin Z, Proceedings of the National Academy of Sciences 104 (52) (2007) 20719–20724.

[118] P. Broz, S. Driamov, J. Ziegler, N. Ben-Haim, S. Marsch, W. Meier, P. Hunziker, Toward intelligent nanosize bioreactors: a pH-switchable, channel-equipped, functional polymer nanocontainer, Nano Letters 6 (10) (2006) 2349–2353.

[119] M. Garni, T. Einfalt, M. Lomora, A. Car, W. Meier, C.G. Palivan, Artificial organelles: reactions inside protein-polymer supramolecular assemblies, Chimia 70 (6) (2016) 424–427.

[120] A. Belluati, V. Mikhalevich, S. Yorulmaz Avsar, D. Daubian, I. Craciun, M. Chami, W.P. Meier, C.G. Palivan, How do the properties of amphiphilic polymer membranes influence the functional insertion of peptide pores? Biomacromolecules 21 (2) (2020) 701–715.

[121] R. Goers, J. Thoma, N. Ritzmann, A. Di Silvestro, C. Alter, G. Gunkel-Grabole, D. Fotiadis, D.J. Müller, W. Meier, Optimized reconstitution of membrane proteins into synthetic membranes, Communications Chemistry 1 (1) (2018) 35.

[122] T. Einfalt, R. Goers, I.A. Dinu, A. Najer, M. Spulber, O. Onaca-Fischer, C.G. Palivan, Stimuli-triggered activity of nanoreactors by biomimetic engineering polymer membranes, Nano Letters 15 (11) (2015) 7596–7603.
[123] R. Stoenescu, A. Graff, W. Meier, Asymmetric ABC-triblock copolymer membranes induce a directed insertion of membrane proteins, Macromolecular Bioscience 4 (10) (2004) 930–935.
[124] G. Njikang, D. Han, J. Wang, G. Liu, ABC triblock copolymer micelle-like aggregates in selective solvents for A and C, Macromolecules 41 (24) (2008) 9727–9735.
[125] E.V. Konishcheva, U.E. Zhumaev, W.P. Meier, PEO-b-PCL-b-PMOXA triblock copolymers: from synthesis to microscale polymersomes with asymmetric membrane, Macromolecules 50 (4) (2017) 1512–1520.
[126] D. Daubian, A. Fillion, J. Gaitzsch, W. Meier, One-pot synthesis of an amphiphilic ABC triblock copolymer PEO-b-PEHOx-b-PEtOz and its self-assembly into nanoscopic asymmetric polymersomes, Macromolecules 53 (24) (2020) 11040–11050.
[127] I. Canton, G. Battaglia, Endocytosis at the nanoscale, Chemical Society Reviews 41 (7) (2012) 2718–2739.
[128] F. Itel, M. Chami, A. Najer, S. Lorcher, D.L. Wu, I.A. Dinu, W. Meier, Molecular organization and dynamics in polymersome membranes: a lateral diffusion study, Macromolecules 47 (21) (2014) 7588–7596.
[129] A. Sharma, U.S. Sharma, Liposomes in drug delivery: progress and limitations, International Journal of Pharmaceutics 154 (2) (1997) 123–140.
[130] E. Beltrán-Gracia, A. López-Camacho, I. Higuera-Ciapara, J.B. Velázquez-Fernández, A.A. Vallejo-Cardona, Nanomedicine review: clinical developments in liposomal applications, Cancer Nanotechnology 10 (1) (2019) 11.
[131] L. Ruiz-Perez, L. Messager, J. Gaitzsch, A. Joseph, L. Sutto, F.L. Gervasio, G. Battaglia, Molecular engineering of polymersome surface topology, Science Advances 2 (4) (2016) e1500948.
[132] J. Gaitzsch, V. Chudasama, E. Morecroft, L. Messager, G. Battaglia, Synthesis of an amphiphilic miktoarm star terpolymer for self-assembly into patchy polymersomes, ACS Macro Letters 5 (3) (2016) 351–354.
[133] C. Contini, R. Pearson, L. Wang, L. Messager, J. Gaitzsch, L. Rizzello, L. Ruiz-Perez, G. Battaglia, Bottom-up evolution of vesicles from disks to high-genus polymersomes, iScience 7 (2018) 132–144.
[134] S.D. Zhang, H.J. Sun, A.D. Hughes, B. Draghici, J. Lejnieks, P. Leowanawat, A. Bertin, L.O. De Leon, O.V. Kulikov, Y.C. Chen, D.J. Pochan, P.A. Heiney, V. Percec, "Single-single" amphiphilic Janus dendrimers self-assemble into uniform dendrimersomes with predictable size, ACS Nano 8 (2) (2014) 1554–1565.
[135] Q. Xiao, J.D. Rubien, Z.C. Wang, E.H. Reed, D.A. Hammer, D. Sahoo, P.A. Heiney, S.S. Yadavalli, M. Goulian, S.E. Wilner, T. Baumgart, S.A. Vinogradov, M.L. Klein, V. Percec, Self-sorting and coassembly of fluorinated, hydrogenated, and hybrid Janus dendrimers into dendrimersomes, Journal of the American Chemical Society 138 (38) (2016) 12655–12663.
[136] R.S. Rawat, Dense plasma focus - from alternative fusion source to versatile high energy density plasma source for plasma nanotechnology, Journal of Physics: Conference Series 591 (2015) 012021.

[137] K. Kızılbey, Optimization of rutin-loaded PLGA nanoparticles synthesized by single-emulsion solvent evaporation method, ACS Omega 4 (1) (2019) 555–562.
[138] S. Desgouilles, C. Vauthier, D. Bazile, J. Vacus, J.-L. Grossiord, M. Veillard, P. Couvreur, The design of nanoparticles obtained by solvent evaporation: a comprehensive study, Langmuir 19 (22) (2003) 9504–9510.
[139] T. Niwa, H. Takeuchi, T. Hino, N. Kunou, Y. Kawashima, Preparations of biodegradable nanospheres of water-soluble and insoluble drugs with D,L-lactide/glycolide copolymer by a novel spontaneous emulsification solvent diffusion method, and the drug release behavior, Journal of Controlled Release 25 (1) (1993) 89–98.
[140] J.P. Rao, K.E. Geckeler, Polymer nanoparticles: preparation techniques and size-control parameters, Progress in Polymer Science 36 (7) (2011) 887–913.
[141] T. Jung, W. Kamm, A. Breitenbach, E. Kaiserling, J.X. Xiao, T. Kissel, Biodegradable nanoparticles for oral delivery of peptides: is there a role for polymers to affect mucosal uptake? European Journal of Pharmaceutics and Biopharmaceutics 50 (1) (2000) 147–160.
[142] J.M. Barichello, M. Morishita, K. Takayama, T. Nagai, Encapsulation of hydrophilic and lipophilic drugs in PLGA nanoparticles by the nanoprecipitation method, Drug Development and Industrial Pharmacy 25 (4) (1999) 471–476.
[143] M. Chidambaram, K. Krishnasamy, Modifications to the conventional nanoprecipitation technique: an approach to fabricate narrow sized polymeric nanoparticles, Advanced Pharmaceutical Bulletin 4 (2) (2014) 205–208.
[144] Y. Sasaki, N. Konishi, M. Kasuya, M. Kohri, T. Taniguchi, K. Kishikawa, Preparation of size-controlled polymer particles by polymerization of O/W emulsion monomer droplets obtained through phase inversion temperature emulsification using amphiphilic comb-like block polymers, Colloids and Surfaces A: Physicochemical and Engineering Aspects 482 (2015) 68–78.
[145] B. Herranz-Blanco, M.A. Shahbazi, A.R. Correia, V. Balasubramanian, T. Kohout, J. Hirvonen, H.A. Santos, pH-switch nanoprecipitation of polymeric nanoparticles for multimodal cancer targeting and intracellular triggered delivery of doxorubicin, Advanced Healthcare Materials 5 (15) (2016) 1904–1916.
[146] L. Palanikumar, S. Al-Hosani, M. Kalmouni, V.P. Nguyen, L. Ali, R. Pasricha, F.N. Barrera, M. Magzoub, pH-responsive high stability polymeric nanoparticles for targeted delivery of anticancer therapeutics, Communications Biology 3 (1) (2020) 95.
[147] C.I.C. Crucho, M.T. Barros, Polymeric nanoparticles: a study on the preparation variables and characterization methods, Materials Science and Engineering: C 80 (2017) 771–784.
[148] W.-M. Wan, C.-Y. Hong, C.-Y. Pan, One-pot synthesis of nanomaterials via RAFT polymerization induced self-assembly and morphology transition, Chemical Communications (39) (2009) 5883–5885.
[149] T. Marante, C. Viegas, I. Duarte, A.S. Macedo, P. Fonte, An overview on spray-drying of protein-loaded polymeric nanoparticles for dry powder inhalation, Pharmaceutics 12 (11) (2020).
[150] G. Battaglia, A.J. Ryan, The evolution of vesicles from bulk lamellar gels, Nature Materials 4 (11) (2005) 869–876.

[151] G. Battaglia, A.J. Ryan, Pathways of polymeric vesicle formation, Journal of Physical Chemistry B 110 (21) (2006) 10272–10279.
[152] J.E. Bartenstein, J. Robertson, G. Battaglia, W.H. Briscoe, Stability of polymersomes prepared by size exclusion chromatography and extrusion, Colloids and Surfaces A: Physicochemical and Engineering Aspects 506 (2016) 739–746.
[153] S.T. Poschenrieder, S.K. Schiebel, K. Castiglione, Polymersomes for biotechnological applications: large-scale production of nano-scale vesicles, Engineering in Life Sciences 17 (1) (2017) 58–70.
[154] S.F.M. van Dongen, H.P.M. de Hoog, R.J.R.W. Peters, M. Nallani, R.J.M. Nolte, J.C.M. van Hest, Biohybrid polymer capsules, Chemical Reviews 109 (11) (2009) 6212–6274.
[155] A. Najer, D.L. Wu, D. Vasquez, C.G. Palivan, W. Meier, Polymer nanocompartments in broad-spectrum medical applications, Nanomedicine 8 (3) (2013) 425–447.
[156] C.G. Palivan, O. Fischer-Onaca, M. Delcea, F. Itel, W. Meier, Protein-polymer nanoreactors for medical applications, Chemical Society Reviews 41 (7) (2012) 2800–2823.
[157] X. Zhang, W. Fu, C.G. Palivan, W. Meier, Natural channel protein inserts and functions in a completely artificial, solid-supported bilayer membrane, Scientific Reports 3 (2013) 1–7.
[158] D. Wu, M. Spulber, F. Itel, M. Chami, T. Pfohl, C.G. Palivan, W. Meier, Effect of molecular parameters on the architecture and membrane properties of 3D assemblies of amphiphilic copolymers, Macromolecules 47 (15) (2014) 5060–5069.
[159] S.Y. Yu, T. Azzam, I. Rouiller, A. Eisenberg, "Breathing" vesicles, Journal of the American Chemical Society 131 (30) (2009) 10557–10566.
[160] E. Konishcheva, D. Häussinger, S. Lörcher, W. Meier, Key aspects to yield low dispersity of PEO- b -PCL diblock copolymers and their mesoscale self-assembly, European Polymer Journal 83 (2016) 300–310.
[161] P.R. Makgwane, S.S. Ray, Synthesis of nanomaterials by continuous-flow microfluidics: a review, Journal of Nanoscience and Nanotechnology 14 (2) (2014) 1338–1363.
[162] G.F. Christopher, S.L. Anna, Microfluidic methods for generating continuous droplet streams, Journal of Physics D Applied Physics 40 (19) (2007) R319–R336.
[163] Z. Toprakcioglu, P.K. Challa, D.B. Morse, T. Knowles, Attoliter protein nanogels from droplet nanofluidics for intracellular delivery, Science Advances 6 (6) (2020) eaay7952.
[164] H.C. Shum, J.-W. Kim, D.A. Weitz, Microfluidic fabrication of monodisperse biocompatible and biodegradable polymersomes with controlled permeability, Journal of the American Chemical Society 130 (29) (2008) 9543–9549.
[165] E.C. dos Santos, A. Belluati, D. Necula, D. Scherrer, C.E. Meyer, R.P. Wehr, E. Lörtscher, C.G. Palivan, W. Meier, Combinatorial strategy for studying biochemical pathways in double emulsion templated cell-sized compartments, Advanced Materials 32 (48) (2020) 2004804.
[166] D.J. Beebe, G.A. Mensing, G.M. Walker, Physics and applications of microfluidics in biology, Annual Review of Biomedical Engineering 4 (1) (2002) 261–286.
[167] N.-T. Nguyen, Z. Wu, Micromixers—a review, Journal of Micromechanics and Microengineering 15 (2) (2004) R1–R16.

[168] T. Nakamura, M. Kawai, Y. Sato, M. Maeki, M. Tokeshi, H. Harashima, The effect of size and charge of lipid nanoparticles prepared by microfluidic mixing on their lymph node transitivity and distribution, Molecular Pharmaceutics 17 (3) (2020) 944–953.
[169] S.J. Shepherd, C.C. Warzecha, S. Yadavali, R. El-Mayta, M.-G. Alameh, L. Wang, D. Weissman, J.M. Wilson, D. Issadore, M.J. Mitchell, Scalable mRNA and siRNA lipid nanoparticle production using a parallelized microfluidic device, Nano Letters 21 (13) (2021) 5671–5680.
[170] L. Brown, S.L. McArthur, P.C. Wright, A. Lewis, G. Battaglia, Polymersome production on a microfluidic platform using pH sensitive block copolymers, Lab on a Chip 10 (15) (2010) 1922–1928.
[171] T.A. Balbino, N.T. Aoki, A.A.M. Gasperini, C.L.P. Oliveira, A.R. Azzoni, L.P. Cavalcanti, L.G. de la Torre, Continuous flow production of cationic liposomes at high lipid concentration in microfluidic devices for gene delivery applications, Chemical Engineering Journal (Lausanne) 226 (2013) 423–433.
[172] U. Bulbake, S. Doppalapudi, N. Kommineni, W. Khan, Liposomal formulations in clinical use: an updated review, Pharmaceutics 9 (2) (2017).
[173] C. Dobrowolski, K. Paunovska, M.Z.C. Hatit, M.P. Lokugamage, J.E. Dahlman, Therapeutic RNA delivery for COVID and other diseases, Advanced Healthcare Materials (2021) 2002022.
[174] D. Bobo, K.J. Robinson, J. Islam, K.J. Thurecht, S.R. Corrie, Nanoparticle-based medicines: a review of FDA-approved materials and clinical trials to date, Pharmaceutical Research 33 (10) (2016) 2373–2387.
[175] A. Akinc, M.A. Maier, M. Manoharan, K. Fitzgerald, M. Jayaraman, S. Barros, S. Ansell, X. Du, M.J. Hope, T.D. Madden, B.L. Mui, S.C. Semple, Y.K. Tam, M. Ciufolini, D. Witzigmann, J.A. Kulkarni, R. van der Meel, P.R. Cullis, The Onpattro story and the clinical translation of nanomedicines containing nucleic acid-based drugs, Nature Nanotechnology 14 (12) (2019) 1084–1087.
[176] N. Dammes, D. Peer, Paving the road for RNA therapeutics, Trends in Pharmacological Sciences 41 (10) (2020) 755–775.
[177] B. Braun, Etomidat-®Lipuro 2 mg/ml Emulsion zur Injektion, Fachinformation zur Zulassung 004548–38342 (2017).
[178] B. Braun, Diazepam-Lipuro 10 mg/2 ml Emulsion zur Injektion, Fachinformation zur Zulassung 002515–Y878 (2006).
[179] B. Braun, EUA 96 Propofol Lipuro-Fact-Sheet-Hcp, US Food and Drug Admistration, USA, 2021.

4

Nanoparticle characterisation and standardisation

Yiwen Pei, Charles A. Clifford and Caterina Minelli

Chemical and Biological Sciences Department, National Physical Laboratory, Teddington, United Kingdom

Abbreviations

AF4	Asymmetric flow field flow fractionation
AFM	Atomic force microscopy
BET	Brunauer–Emmett–Teller
CLS	Centrifugal liquid sedimentation
DLS	Dynamic light scattering
ELS	Electrophoretic light scattering
IEC	International electrotechnical commission
ISO	International organization for standardisation
PEG	Polyethylene glycol
PTA	Particle tracking analysis
SAXS	Small-angle X-ray scattering
SEM	Scanning electron microscopy
SI	International system of units
SIMS	Secondary ion mass spectroscopy
spICP-MS	Single-particle inductively coupled-plasma mass spectrometry
SRS	Stimulated Raman scattering
STEM	Scanning transmission electron microscopy
TEM	Transmission electron microscopy
Tris	Tris(hydroxymethyl)aminomethane
TRPS	Tunable resistive pulse sensing
UV-Vis	Ultraviolet-visible spectrophotometer
VAMAS	Versailles project on advanced materials and standards
XPS	X-ray photoelectron spectroscopy

1. Introduction

With an increasing rate of innovation in nanotechnology for infection prevention and control [1,2], accurate and reliable measurements of nanoparticle properties are required to support the development, manufacturing and testing of formulated end products. There is growing demand [3] for characterisation techniques

Nanotechnology Tools for Infection Control. https://doi.org/10.1016/B978-0-12-823994-0.00007-4

that measure critical properties relevant to nanoparticle performance, including size, shape, zeta-potential and chemistry.

Understanding the properties and behaviour of particles in biological systems is particularly important since it helps scientists to predict the performance and ensure the safety of nanoparticle-based products during their uses. However, biological systems are complex, and a range of analytical methods are typically required for a comprehensive analysis of nanoparticles within these systems. Accurate nanoparticle characterisation in biological systems, such as cells and tissues, requires a relatively high level of skill and know-how in terms of sample preparation, instrument set-up and data interpretation.

This chapter is concerned not only with measurement and standardisation of nanoparticles with antimicrobial properties but also provides guidance to help select the most appropriate techniques for nanoparticle characterisation along with some considerations for sample preparation. This chapter concludes with an overview of international standardisation activities in nanotechnologies with a focus on standards for particle characterisations, and a brief survey of measurement standards for antimicrobial properties. Characterisation and standardisation of nanoparticles for other applications can be found elsewhere [4–6].

2. Sample preparation

2.1 Sampling

Nanoparticle samples often have a large distribution of particle size, shape, surface area, density and composition. The segregation of particles based on their properties occurs during sample storage, transport and handling due to the free-flowing behaviour of powder material as well as sedimentation in colloidal suspension. Therefore, thorough sample mixing and splitting is essential before sampling to obtain measurement results that are representative of the entire sample [7]. Inappropriate mixing and sampling procedures can result in a non-representative portion of sample being measured. This type of error is especially significant for heterogenous systems, such as nanoparticles with a wide particle size and shape distribution. Documentary standards ISO 14488:2007 and ISO 8213:1986 provide useful guidance and detailed requirements for sampling and sample splitting of particles, including for industrial uses [8]. General guidance on particle sampling and sample splitting techniques as well as dispersing procedures for nanoparticle suspensions can be found in other international organisation for standardisation (ISO) documents [7,9]. ISO 20579-4:2018 provides instructions on how to report the history, preparation, handling and mounting of nanoparticles prior to surface chemical analysis [10].

For nanoparticle colloidal suspensions, it is essential to minimise the occurrence of unintended and uncontrolled particle agglomeration. Ultrasonic treatment, also called sonication, during sample preparation is frequently used to reduce agglomeration of nanoparticles in liquid. However, this process can also induce agglomeration and/or cause sample damage depending on the nature of material. Gentle swirling or vortexing offers milder treatment for delicate samples, such as polymeric drug carriers. The application of surfactants, polymers or oligomers which form a coating on particles is a common strategy to prevent agglomeration during manufacturing by introducing steric hindrance or surface charge at the particle surface to minimise contact between nanoparticles or to increase repulsive interactions.

It is best practice to validate the sample preparation and measurement methods with reference materials similar to the sample under study, where these are available. The number of measurement repeats required to obtain statistically valid measurement results depends upon several factors, including material type, measurands and measurand spread, sample preparation process and target measurement uncertainty. For example, for imaging techniques measuring particle size, this number typically ranges from a couple of hundreds to a couple of thousands of nanoparticles that need to be measured and reported [11]. For measurements in suspensions, at least three to five replicated measurements are typically required to obtain statistically representative results. It is then best practice to assess method variability due to day-to-day variations in instrument conditions or different analysts. Interlaboratory comparisons are particularly useful to assess method repeatability and measurement reproducibility and identify sources of variability.

2.2 Powder samples

Depending on the nature of the materials and the measurement technique, the preparation of powder samples can be complex. Rigorous risk assessment should be performed aimed at eliminating the risks of inhalation of nanomaterials during handling. Guidance on how to handle powder samples can be found in ISO 14887:2000, ISO 14703:2008 and ISO 14488:2007 [7,9,12].

Nanoparticle powder sample preparation depends on the technique used. Powder samples are sometimes dispersed in liquids for analysis, or deposited onto a substrate from powders or dispersions, or compacted into a pellet. The use of imaging techniques such as scanning electron microscopy (SEM) and atomic force microscopy (AFM) for the analysis will typically require the preparation of discrete particles onto a substrate, which can be achieved through deposition of a controlled dilution of the nanoparticle suspensions [11]. The selection of a suitable substrate is a critical step in particle analysis. The main objective is to generate a uniform distribution of nanoparticles across the entire measurement substrate. Selective particle–substrate interactions should be avoided to ensure unbiased sample deposition. Generally, a good substrate is clean, uniform and flat over the measurement area and produces a low signal with good contrast with respect to the samples [13]. Several common methods for depositing nanoparticles on substrates can be found in the literature [14] and ISO documentations [15,16].

2.3 Colloidal samples

Sample preparation of nanoparticles in liquids usually involves sample dilution to obtain the optimal concentration for the analytical technique. Where there is a need to know the concentration of nanoparticle suspensions with accuracy, it is recommended to perform the dilution gravimetrically to minimise uncertainties in the dilution factor. However, if volumetric dilutions are used, it is important to ensure that pipettes are well maintained and regularly calibrated. General guidance on samples preparation for nanoparticle suspensions can be found in the literature [17].

3. Measurements of nanoparticle properties

3.1 Size

It is well-documented [18–21] that the size of nanoparticles plays a significant role in their interactions with living cells, influencing cell uptake efficiency, cytotoxicity, internalisation pathway selection and intracellular localisation. For antimicrobial applications, the size of nanoparticles is critical for the success of targeted bactericidal effects [22]. Due to their high surface to volume ratio, nanoparticles with small particle size (<10 nm) are often associated with direct interaction with bacterial membranes [23] and faster release of active ingredients [24,25], leading to improved antimicrobial efficiency [26,27]. In addition, for inorganic nanoparticles, previous work [28] has shown that the electronic structure of a nanoparticle surface can change as a function of its size, which ultimately affects their surface reactivity. Therefore, accurate and robust measurement of nanoparticle size and size distribution is of great importance in predicting their performance and effectiveness in antimicrobial applications. A large number of techniques have been employed to measure the size and size distribution of various nanoparticle products for infection control, including gold [29,30], silver [20,31,32], copper [33,34], metal oxide [19,35], polymer [36–38] and others [39,40].

Table 4.1 provides an overview of commonly used methods for measuring nanoparticle size and size distribution. The use of these techniques is supported by a number of documentary standards published by ISO and ASTM. The size of nanoparticles can be measured by techniques that either measure individual particles (known as *particle-by-particle* techniques) or process the total signal from a collection of particles (known as *ensemble* techniques) to determine particle size. As shown in Table 4.1, commonly used particle-by-particle techniques include AFM, SEM, transmission electron microscopy (TEM), tunable resistive pulse sensing (TRPS), particle tracking analysis (PTA) and single-particle inductively coupled-plasma mass spectrometry (spICP-MS). Ensemble techniques include small-angle X-ray scattering (SAXS), centrifugal liquid sedimentation (CLS) and dynamic light scattering (DLS). Generally, ensemble techniques detect signals from a population of particles and provide good sample statistics. However, the measurement accuracy of these techniques may suffer from limitations arising from the assumption of other particle characteristics such as refractive index and density. In addition, broad nanoparticle size distributions or agglomerates can introduce biases in the measurement results because of complicated sensitivity changes across the particle size range. In particle-by-particle methods, this problem is partially mitigated by measuring the signals from individual particle. For this reason, these methods tend to have higher resolution in size with respect to the ensemble methods. However, imaging methods such as electron microscopy and AFM are low throughput and can be time-consuming to achieve statistically significant measurement results. It is worth noting that SEM, TEM and AFM require particles to be deposited onto a substrate. SEM and TEM require a high vacuum system, while all the other methods measure nanoparticles in liquids, with the exception of SAXS and AFM which can perform analysis both in air and in liquids.

Table 4.1 A list of commonly used techniques for nanoparticles size and size distribution measurement, with information on the underpinning physical principle, their measurand and the selected reference ISO and ASTM documentary standards.

Technique	Type	Physical principle	Measurand	Standard
AFM	Particle-by-particle	Surface—probe interaction	Particle height	ISO 13095:2014 ASTM E2859-11
SEM		Electron optics	2D rotational-averaged projected diameter	ISO 19749:2021
TEM		Electron optics	2D rotary projected diameter	ISO 21363:2022 ISO/TS 22292:2021
TRPS		Coulter counter	Spherical volume equivalent diameter	ISO 13319:2007
PTA		Light scattering	Spherical equivalent translatory diffusion hydrodynamic diameter	ISO 19430:2016 ASTM E2834-12
spICP-MS		Mass spectrometry	Spherical mass equivalent diameter	ISO/TS 19590:2017
DLS	Ensemble	Light scattering	Spherical equivalent translatory diffusion hydrodynamic diameter	ISO 22412:2017 ASTM E2490-09 ASTM E3247-20
CLS		Sedimentation and light scattering	Spherical equivalent Stokes' diameter	ISO 13318-1:2001 ISO 13318-2:2007 ISO 13318-3:2004
SAXS		X-ray scattering	Spherical electron density equivalent diameter	ISO 17867:2020

3.1.1 AFM

AFM is the principal member of the scanning probe microscopy family. It has been used to provide information on the 3D morphology and mechanical properties of particles, as well as cells and bacterial membranes. AFM has the capability to measure various types of materials, including biological and non-conductive samples, in a wide range of environments (air, vacuum and liquid). Other advantages include high spatial resolution, potentially down to atomic resolution, the ability to simultaneously acquire 3D images with for example mechanical or electrical properties and the possibility of investigating molecular interactions. With these unique features, AFM has become a useful tool for morphological analysis of nanoparticles for antimicrobial applications [41], as well as biological membranes treated with antimicrobial agents [42].

The operational principle of AFM is based on measuring interactions between the probe tip and the sample surface. Typically, a cantilever equipped with a sharp silicon or silicon nitride-based probing tip is scanned across a specimen surface. During scanning, the cantilever is deflected in response to the force between the probe tip and the sample, the deflection is detected via an optical beam and four quadrant photodiodes. An AFM image is acquired by rastering the sample relative to the probing tip or vice versa. Based on the nature of the probe–surface interactions (attractive or repulsive), three operational modes are commonly used: (1) contact mode – the sample is scanned while the tip essentially maintains contact with the sample surface at all time; (2) non-contact mode – the tip oscillates at a frequency that is slightly above the cantilever's resonance frequency, and the sample surface topography is detected by measuring changes in resonance frequency; (3) intermittent contact mode (also known as tapping mode) – the tip attached to an oscillating cantilever that intermittently contacts the surface at the lowest point in the oscillation, and the sample surface topography is detected based on changes in the oscillation amplitude [43].

In addition to visualising and quantifying the morphology of nanoparticles, AFM is also suited to measure their mechanical properties [44]. However, accurate nanomechanical measurements for soft nanoparticles can be challenging due to the likelihood of measurement artefacts caused by substate stiffness [4]. Detailed information of scanner and probing tip-related artefacts in AFM can be found in ASTM E2382 [45]. Descriptive and quantitative representation of particle shape and morphology with examples of methods to present shape distribution data are provided in ISO 9276-6 [13]. In order to achieve a more comprehensive description of a particle system, information on particle size should be used together with shape and morphological information. ASTM E2859 gives a comprehensive guide for size measurement of nanoparticle using AFM [46].

3.1.2 Electron microscopies

SEM is a vacuum-based technique that provides high resolution size and morphological information of nanoparticles. In SEM analysis, a primary electron beam is employed to scan the surface of a specimen generating secondary electrons and/or backscattered electrons that are detected to form an image of a sample. It should be noted that the SEM image is a two-dimensional (2D) representation of the three-dimensional (3D) objects from a certain viewing angle [4]. SEM image-based particle size measurements determine a parameter, the circular equivalent diameter in a projected 2D image, which is often assumed to be equivalent to the equivalent spherical diameter of 3D particles. Conventional SEM typically operates at high accelerating voltages (e.g. 5–30 kV) and often requires non-conducting samples to be coated with a thin layer of conductive metals, such as gold, palladium and chromium for imaging. Depending on the resolving power of the SEM instrument, it is sometimes possible to measure particle size and size distribution below 10 nm [11]. While SEM can provide both size and shape of nanoparticles, its main drawback for particle sizing is the relative long measurement time due to processing required for image acquisition and analysis [47].

In TEM analysis, an electron source is used to generate a primary electron beam which is projected onto a sample specimen through a set of electromagnetic lenses and apertures. The selection of the TEM acquisition mode is of great importance for obtaining the data of interest. Bright field-TEM mode is commonly used to provide fast and easy shape analysis of nanoparticles. For the analysis of sensitive materials, such as soft matter and degradable polymers, care needs to be taken to ensure that the sample is not altered due to electron beam damage during image acquisition [48]. It is recommended to perform a series of beam damage studies on the sample of interest prior to the analysis. TEM provides high spatial resolution and like SEM projected 2D images with the option to reconstruct 3D images of nano-objects. Both TEM and SEM can be operated in scanning mode where the primary electron beam is focussed into a subnanometre sized probe and rastered over the sample specimen. In high-resolution scanning-TEM (STEM) mode, spatial resolution can reach 0.1 nm when a corrected nanosized illuminating electron probe is used. One advantage of STEM analysis is the high contrast of annular dark-field images, which allows imaging samples without the need for staining [4]. There are several factors which may impact the TEM measurement uncertainties for particle size and shape distribution, such as number of particles and minimum particle area. Although it can be sample dependent, the ISO standard (ISO 21362:2020) suggests that the users should acquire at least 500 particles per sample to obtain accurate measurements [13].

3.1.3 TRPS

TRPS measures particle size, concentration and zeta-potential in conductive liquids and is suitable for particles ranging from nominally 40 nm to hundreds of micrometres in diameter. Based on the Coulter principle, TRPS measures a reduction in ionic current (known as a 'resistive pulse') across a single pore in a membrane as the particle analyte travels through the pore. The height, width and frequency of these resistive pulses provide the information required to determine particle volume, zeta-potential and total number concentration relative to a calibrant particle sample with known properties. The calibrant is required because the aperture geometry can be adjusted for each sample by stretching the membrane and the resulting geometry is therefore unknown. The aperture needs to be calibrated with reference materials, ideally spherical particles of known diameter, zeta potential and number concentration traceable to the International System of Units (SI). Such certified reference materials do not currently exist, but companies are typically able to provide reference test particles as calibrants. Unlike light scattering-based techniques, such as DLS and PTA, TRPS does not require the analyte species to absorb or scatter light. As such, TRPS is suitable for measuring particles regardless of their light scattering properties, including biological relevant nanocomposites, bacteria, cells and microorganisms, which often have a relatively similar refractive index compared to their dispersion media. It is worth noting that conductive aqueous electrolyte is often required as the dispersant to establish a baseline current, which may impair the stability of nanoparticles. For this reason, when the dispersant is altered for TRPS analysis, sample stability should be examined using other particle sizing techniques such as DLS. Several review articles [49,50] and a documentary standard [51] detail the use of TRPS for the analysis of nanoparticles.

3.1.4 Scattering-based methods

DLS [52–54] has been widely utilised to characterise the size and size distribution of nanoparticle suspensions. The technique measures the translational diffusion coefficient of particles that are subject to Brownian motion by measuring the intensity fluctuations of a laser caused by scattering events with particles. Because smaller particles move faster under Brownian motion, they also result in more rapid fluctuation with respect to larger particles. A number of approaches exist to enable the determination of the hydrodynamic size of the nanoparticles from these data, which typically assume that the particles are perfect solid spheres. One of the most common analysis methods is the cumulant method, which determine the average size (called Z-average) and polydispersity index of the particle population from the fit of the scattered intensity correlation function using the Stokes–Einstein theory [55,56]. DLS is applied to particles typically in the size range around 1 nm–10 μm in diameter.

PTA [57,58] measures particle size in a similar fashion, with the exception that the scattered light from individual particles is visualised using microscopy and recorded over time. By tracking the movements of individual nanoparticles, the diffusion coefficient is estimated from the sequence of displacements in the images and the hydrodynamic size of individually tracked particles is then calculated. The size range measurement for PTA is approximately 10 nm–1 μm in diameter, depending upon the light-scattering properties of the analyte.

Thanks to its relative short wavelength (typically below 1 nm), X-rays are well-suited for nanoparticle characterisation. SAXS is capable of measuring size, size distribution, concentration, surface area and in some cases the internal structure of spherical nanoparticles. This technique can be applied to heterogenous systems containing multiple phases with different electron density.

When electromagnetic radiation passes through matter, a small fraction of the irradiation is scattered in the forward direction with a small deflection to form a scattered radiation intensity profile. Based upon this information, the mean particle size can be determined from either classic Guinier analysis or curve-fitting depending on the sample shape. As an ensemble method, SAXS can be utilised to investigate nanoparticle properties by averaging the collected information over a large number of nanoparticles. One of the great advantages of SAXS is its ability to measure nanoparticles in real time and within realistic sample environments without extensive sample preparation. Further aspects of nanoparticle characterisation using SAXS can be found in recent literature [4,59] and standard documentations [60].

3.1.5 CLS

CLS is a type of analytical centrifuge used to measure high-resolution size distribution of colloidal particles, with information on particle dispersity and/or agglomeration [61]. The method is highly precise and can also be used to measure the density of particles, as well as their relative concentration. Current commercially available CLS instruments have either a disc or a number of cuvettes containing a dispersion of the particle sample in a liquid of different density. While rotating, the particles separate based on their size and density. During rotation, the particles traverse a light beam and the optical attenuation is measured by a photodetector, as a function of sedimentation time. This information is converted in a size distribution, for some models with the aid of a particle calibrant of known size and density. CLS instruments exist with different types of light sources, typically in the visible range but also extending to the near infra-red and X-rays. The choice of the light source is generally dictated by the sample of interest.

3.1.6 spICP-MS

This technique can detect single particles containing inorganic elements or tags detected by ICP-MS at very low concentrations and measure nanoparticle size, size distribution and number concentration simultaneously. In spICP-MS, a dilute aqueous suspension of nanoparticles is introduced continuously to a standard ICP-MS set-up which can collect ion signals at high time resolution, allowing detection of single particles as discrete events. As the constituents of the nanoparticles are atomised and ionised by plasma, a discrete pulse of atomic ions is generated and detected by a calibrated mass spectrometer. This results in a signal at a specific mass-to-charge ratio lasting on the order of a few hundreds of microseconds above a continuous background signal [62]. The pulse area is proportional to the mass of a nanoparticle which can then be used to calculate the spherical-equivalent particle diameter and number-based size distribution of nanoparticles. The frequency of the pulse can be related to nanoparticle number concentration. However, these calculations require careful calibration of the system using a reference nanoparticle ideally made of the same material [63].

3.1.7 General considerations

While it is best practice to measure the size distribution of particles with multiple methods, it is not straightforward to perform comparative evaluation of these techniques due to the differences in the sample preparation conditions and the underpinning physical measuring principles, which means that different techniques measure different particle characteristics or measurands and hence different particle sizes. For instance, SEM provides the circular equivalent diameter in a projected image and AFM the size is measured by the interactive forces between the sample and the probe tip. Both DLS and PTA measure the hydrodynamic spherical-equivalent diameter, TRPS provides the volume-based spherical equivalent diameter. Particle size measured by SEM is often referred as the 'core' size of nanoparticles, while the hydrodynamic size measured by DLS contains a hydration shell consisting of the water and other molecules surrounding the particles. Therefore, when analysing the same sample, it is not uncommon to observe larger particle sizes using liquid-based techniques such as DLS and PTA in comparison to the vacuum-based SEM. In addition, the size distribution of nanoparticles measured by a technique depends upon the type of method used, e.g. particle-by-particle techniques provide number-based size distribution, whereas, for example, DLS provides a scattered light intensity-based distribution. When comparing different techniques, it is important to compare the same type of particle distribution. It is often possible to transform the measured size distribution into a number-based size distribution. However, it is important to be aware of the assumptions about materials properties (e.g. refractive index, density, geometry) underpinning this transformation and of any associated uncertainties.

In terms of sample preparation, a protocol needs to be developed and optimised for each specific measurement method. For liquid-based methods, the concentration of the particle analyte needs to be adjusted to the working range of the instrument by dilution or concentration of the sample. Sample concentration can be achieved by means of centrifugation-assisted sample filtration. In some cases, for example TRPS, the sample may require transferring to a different dispersion medium. Imaging-based methods require the deposition of the particles upon a suitable substrate and, in most cases such as measurements in air and vacuum, require drying the sample. In this task, it is important to ensure that any salts or molecules that are not bonded to the particles are removed from the dispersion before the deposition. This is typically achieved through cycles of centrifugation-aided precipitation or filtration and redispersion of the materials in clean dispersant, or through dialysis. Sample preparation methods, thus, can vary in terms of complexity and time and necessitate a procedure to ensure that the analysed sub-set of particles is representative of the entire sample. It is also essential to ensure that sample preparation conditions do not affect the physical and chemical properties of nanoparticles prior to the analysis, or at least be aware of the possibility that they can.

Nanoparticles tend to agglomerate in buffer solutions with high ionic strength. This is due to a reduction in length of the electrical double layer and the related reduction of effective surface charge. It is known that anti-bacterial effectiveness is associated with their state of agglomeration since the occurrence of agglomeration/aggregation can decrease the surface to volume ratio, resulting in a detrimental effect on antibacterial performance. In addition, aggregates can decrease the dose of active ingredients released from nanoparticle formulations in killing bacteria [64,65]. Agglomeration/aggregation in nanoparticles can drastically increase the polydispersity of particles and generally poses a challenge for accurate size measurements of the isolated, individual particles. For the user to select an appropriate size measurement technique, it is important to consider the performance and measurement outcome of the various methods in the presence of particle agglomeration. DLS measurement results, for example, may be biased towards the larger nanoparticles or particle agglomerates in the sample because, for Rayleigh-scattering, the intensity of the scattered light follows a sixth power law with the size of a particle. In the presence of agglomeration, high resolution methods such as analytical centrifugation and field flow fractionation are particularly useful, because the particles are separated based on their size and density before reaching the detector. Selection of appropriate high-resolution particle-by-particle techniques, such as SEM, PTA and TRPS, can also provide quantitative information on particle agglomeration because of their ability to measure individual particles or particle agglomerates.

3.1.8 Examples

Various sizing techniques have been employed to measure a range of antimicrobial nanoparticles with different characteristics to understand their performance and mechanism in infection control [29,39,66–68]. For example, TEM has shown [29,39] to be particularly useful to characterise small nano-objects (e.g. below 40 nm) and differentiate monodisperse nanoparticles with very similar sizes. Using this technique, Docherty et al. have successfully demonstrated that a subtle change in particle size (<1 nm) can drastically affect the interactions between sub 10 nm palladium nanospheres and biological cells, leading to significant impact on their antimicrobial effectiveness [39]. Furthermore, for complex nanoparticles with internal structures such as core–shell particles, techniques such as electron microscopy and SAXS have been shown to be particularly useful to characterise nanoparticle's core, assuming the total collapsing of the corona. These techniques can also be combined with liquid techniques such as DLS to measure characteristics of a particle corona (e.g. hydrated shell thickness in liquids). For instance, using TEM analysis, Liang et al. [29] found that an increase in the core size of gold nanoparticles from 2 to 6 nm in diameter, enhanced the potency of antimicrobial activity, efficiently disrupting the cell membrane of targeted bacteria, as shown in Fig. 4.1A. They concluded that the greater bacterial killing capability is likely caused by more

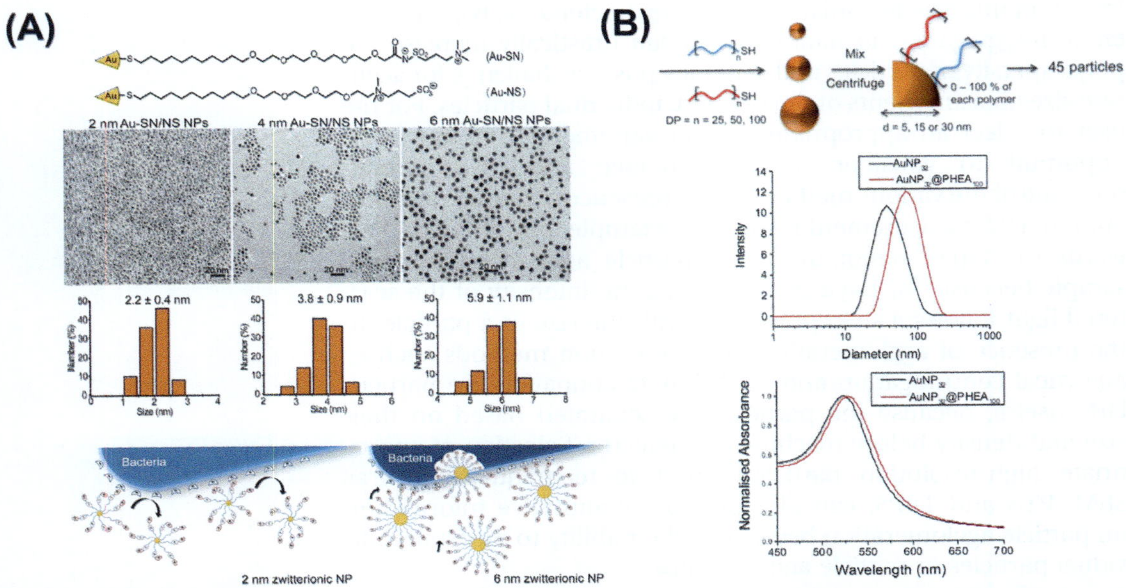

Figure 4.1 (A) Chemical structure of core–shell zwitterionic gold nanoparticles; TEM-determined nanoparticle size distribution and schematic illustration of interaction mechanism between bacteria membrane with 2 and 6 nm (in diameter) zwitterionic nanoparticle [29]; (B) schematic synthetic procedure for producing a library of polymer-grafted gold nanoparticles, DLS and UV-vis analysis before and after functionalisation of 32 nm (in diameter) gold nanoparticle with poly(*N*-hydroxyethyl acrylamide) on the surface [66]. (A) Reprinted with permission from Huo et al. [29]; (B) Adopted from Richards et al. [66].

densely packed zwitterionic corona in larger particles which enhance the interactions between nanospheres and bacterial membranes. For polydisperse samples, it is not uncommon to make use of several complimentary techniques to obtain accurate size information of nanoparticles. Based on DLS analysis, Gibson et al. [66] successfully estimated the corona thickness of a library of 45 distinct polycation-grafted gold nanoparticles in water. Subsequently, they assessed the colloidal stability of cationic polymer-coated gold nanospheres in both saline and complex biological media by comparing DLS with ultraviolet-visible spectrophotometer (UV-Vis) spectroscopy and TEM analysis, as shown in Fig. 4.1B. Kvitek and co-workers have utilised DLS, TEM and AFM to characterise and identify the aggregation state of silver bromide nanoparticles in the presence of polymer additives, ranging between 8 and 40 nm in diameter [67]. Using a combination of SEM, DLS and CLS, Epple et al. performed the size analysis of silver nanoparticles with different size and shape to assess the morphological impact on dissolution kinetics and the biological effect on cells [68].

3.2 Morphology

The surface area of nano-objects available for interaction with bacterial membrane will depend on not only their size but also their shape. The morphology of a nano-object can therefore affect their antibacterial efficiency and bacterial killing capability. Generally, if there is little difference in size between nanoparticles, those with larger surface area are more likely to interact with the bacterial cell wall and hence cause cell damage and finally, kill the bacteria [69]. It is also found that certain morphologies can optimise the distribution and facilitate the dissolution of active ingredients to enhance the antibacterial activity [23]. Due in part to their higher specific surface area non-spherical particles, such as rod- or disk-shaped nano-objects, have become attractive candidates in the design of antimicrobial agents [70]. Studies [71–74] have shown enhanced cell uptake and binding capability using rod-like particles compared to spherical ones. The techniques of gas adsorption analysis and nuclear magnetic resonance proton relaxation are used to measure the specific surface area of nano-objects in air and liquids respectively [75]. Techniques like AFM, electron microscopy and SAXS are particularly useful in characterising various nano-objects with complex structures. TEM and SEM provide invaluable information on particles' lateral size while AFM is capable of quantifying both lateral size and thickness of nanoparticles in air and liquids. SAXS is particularly useful in measuring nano-objects with characteristic lengths typically ranging from 1 to 100 nm. For polydisperse nano-objects, both TEM [76] and AFM [77] analysis have shown their usefulness in measuring the morphology and shape distribution of various functional nanostructures. For example, TEM has been utilised to locate and quantify silver nanoparticles in self-assembled organic-inorganic hybrid nanofibers which possess bacteriostatic effects against *E. coli* [78].

3.3 Surface composition characteristics

Surface compositional characteristics of nanoparticles, such as surface charge and chemistry, have a profound impact on colloidal stability, particle–cell interactions, and their performance as antimicrobial agents. Meyer and co-workers [79] have demonstrated the adsorption of cationic peptide-based nanoparticles to cell surfaces via electrostatic interactions between cationic ε-Poly-L-lysine and the phospholipid head groups of the cell membrane in *E. coli*. The strength of this particle–cell interaction determines how easily the nanoparticles enter cell membranes to cause damage: the cell membrane of *E. coli* exhibited higher nanoparticle permeability than that of *L. innocua* due to its stronger net negative charge. Maas et al. [80] have reported the impact of surface chemistry on the performance of antimicrobial nanodiamonds. They found that nanodiamonds with various reactive functional groups on the surface can form covalent bonds with adjacent proteins and molecules on cell walls to cause a disorder of bacterial metabolism and eventually kill bacteria.

3.3.1 Zeta-potential

Surface charge has significant implications on controlling the interactions between nanoparticles and the surrounding biological environment. For example, the formation of a protein corona on the surface of the nanoparticles and the probability of nanoparticle uptake by various types of bacteria cells largely depend on the nanoparticle surface charge. A typical measure of surface charge is given by ζ-potential (zeta-potential), which is the electric potential difference between the dispersion medium and the stationary layer of fluid attached to the dispersed particle [81]. From a theoretic point of view, it is the electrical potential at the slipping plane of an interfacial double layer. ζ-potential can be used as an indicator for colloidal stability. For charge-stabilised particles, ζ-potential magnitudes of 30 mV or higher are representative of a stable colloidal system. ζ-potential is useful in identifying biological analytes carrying different surface charge when their sizes are comparable. In addition, ζ-potential can be used to study the adsorption of molecules and ions on particles in contact with liquids. It should be noted that ζ-potential is not a directly measurable parameter but can be calculated from other measurands by applying an appropriate theory. The environment that particles reside in (e.g. pH, concentration, and ionic strength) plays a significant role on their ζ-potential and should always be indicated with any ζ-potential value. The method for the measurement of ζ-potential is described in several documentary standards [81–84].

One of the common techniques for measuring ζ-potential of nanoparticles in liquid dispersions is based upon electrophoresis where the equipment is typically equipped with optical detectors for monitoring the motion of nanoparticles. This method is mostly suitable for dilute systems, for example, approximately 1.0 wt% or lower concentrations of nanoparticles in liquid. Electrophoresis refers to the motion of electrically charged nanoparticles relative to a fluid when applying a spatially uniform electric field. Specifically, velocity of the nanoparticles is proportional to the applied electrical filed strength and the proportional coefficient is defined as electrophoretic mobility (μ).

The electrophoretic mobility is commonly used to calculate ζ-potential of particles [82]. The velocity of the particles can be determined using the electrophoretic light scattering (ELS) technique through a laser Doppler arrangement. In ELS analysis, a suspension of nanoparticles with a specific surface charge is placed into an electrochemical cell equipped with a pair of electrodes at a known fixed distance apart. When a potential is applied between the electrodes, particles carrying a net electric charge are drawn towards the electrode of opposite sign due to the electrophoresis process. As a result, the frequency of light scattered by particles will be shifted due to the Doppler effect. The distribution of particle electrophoretic mobility can be determined from the frequency shift. ELS analysis can measure both the velocity and the direction of the moving particles in the frame of reference associated with the measurement cell. ELS generally provides rapid, accurate, and highly reproducible ζ-potential measurements of nanoparticles suspended in either aqueous or nonaqueous media without the need to use calibrants. Detailed methods for measuring electrophoretic mobility using optical means and for calculating ζ-potential can be found in ISO 13099-2 [83].

TRPS offers an alternative approach to measure particle electrophoretic mobility on a particle-by-particle basis and simultaneously measure their size. In order to achieve accurate and reliable particle ζ-potential measurements by TRPS, the instrument settings should ensure that the electrophoretic forces are the dominant contribution to the particle transport mechanism. The same settings must be used to measure a particle calibrant with known ζ-potential, relative to which the measurement is done. One instrument manufacturer (Izon Science) reconmends that the pressure range applied during ζ—potential measurements is set to 10-fold lower than size and concentration measurements. Like ELS, the electrophoretic mobility needs to be measured in an aqueous media with moderate electrolyte concentrations. The most widely used theory of electrophoresis is the Smoluchowski approach [85].

$$\zeta = \frac{\eta\mu}{\varepsilon} \tag{4.1}$$

where η and ε are, respectively, the dynamic viscosity of the electrolyte and the dielectric constant. To date, several TRPS protocols [86,87] have been written to measure ζ-potential of individual particles.

3.3.2 Surface chemistry

Chemical composition of nanoparticles is often erroneously assumed rather than measured. The chemistry of the outmost layers of nanoparticles is critically important for many functional properties, including wettability, conductivity and chemical reactivities of particles. It is well-documented [80] that surface chemistry of nanoparticles plays a significant role in the particle–cell interactions for antimicrobial applications. To perform surface chemical analysis, it becomes appropriate to use surface sensitive techniques such as X-ray photoelectron spectroscopy (XPS) and secondary ion mass spectroscopy (SIMS) that gathers information from only the outmost layers of nanoparticles so that bulk signal does not dominate the data. XPS makes use of the photoelectric effect to measure the binding energy of the electrons ejected from the sample by illuminating it with X-rays. In XPS analysis, the energy required for an electron to be ejected from the surface of the sample has two contributions: the binding energy of electron in the atom, E_b and the energy required to leave the sample surface, φ, which is also called the electron work function and has a typical energy of ~5 eV. The kinetic energy, E, of unscattered and elastically scattered electrons in XPS is then given by the following equation:

$$E = hv - E_b - \varphi - c \tag{4.2}$$

where hv is the energy of the X-ray photon and c is the electric potential of the surface relative to the spectrometer. Identifying elements on the sample surface using XPS is relatively straightforward because each element has well-known and tabulated value of E_b for its core-level electrons. XPS can provide quantitative elemental composition as well as binding state information.

SIMS offers an alternative approach to study the chemistry of nanoparticle samples. In SIMS, a focussed primary ion beam is used to bombard a sample's surface. The resultant impact causes a release of secondary ions from the surface which are then analysed in a mass analyser [88]. SIMS is inherently surface sensitive, providing information typically from the top 1–3 nm of a sample with a lateral resolution in the cellular range <10 μm. Time-of-flight SIMS (TOF-SIMS) can analyse both organic and inorganic nanoparticle measurements. Whilst SIMS offers high chemical specifications, it is not generally quantitative. It can also suffer from the so-called matrix effect [89] (the dependence of the signal strength of an analyte on its chemical environment in the sample) and may require calibration with other surface analysis techniques such as XPS to achieve measurement accuracy. Controlled materials sputtering coupled with TOF-SIMS or XPS affords an alternative strategy to electron microscopy for carrying out chemical depth profiling and has been used to study the internal structure of various nanoparticle samples [90–92]. Equipped with gas cluster ion beam sputtering process, XPS and SIMS analysis can provide chemical depth profiling of complex organic and inorganic samples. Argon cluster ions are one of the commonly used gas cluster ion beam for treating organic materials and is capable of achieving depth resolutions of 5 nm for flat, uniform layers [93]. However, limited studies have so far been performed on topographic samples, including nanoparticles. A good understanding of the sputtering behaviour of nanoparticles is critical to achieve meaningful depth profiles. In particular, it is critically important to measure the change in material shape as it can affect both the apparent sputtering rate and the depth resolution. Seah et al. demonstrated [91] that metallic particles, such as gold nanospheres, are prone to melting under the argon cluster beam irradiation designed to etch the sample for chemical depth profiling. Pei and co-workers [90] described in detail the sputtering behaviour of polystyrene submicron-sized particles. They found there is a significant difference in the sputtering yield between isolated nanoparticles and congregated ones due to a shadowing effect. Based on these observations, they developed a geometric model and used XPS sputter depth profiling with argon cluster ions to perform chemical depth profiling of polymeric core-shell nanoparticles, as shown in Fig. 4.2A. It has been shown that SIMS provided high resolution chemical distributions over several layers of nanoparticles which can be nicely correlated to the structure acquired using SEM analysis (Fig. 4.2B and D). However, due to matrix effects in SIMS, calibration is required using XPS data to obtain quantitative chemical analysis of nanoparticles (Fig. 4.2C). It is worth noting that this approach is complementary to electron microscopy. Argon cluster sputtering assisted XPS and SIMS analysis can provide chemistry and structural properties of nanoparticles, including shell thickness, size, quantity and distribution of particle core.

3.4 Other properties

There are techniques that can be used to measure additional properties of antimicrobial nanoparticles, such as porosity, specific surface area and particle number concentration. Porous nanoparticles can provide a substantial increase in their surface-to-volume ratio which may significantly impact their bacterial killing capabilities. Specific surface area can be determined using gas adsorption analysis under controlled temperature and pressure conditions and the Brunauer–Emmett–Teller (BET) theory [94].

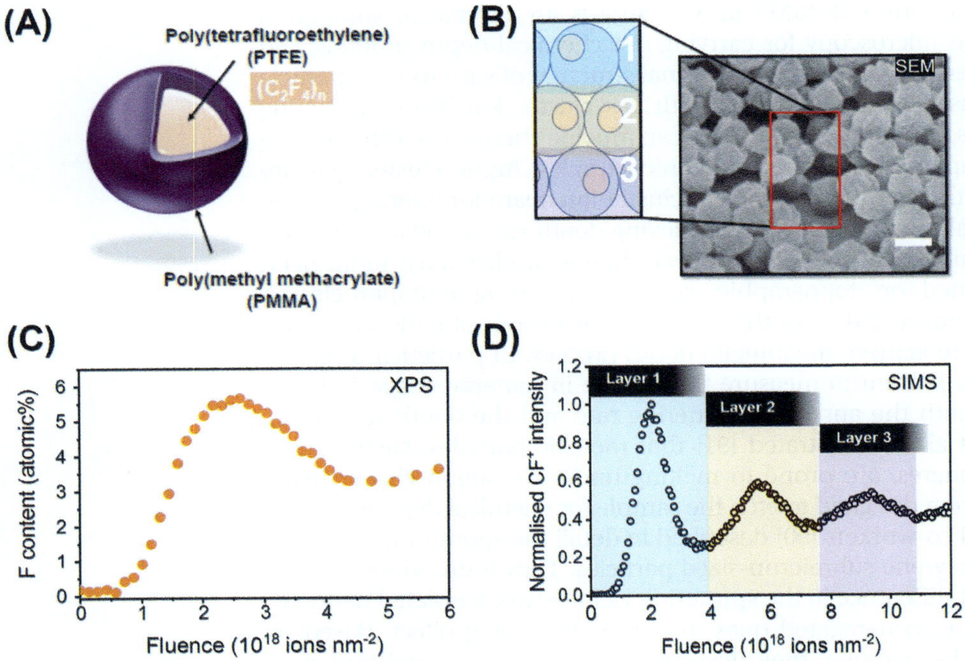

Figure 4.2 Characterisation of the internal chemical distribution of poly(tetrafluoroethylene)-poly(methyl methacrylate) core–shell nanoparticles using XPS and SIMS analysis coupled with argon cluster sputtering: (A) Schematic of the internal structure of heterogeneous polymer nanoparticles; (B) sample structure after initial argon cluster sputtering consist of several layers of the nanoparticles; (C) XPS depth profile plotting the equivalent homogeneous concentration of fluorine against argon cluster ion fluence; (D) SIMS depth profile plotting normalised CF^+ secondary ion intensity against argon cluster ion fluence. Scale bar = 100 nm [90].

Another important feature which can affect the loading of active ingredient and hence the performance of bactericidal nanoparticles is nanoparticle number concentration. There are a range of measurement methods that can be utilised to measure the particle number concentration, including PTA, CLS, TRPS and, in the case of gold nanoparticles, UV-Vis. The selection of techniques depends on a variety of factors, such as the type of samples (organic versus inorganic), whether or not the analytes scatter light efficiently, and nanoparticle concentration range among others (see Section 2). It should be noted that no single nanoparticle characterisation method can provide answers to all the questions with regards to nanoparticle size, shape, zeta potential and chemical compositions. A combination of complementary techniques should be used to characterise nanoparticles with antibacterial capabilities.

3.5 Measuring nanoparticles in biological environments

Applying nanotechnology to medicine and biotechnology often necessitates nanomaterials and nanostructured surfaces interfacing with biological environments, such as serum, blood, cells and tissues. It is important to measure nanoparticles in the environment intended for use. This significantly increases complexity and poses substantial analytical challenges.

When nanoparticles are introduced into a biological environment, proteins from the media tend to adsorb at the nanoparticle's surfaces forming a so-called 'protein corona' [95–97]. This is a dynamic process and the chemical composition of the corona changes with time. In the initial step, the most abundant proteins, typically albumin, cover the surface of the particles. However, other higher affinity proteins may displace albumin and become strongly adsorbed to the particle surface over time, a process which is known as the Vroman effect [98]. On a short timescale, a 'soft' protein corona develops, where proteins are loosely bound via weak protein–protein interactions with low affinity to the nanoparticle surfaces [96]. Within hours, however, the proteins with higher affinity to the particle surface form a more stable 'hard' corona. This defines the biological identity of the particles. For in vivo applications, the make-up of the protein corona of nanoparticles impacts their interactions with the reticuloendothelial system and therefore their circulation time and clearance mechanism within the body [99,100].

The surface chemistry and surface charge of the nanoparticles influence the type and quantity of proteins that adsorb at their surface. In fact, there are several chemical strategies that are routinely employed to prevent, or delay, surface protein adsorption, the most common being the covalent binding of polyethylene glycol (PEG) molecules to particle surfaces. The ability of PEG coatings to resist protein adsorption relates to the conformation of the individual polymer chains and their packing density on the surface [101,102]. Due to its hydrophilicity, the formation of a large hydration shell shields the particle surface from the adsorption of proteins. PEG coatings also sterically stabilise the particles hindering their agglomeration [103]. However, it has been shown that PEG coatings in biological environments will sometimes adsorb proteins [101,104].

The formation of protein corona around nanoparticles causes an increase in their hydrodynamic size and a change in their average density. Additionally, protein–protein interactions can lead to particle agglomeration. This is in addition to the obvious changes in their surface properties, for example, in terms of surface chemistry and charge. These changes can be measured with the same analytical methods that are utilised for the characterisation of the pristine particles, although sample preparation and measurement protocols need to be optimised on a case-by-case basis. In general, there are two types of approaches to measure nanoparticles in liquid-based complex matrices. The first approach consists of measuring the particles within their biological matrix. This is possible under the assumption that the analytical capability can handle any background signal caused by the matrix, for example due to the presence of proteins in solution. In the second approach, particles are separated from the biological matrix before measurement. In this case, it is important that the separation protocols are optimised so that they do not alter the state of the particles, for example in terms of the nature of the protein corona or the level of agglomeration. Furthermore, due to the typical agglomeration occurring to the particles in these media, methods that allow for separation and fractionation of the samples are particularly useful to improve the quality and meaningfulness of the measurements.

Fig. 4.3 [105] shows an example of size distribution and ζ-potential measurements of silica particles after incubation in 50 mM tris(hydroxymethyl)aminomethane hydrochloride, pH 7.4 (Tris buffer) and 10% (v/v) foetal bovine serum in Eagle's minimum essential medium (serum). According to the DLS measurements, silica nanoparticles dispersed in Tris buffer and serum exhibit in both cases a monomodal peak, but with different peak shapes and positions. These results can be interpreted as a change of hydrodynamic diameter of the particles due to the absorption of protein at their surface or as an increased particle agglomeration or both. TRPS has higher size resolution than the DLS method and allows for deeper insights into the changes in the particle sizes upon introduction into serum media. As shown in Fig. 4.3A, TRPS measurements show a shift in the modal diameter of the size distribution accompanied by a broadening of the peak, which is consistent with the formation of a protein corona of approximately 5 nm in thickness. Some peaks at larger diameters are also visible and more pronounced for the particles in serum, indicating the presence of agglomeration. This behaviour can be seen more clearly in Fig. 4.3B, where the results of TRPS measurements are shown on a particle-by-particle basis. Whilst most of the particles in Tris buffer have diameters between 60 and 100 nm, the diameter of the particles in the serum medium ranges from 50 to 350 nm. Fig. 4.3B also shows the change in

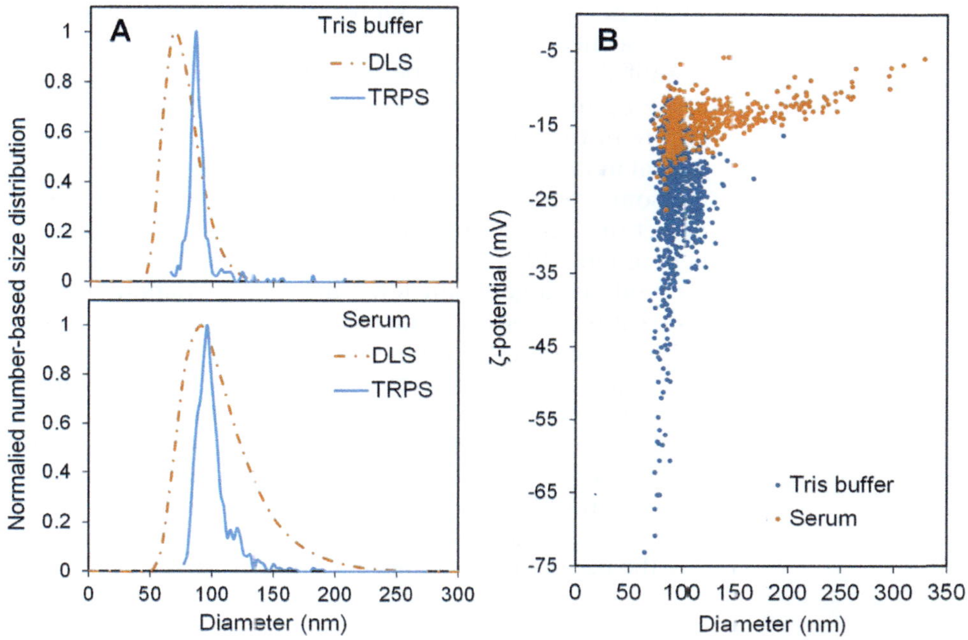

Figure 4.3 (A) Number-based size distribution as measured by DLS and TRPS of silica particles dispersed in 50 mM tris(hydroxymethyl)aminomethane hydrochloride, pH 7.4 (Tris buffer, top) and 10% (v/v) foetal bovine serum in Eagle's minimum essential medium (serum, bottom); (B) TRPS analysis of the same samples showing particle-by-particle results of the measurement of particle diameter and ζ-potential (particles in Tris buffer in blue and in serum in orange) [105].

ζ-potential for the same particles. The silica particles in Tris-buffer appear to have a spread of values of surface ζ-potential, while the particles in serum, i.e. whose surface is coated by the protein corona, appear to have a more homogeneous charge at the surface, with a ζ-potential value around −15 mV.

Recently, the European Nanomedicine Characterisation Laboratory and the US National Cancer Institute Nanotechnology Characterization Laboratory have jointly developed a standard operating procedure for assessing nanoparticle medical products in liquid dispersions using multiple techniques with a special focus on nanoparticle size distribution measurement in complex biological environment. In this documentation, there is strong emphasis on emerging techniques such as asymmetric flow field flow fractionation (AF4)-DLS-multi angle light scattering [106].

The analysis of nanoparticles in solid biological matrices is typically achieved through some type of microscopy (SEM,

TEM) or spectroscopy. Optical-based spectroscopies, such as fluorescence and Raman spectroscopy, generally detect the chemical signature of the particles, or that of a chemical label attached to them. In such methods, for detection, the chemical nature of the particles must be different to the surrounding biological matrix. Depending on the materials the particles are made of, some types of non-linear optical spectroscopies can also detect the particles by photothermal lensing or second harmonic generation [107]. In general, the lateral resolution of optical methods is larger than few hundreds of nanometres and their application is useful to identify the distribution of the nanoparticles in the sample, rather than the measurement of the physical properties of the particles. Fig. 4.4A shows an example of non-linear optical spectroscopy imaging of metal nanoparticles in a rat skin section using three different modalities, namely: stimulated Raman scattering (SRS) (red), second harmonic generation (green) and photothermal lensing (cyan hot). The different colours in the image show different chemical entities in the skin sample, the nanoparticles being in cyan hot. Note that the sample was

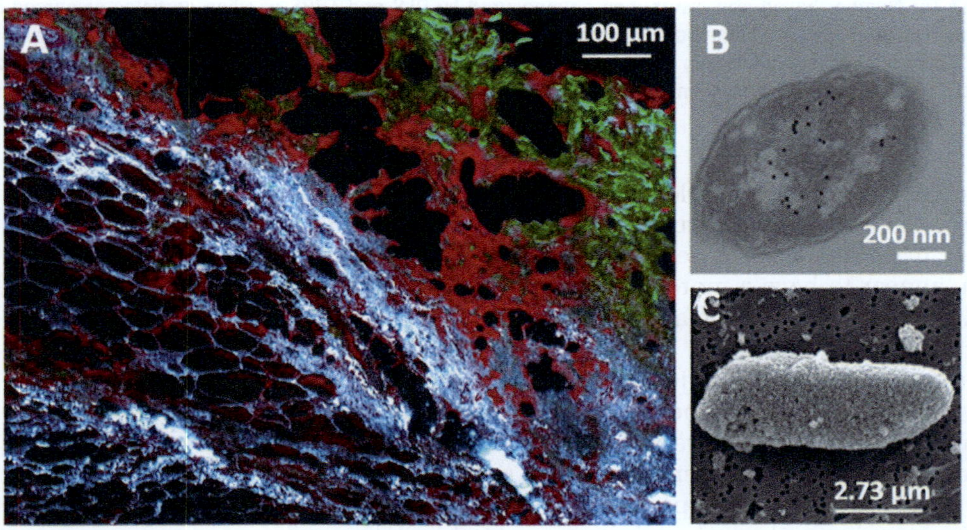

Figure 4.4 (A) SRS and second harmonic generation microscopy composite image of a rat skin section containing metallic particles. SRS contrast for CH_2 stretching is shown in red, and off-resonance signals at 2770 cm^{-1} are overlaid in cyan hot, revealing the distribution of the metal particles based on their strong signals due to absorption and photothermal lensing. Collagen (green) is visualised using SHG [107]. (B) TEM image of *M. luteus* treated by surface-modified gold nanoparticles [108]. (C) SEM image of *E. coli* O157:H7 cell incubated with antibody-conjugated nanoparticles [109]. (A) Reproduced from Tsikritsis et al. [107]; (B) Adopted with permission from Yang et al. [108] (C) Adopted from Zhao et al. [109].

free from optical or fluorescent probes or other types of imaging labels or contrast enhancers.

Electron microscopies afford higher lateral resolution and are used to locate the nanoparticles within the biological media. Fig. 4.4B and C show examples of nanoparticles with bacteria by transmission and scanning electron microscopies respectively. As seen for example in these figures, particles with higher electron density, typically metallic, offer high contrast with respect to organic materials and can in principle be easily identified. However, this is not the case where staining is used to generate contrast in imaging of biological samples, in which case further chemical analysis may be employed to identify the particles. Furthermore, the impact of the staining procedure on the distribution and morphology of the particles needs assessing. The identification and localisation of nanoparticles of organic, as opposed to inorganic, nature within biological matrices is more challenging because of the lack of contrast between the particles and the surrounding environment.

A final consideration on microscopy methods is the need to evaluate variability within the same sample and across sample repeats and ensure results are statistically valid. A number of control samples will typically be necessary to assess the robustness of the method from both a biological and metrological point of view. Furthermore, a sufficient number of particles need to be measured for statistically relevant results.

4. Considerations when selecting a technique

The selection of appropriate techniques for measuring nanoparticle samples requires users to consider a number of factors, some of which are discussed below.

4.1 Sample type

All the techniques described in this chapter can be applied to a large variety of material types, including organic, inorganic and biological particles. Several of the techniques that operate in suspension, such as DLS, detect aspects of light extinction and thereby require nanoparticles to absorb or scatter light at the wavelength of the light source applied. For particles and suspending medium with relatively low differential scattering cross section, techniques based on alternative principle of detection can be employed. For example, TRPS is used to characterise nanoparticles in electrolytes using electrical signals, instead of scattered light, and spICP-MS perform mass spectrometry on a particle-by-particle basis and measure the mass of inorganic elements within.

4.2 Sample state

Nanoparticle samples can be either measured in the liquid form as suspensions or in the solid state as dry powders. A user's selection of a technique largely depends on the state of the analyte of interest. Liquid-based methods typically have specific requirements on the sample particle concentration and the characteristics of the dispersant (e.g. ionic strength). For meaningful measurements, the sample need to be prepared in order to meet these criteria. Microscopy methods require the sample to be deposited onto a suitable substrate either from dry powder or dispersion. Some of them, such as AFM, are capable of measuring nanoparticles both in air as powders and in liquid as dispersions. Surface chemical analysis techniques like XPS and SIMS require dispersions to be deposited on a substrate from solution. Alternatively, nanoparticles powders can be pressed into films or pellets.

4.3 Sample quantity

The quantity of sample required for a method can be an important factor in selecting a technique, especially when dealing with samples that are expensive, toxic or available only in limited quantity. The minimum amount of sample required for a measurement is related to both the minimal sample volume accepted by an instrument and the nanoparticle concentration required by the selected technique. For methods that perform a chemical measurement of the nanoparticles (XPS and SIMS), it is important to consider the concentration and amount of the element or molecule of interest in the sample with respect to the instrument sensitivity for the same element or molecule.

4.4 Accuracy and precision

The required accuracy and precision with which nanoparticle properties must be known drives significantly the choice of the method to apply. In many practical applications, the users' choice is largely dependent upon the aim of the measurement. For example, for product development, it is usually preferable for users to know sample properties with accuracy, whereas the precision of a technique is more valued for quality assurance and quality control purposes. In general, techniques that require minimal sample preparation and negligible requirement of user input (e.g. manual setting of signal thresholds) tend to be more precise. The sources of uncertainty impacting on the accuracy and precision of different techniques, along with the limit of detection, are widely discussed in related documentary standards and some aspects will be covered in the later sections of this chapter. It should be noted that the methods and tools utilised for sample preparation and transfer can also have significant impact on the method accuracy and precision. It is best practice to validate accuracy and precision of a method using traceable certified reference materials with known nanoparticle properties according to standard documentation.

5. Standardisation

This section provides an overview of the documentary standardisation process. It describes what it is and how it works. Details of standards and standardisation bodies in nanotechnologies are described. An overview of the standards in antimicrobial properties and measurements are also highlighted.

5.1 What, why and how

A standard, for the purposes of this chapter, is a documentary standard as opposed to a reference material of a known specific property. International Organization for Standardisation (ISO) defines this as a '*document, established by consensus and approved by a recognised body, that provides for common and repeated use, rules, guidelines or characteristics for activities or their results, aimed at the achievement of the optimum degree of order in a given context*' [110]. Hence, a standard is developed by technical experts in a committee such as ISO, International Electrotechnical Commission (IEC) or ASTM International (formerly known as the American Society for Testing Materials International) who come to an agreement on the text of the standard.

A standard represents the best practice in a particular field, it allows repeatable and reliable measurements to be made and allows comparisons between different laboratories and

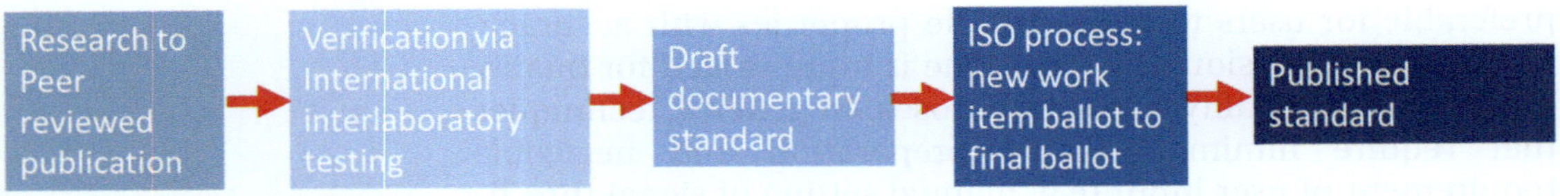

Figure 4.5 A flow chart of the typical development of a measurement-based documentary standard.

instruments. Standards are voluntary but often can become the basis of regulations or referred to in regulatory guidelines.

The typical process leading to a published measurement and characterisation standard is outlined in Fig. 4.5. Here, one laboratory develops and publishes a method. A protocol, the basis of a standard, is then tested and refined via international interlaboratory studies. These interlaboratory studies are often organised under the auspices of Versailles Project on Advanced Materials and Standards (VAMAS) [111], an international prenormative organisation. Once the interlaboratory study is completed, a new work item ballot in, for example, ISO ensues followed by the various other ballot stages. At each stage technical experts from contributing countries have opportunities to comment and agree on the text. Publication then follows. In some cases, for example, within ASTM International, an interlaboratory comparison among selected expert laboratories also takes place before the final publication of the standard, as a way to test and consolidate operating procedures described in the standards [112].

5.2 International standardisation in nanotechnologies

There are a number of different international standards committees in the nanotechnologies. These committees are summarised in Table 4.2. Lists of published standards from each committee shown in Table 4.2 can be found on the web page of each committee.

ISO/TC 229 nanotechnologies is the largest standards committee in the nanotechnologies field and contains working groups on (i) terminology and nomenclature, (ii) measurement and characterisation, (iii) health, safety and environmental aspects of nanotechnologies, (iv) material specifications and (v) products and applications.

Terminology standards are essential to allow people from different backgrounds and areas to use a common clear set of terms and definitions to avoid misunderstandings and mistakes.

Table 4.2 International standardisation committees in nanotechnologies.

Committee	Membership type and number[a]	Number of published standards[a]	Number of standards under development[a]
ISO/TC 229 Nanotechnologies	Country-based (39 members, 18 observers)	100	33
IEC/TC113 Nanotechnology for electrotechnical products and systems	Country-based (16 members, 19 observers)	67	61
ASTM International TC E56 Nanotechnology	Individual membership (over 168 members)	32	14

[a]As of December 2022.

In terms of terminology in nanotechnology, ISO/TC 229 has published a 13-part series of standards in terminology (ISO TS 80004 series). This series include terms and definitions in measurement, materials, coatings and characterisation as well as defining key core terms including nanoscale, nano-object and nanotechnology.

In measurement and characterisation, ISO/TR 18196:2016 'Nanotechnologies – Measurement technique matrix for the characterisation of nano-objects' provides an overview of the measurands or properties that are required to characterise nano-objects, including size, shape, charge and chemistry. It links these properties to the different measurement techniques. A detailed description of the key measurands can be found in ISO/TS 23302:2021 'Nanotechnologies – Requirements and recommendations for the identification of measurands that characterise nano-objects and materials that contain them'.

There are specific standards on the measurement techniques, these are highlighted further in Section 5 of this chapter. These are general measurement standards for a particular technique for the analysis of any sample. Alternatively, sometimes there are standards that are specific to a material using one or more different techniques. These standards are developed in ISO/TC 229, ISO/TC 24/SC 4 particle characterisation, ISO/TC 201 surface chemical analysis and ISO/TC 202 microbeam analysis.

5.3 International standardisation in antimicrobial properties

The technical committee ISO/TC 330 on surfaces with biocidal and antimicrobial properties was formed in 2020. Its scope is the standardisation of test methods used to assess the biocidal performance and efficacy of any surfaces with antimicrobial activities, including their compatibility with different families of disinfectants and cleaning agents. Such methods aim at evaluating the biocidal activity (i.e. that which irreversibly inactivates microorganism) and at differentiating it from the biostatic activity (i.e. the inhibition of the growth of microorganisms). This field covers the assessment of surfaces displaying intrinsic biocidal properties and of surfaces processed by any means so as to deliver biocidal properties under normal environmental conditions for the intended application. The field targets only surfaces, regardless of their final use. Areas of interest may include medical and veterinary applications, aerospace, agriculture, food, hygiene and other industrial fields, institutional and domestic applications. ISO/TC 330 does not cover toxicological and ecotoxicological surface testing methods, disinfection processes, antimicrobial activities of textile and porous products (including footwear), photocatalysis and nanotechnologies, excepting nano-enhanced/nano-enabled biocidal performance.

The first standard published by ISO/TC 330 is ISO 7581:2023 Evaluation of bactericidal activity of a non-porous antimicrobial surface used in a dry environment'. The document specifies the test conditions and the levels of activity with which non-porous surfaces shall comply in order to justify a claim of bactericidal activity. It defines a protocol to validate the bactericidal character of a surface and to measure its performance. It is not used to substantiate cleaning or disinfecting properties.

Other ISO standards that are relevant include

- ISO 22196:2011 'Measurement of antibacterial activity on plastics and other non-porous surfaces'.
- ISO 20743:2021 'Textiles — Determination of antibacterial activity of textile products'.

6. Conclusion and perspectives

The increasing complexity in nanomaterial design and the growth of their application in tackling global problems of infectious diseases require continuous progress in nanoparticle characterisation. There are several critical properties of nanoparticles that are intimately connected with the performance of end-products and their effects on health and the environment: particle size and size distribution, shape, surface topography, surface charge and chemical composition. Accurate and reliable measurement of these properties will underpin the rapid growing development of advanced nanomaterials. In addition, documentary standards and analysis protocols are increasingly required to accurately measure the properties of nanoparticles repeatably, ensuring the nanoparticles are manufactured within specified tolerances to achieve optimal performance of the end-products and accelerate regulatory approval. In this chapter, we provided description and comparison of a range of analytical tools for the characterisation of antimicrobial nanoparticles. Through the comprehensive summary of methods, we demonstrated the use of each technique, their advantages and drawbacks and how to achieve accurate and reliable measurements using relevant standard documentations. We also emphasised the importance of combining complementary techniques to obtain a full picture of numerous features associated with nanomaterials in complex biological environment.

With increasing complexity in material design, development of novel analytical approaches for nanoparticle characterisation under physiological conditions is urgently required to improve the understanding in the mechanisms of the bactericidal and fungicidal actions. In addition, inline measurements under the operating conditions will be needed to support the scale-up manufacturing and quality control of end-products. We expect that continuous growth in nanoparticle metrology and standardisation to drive innovations in this area, leading to cheaper and more effective antimicrobial products in the market to combat antimicrobial resistance and infectious diseases.

References

[1] A.R. Kirtane, M. Verma, P. Karandikar, J. Furin, R. Langer, G. Traverso, Nanotechnology approaches for global infectious diseases, Nature Nanotechnology 16 (2021) 369–384.
[2] L. Kumar, M. Bisen, K. Harjai, S. Chhibber, S. Azizov, H. Lalhlenmawia, D. Kumar, Advances in nanotechnology for biofilm inhibition, ACS Omega 8 (2023) 21352–22255.
[3] S. Xie, Y. Tao, Y. Pan, W. Qu, G. Cheng, L. Huang, D. Chen, X. Wang, Z. Liu, Z. Yuan, Biodegradable nanoparticles for intracellular delivery of antimicrobial agents, Journal of Controlled Release 187 (2014) 101–117.
[4] W. Unger, V.D. Hodoroaba, A. Shard, Characterization of Nanoparticles: Measurement Processes for Nanoparticles, Elsevier, 2019.

[5] M.M. Modena, B. Rühle, T.P. Burg, S. Wuttke, Nanoparticle characterization: what to measure? Advanced Materials 31 (2019) 1901556.

[6] S. Mourdikoudis, R.M. Pallares, N.T.K. Thanh, Characterization techniques for nanoparticles: comparison and complementarity upon studying nanoparticle properties, Nanoscale 10 (2018) 12871–12934.

[7] ISO 14488:2007 Particulate materials — Sampling and sample splitting for the determination of particulate properties.

[8] ISO 8213:1986 Chemical products for industrial use — Sampling techniques — Solid chemical products in the form of particles varying from powders to coarse lumps.

[9] ISO 14887:2000 Sample preparation — Dispersing procedures for powders in liquids.

[10] ISO 20579-4:2018 Surface chemical analysis — Guidelines to sample handling, preparation and mounting. Part 4: Reporting information related to the history, preparation, handling and mounting of nano-objects prior to surface analysis.

[11] ISO 19749:2021 Nanotechnologies — Measurements of particle size and shape distributions by scanning electron microscopy.

[12] ISO 14703:2008 Fine ceramics (advanced ceramics, advanced technical ceramics) — Sample preparation for the determination of particle size distribution of ceramic powders.

[13] ISO 21363:2020 Nanotechnologies — Measurements of particle size and shape distributions by transmission electron microscopy.

[14] R.D. Boyd, A. Cuenat, F. Meli, T. Klein, C.G. Frase, G. Gleber, M. Krumrey, A. Duta, S. Duta, R. Hogstrom, Good practice guide for the determination of the size distributions of spherical nanoparticle samples, 2011.

[15] ISO/TS 24597:2011 Microbeam analysis — Scanning electron microscopy — Methods of evaluating image sharpness.

[16] ISO 29301:2023 Microbeam analysis — Analytical electron microscopy — Methods for calibrating image magnification by using reference materials with periodic structures.

[17] C. Minelli, M. Wywijas, D. Bartczak, S. Nunez, H. Goenaga-Infante, VAMAS TWA34, Project 10: inter-laboratory study of the measurement of number concentration of colloidal nanoparticles: protocol for sample handling, Preparation and Measurements (2018).

[18] K.R. Raghupathi, R.T. Koodali, A.C. Manna, Size-dependent bacterial growth inhibition and mechanism of antibacterial activity of zinc oxide nanoparticles, Langmuir 27 (2011) 4020–4028.

[19] A. Azam, A.S. Ahmed, M. Oves, M.S. Khan, A. Memic, Size-dependent antimicrobial properties of CuO nanoparticles against Gram-positive and-negative bacterial strains, International Journal of Nanomedicine 7 (2012) 3527.

[20] A. Ivask, I. Kurvet, K. Kasemets, I. Blinova, V. Aruoja, S. Suppi, H. Vija, A. Käkinen, T. Titma, M. Heinlaan, Size-dependent toxicity of silver nanoparticles to bacteria, yeast, algae, crustaceans and mammalian cells in vitro, PLoS One 9 (2014) e102108.

[21] L. Shang, K. Nienhaus, G.U. Nienhaus, Engineered nanoparticles interacting with cells: size matters, Journal of Nanobiotechnology 12 (2014) 1–11.

[22] S.M. Dizaj, F. Lotfipour, M. Barzegar-Jalali, M.H. Zarrintan, K. Adibkia, Antimicrobial activity of the metals and metal oxide nanoparticles, Materials Science and Engineering: C 44 (2014) 278–284.

[23] J.R. Morones, J.L. Elechiguerra, A. Camacho, K. Holt, J.B. Kouri, J.T. Ramírez, M.J. Yacaman, The bactericidal effect of silver nanoparticles, Nanotechnology 16 (2005) 2346.
[24] W. Zhang, Y. Yao, N. Sullivan, Y. Chen, Modeling the primary size effects of citrate-coated silver nanoparticles on their ion release kinetics, Environmental Science and Technology 45 (2011) 4422–4428.
[25] A. Ivask, A. ElBadawy, C. Kaweeteerawat, D. Boren, H. Fischer, Z. Ji, C.H. Chang, R. Liu, T. Tolaymat, D. Telesca, Toxicity mechanisms in *Escherichia coli* vary for silver nanoparticles and differ from ionic silver, ACS Nano 8 (2014) 374–386.
[26] Y. Zhang, H. Peng, W. Huang, Y. Zhou, D. Yan, Facile preparation and characterization of highly antimicrobial colloid Ag or Au nanoparticles, Journal of Colloid and Interface Science 325 (2008) 371–376.
[27] O. Choi, Z. Hu, Size dependent and reactive oxygen species related nanosilver toxicity to nitrifying bacteria, Environmental Science and Technology 42 (2008) 4583–4588.
[28] F. Raimondi, G.G. Scherer, R. Kötz, A. Wokaun, Nanoparticles in energy technology: examples from electrochemistry and catalysis, Angewandte Chemie International Edition 44 (2005) 2190–2209.
[29] S. Huo, Y. Jiang, A. Gupta, Z. Jiang, R.F. Landis, S. Hou, X.-J. Liang, V.M. Rotello, Fully zwitterionic nanoparticle antimicrobial agents through tuning of core size and ligand structure, ACS Nano 10 (2016) 8732–8737.
[30] K. Zheng, M.I. Setyawati, D T. Leong, J. Xie, Antimicrobial gold nanoclusters, ACS Nano 11 (2017) 6904–6910.
[31] K. Zheng, M.I. Setyawati, D T. Leong, J. Xie, Antimicrobial silver nanomaterials, Coordination Chemistry Reviews 357 (2018) 1–17.
[32] X. Xie, T. Sun, J. Xue, Z. Miao, X. Yan, W. Fang, Q. Li, R. Tang, Y. Lu, L. Tang, Ag nanoparticles cluster with pH-triggered reassembly in targeting antimicrobial applications, Advanced Functional Materials 30 (2020) 2000511.
[33] J.P. Ruparelia, A.K. Chatterjee, S.P. Duttagupta, S. Mukherji, Strain specificity in antimicrobial activity of silver and copper nanoparticles, Acta Biomaterialia 4 (2008) 707–716.
[34] C. Calabrese, V. La Parola, M.L. Testa, L.F. Liotta, Antifouling and antimicrobial activity of Ag, Cu and Fe nanoparticles supported on silica and titania, Inorganica Chimica Acta (2021) 120636.
[35] S. Elyamny, M. Eltarahony, M. Abu-Serie, M.M. Nabil, A.E.-H.B. Kashyout, One-pot fabrication of Ag@ Ag2O core–shell nanostructures for biosafe antimicrobial and antibiofilm applications, Scientific Reports 11 (2021) 1–13.
[36] L. Giraud, A. Tourrette, E. Flahaut, Carbon nanomaterials-based polymer-matrix nanocomposites for antimicrobial applications: a review, Carbon 183 (2021) 463–483.
[37] M.S. Deepika, R. Thangam, S. Sundarraj, T.S. Sheena, S. Sivasubramanian, J. Kulandaivel, R. Thirumurugan, Co-delivery of diverse therapeutic compounds using PEG–PLGA nanoparticle cargo against drug-resistant bacteria: an improved anti-biofilm strategy, ACS Applied Bio Materials 3 (2019) 385–399.
[38] S.J. Lam, E.H.H. Wong, C. Boyer, G.G. Qiao, Antimicrobial polymeric nanoparticles, Progress in Polymer Science 76 (2018) 40–64.
[39] C.P. Adams, K.A. Walker, S.O. Obare, K.M. Docherty, Size-dependent antimicrobial effects of novel palladium nanoparticles, PLoS One 9 (2014) e85981.

[40] T. Huang, J.A. Holden, D.E. Heath, N.M. O'Brien-Simpson, A.J. O'Connor, Engineering highly effective antimicrobial selenium nanoparticles through control of particle size, Nanoscale 11 (2019) 14937–14951.
[41] T.K. Lind, P. Zielinska, H.P. Wacklin, Z. Urbanczyk-Lipkowska, M. Cárdenas, Continuous flow atomic force microscopy imaging reveals fluidity and time-dependent interactions of antimicrobial dendrimer with model lipid membranes, ACS Nano 8 (2014) 396–408.
[42] P.D. Rakowska, H. Jiang, S. Ray, A. Pyne, B. Lamarre, M. Carr, P.J. Judge, J. Ravi, U.I. M. Gerling, B. Koksch, Nanoscale imaging reveals laterally expanding antimicrobial pores in lipid bilayers, Proceedings of the National Academy of Sciences 110 (2013) 8918–8923.
[43] E. Meyer, Atomic force microscopy, Progress in Surface Science 41 (1992) 3–49.
[44] K. Egami, K. Higashi, K. Yamamoto, K. Moribe, Crystallization of probucol in nanoparticles revealed by AFM analysis in aqueous solution, Molecular Pharmaceutics 12 (2015) 2972–2980.
[45] ASTM E2382-04:2020 Standard guide to scanner and tip related artifacts in scanning tunneling microscopy and atomic force microscopy.
[46] ASTM E2859-11:2017 Standard guide for size measurement of nanoparticles using atomic force microscopy.
[47] W.D. Pyrz, D.J. Buttrey, Particle size determination using TEM: a discussion of image acquisition and analysis for the novice microscopist, Langmuir 24 (2008) 11350–11360.
[48] O. Ersen, I. Florea, C. Hirlimann, C. Pham-Huu, Exploring nanomaterials with 3D electron microscopy, Materials Today 18 (2015) 395–408.
[49] L. Luo, S.R. German, W.-J. Lan, D.A. Holden, T.L. Mega, H.S. White, Resistive-pulse analysis of nanoparticles, Annual Review of Analytical Chemistry 7 (2014) 513–535.
[50] E. Weatherall, G.R. Willmott, Applications of tunable resistive pulse sensing, Analyst 140 (2015) 3318–3334.
[51] ISO 13319-1:2021 Determination of particle size distribution — Electrical sensing zone method. Part 1: Aperture/orifice tube method.
[52] ASTM E2490-09:2021 Standard guide for measurement of particle size distribution of nanomaterials in suspension by photon correlation spectroscopy (PCS).
[53] ASTM E3247-20:2020 Standard test method for measuring the size of nanoparticles in aqueous media using dynamic light scattering.
[54] ISO 22412:2017 Particle size analysis — Dynamic light scattering (DLS).
[55] A. Einstein, Zur theorie der brownschen bewegung, Annalen der Physik 324 (1906) 371–381.
[56] J. Stetefeld, S.A. McKenna, T.R. Patel, Dynamic light scattering: a practical guide and applications in biomedical sciences, Biophysical Reviews 8 (2016) 409–427.
[57] ISO 19430:2016 Particle size analysis particle size analysis — Particle tracking analysis (PTA) method.
[58] ASTM E2834-12:2018, Standard guide for measurement of particle size distribution of nanomaterials in suspension by nanoparticle tracking analysis (NTA).
[59] T. Li, A.J. Senesi, B. Lee, Small angle X-ray scattering for nanoparticle research, Chemical Reviews 116 (2016) 11128–11180.
[60] ISO 17867:2020 Particle size analysis — Small angle X-ray scattering (SAXS).

[61] C. Minelli, V. Kestens, F. Babick, D. Lerche, Centrifugal liquid sedimentation methods, in: C. Contado (Ed.), Particle Separation Techniques, Elsevier, 2022, pp. 541–577.
[62] D. Mozhayeva, C. Engelhard, A critical review of single particle inductively coupled plasma mass spectrometry – a step towards an ideal method for nanomaterial characterization, Journal of Analytical Atomic Spectrometry 35 (2020) 1740.
[63] ISO/TS 19590:2017 Nanotechnologies — Size distribution and concentration of inorganic nanoparticles in aqueous media via single particle inductively coupled plasma mass spectrometry.
[64] C. Levard, E.M. Hotze, G.V. Lowry, G.E. Brown Jr, Environmental transformations of silver nanoparticles: impact on stability and toxicity, Environmental Science and Technology 46 (2012) 6900–6914.
[65] S.K. Misra, A. Dybowska, D. Berhanu, S.N. Luoma, E. Valsami-Jones, The complexity of nanoparticle dissolution and its importance in nanotoxicological studies, Science of the Total Environment 438 (2012) 225–232.
[66] S.-J. Richards, K. Isufi, L.E. Wilkins, J. Lipecki, E. Fullam, M.I. Gibson, Multivalent antimicrobial polymer nanoparticles target mycobacteria and gram-negative bacteria by distinct mechanisms, Biomacromolecules 19 (2018) 256–264.
[67] P. Suchomel, L. Kvitek, A. Panacek, R. Prucek, J. Hrbac, R. Vecerova, R. Zboril, Comparative study of antimicrobial activity of AgBr and Ag nanoparticles (NPs), PLoS One 10 (2015) e0119202.
[68] J. Helmlinger, C. Sengstock, C. Groß-Heitfeld, C. Mayer, T.A. Schildhauer, M. Köller, M. Epple, Silver nanoparticles with different size and shape: equal cytotoxicity, but different antibacterial effects, RSC Advances 6 (2016) 18490–18501.
[69] B. Sadeghi, F.S. Garmaroudi, M. Hashemi, H.R. Nezhad, A. Nasrollahi, S. Ardalan, S. Ardalan, Comparison of the anti-bacterial activity on the nanosilver shapes: nanoparticles, nanorods and nanoplates, Advanced Powder Technology 23 (2012) 22–26.
[70] C. Ferrag, S. Li, K. Jeon, N.M. Andoy, R.M.A. Sullan, S. Mikhaylichenko, K. Kerman, Polyacrylamide hydrogels doped with different shapes of silver nanoparticles: antibacterial and mechanical properties, Colloids and Surfaces B: Biointerfaces 197 (2021) 111397.
[71] P. Decuzzi, M. Ferrari, The adhesive strength of non-spherical particles mediated by specific interactions, Biomaterials 27 (2006) 5307–5314.
[72] S.E.A. Gratton, P.A. Ropp, P.D. Pohlhaus, J.C. Luft, V.J. Madden, M.E. Napier, J.M. DeSimone, The effect of particle design on cellular internalization pathways, Proceedings of the National Academy of Sciences 105 (2008) 11613–11618.
[73] R. Agarwal, V. Singh, P. Jurney, L. Shi, S.V. Sreenivasan, K. Roy, Mammalian cells preferentially internalize hydrogel nanodiscs over nanorods and use shape-specific uptake mechanisms, Proceedings of the National Academy of Sciences 110 (2013) 17247–17252.
[74] X. Liu, F. Wu, Y. Tian, M. Wu, Q. Zhou, S. Jiang, Z. Niu, Size dependent cellular uptake of rod-like bionanoparticles with different aspect ratios, Scientific Reports 6 (2016) 1–10.
[75] S. Marchesini, P. Turner, K.R. Paton, B.P. Reed, A.J. Pollard, Rapid monitoring of graphene exfoliation using NMR proton relaxation, Nanoscale 13 (2021) 14518–14524.

[76] Y. Song, M. Elsabahy, C.A. Collins, S. Khan, R. Li, T.N. Hreha, Y. Shen, Y.-N. Lin, R.A. Letteri, L. Su, Morphologic design of silver-bearing sugar-based polymer nanoparticles for uroepithelial cell binding and antimicrobial delivery, Nano Letters 21 (2021) 4990–4998.
[77] K.P. Bankura, D. Maity, M.M.R. Mollick, D. Mondal, B. Bhowmick, M.K. Bain, A. Chakraborty, J. Sarkar, K. Acharya, D. Chattopadhyay, Synthesis, characterization and antimicrobial activity of dextran stabilized silver nanoparticles in aqueous medium, Carbohydrate Polymers 89 (2012) 1159–1165.
[78] E. Pazos, E. Sleep, C.M. Rubert Pérez, S.S. Lee, F. Tantakitti, S.I. Stupp, Nucleation and growth of ordered arrays of silver nanoparticles on peptide nanofibers: hybrid nanostructures with antimicrobial properties, Journal of the American Chemical Society 138 (2016) 5507–5510.
[79] M. Hyldgaard, T. Mygind, B.S. Vad, M. Stenvang, D.E. Otzen, R.L. Meyer, The antimicrobial mechanism of action of epsilon-poly-l-lysine, Applied and Environmental Microbiology 80 (2014) 7758–7770.
[80] J. Wehling, R. Dringen, R.N. Zare, M. Maas, K. Rezwan, Bactericidal activity of partially oxidized nanodiamonds, ACS Nano 8 (2014) 6475–6483.
[81] ASTM E2865-12:2018 Standard guide for measurement of electrophoretic mobility and zeta potential of nanosized biological materials.
[82] ISO 13099-1:2012 Colloidal systems — Methods for zeta-potential determination. Part 1: Electroacoustic and electrokinetic phenomena.
[83] ISO 13099-2:2012 Colloidal systems — Methods for zeta-potential determination. Part 2: Optical methods.
[84] ISO 13099-3:2014 Colloidal systems — Methods for zeta potential determination. Part 3: Acoustic methods.
[85] M.V. Smoluchowski, Contribution to the theory of electro-osmosis and related phenomena, Bulletin International de l'Académie des Sciences de Cracovie 3 (1903) 184–199.
[86] R. Vogel, W. Anderson, J. Eldridge, B. Glossop, G. Willmott, A variable pressure method for characterizing nanoparticle surface charge using pore sensors, Analytical Chemistry 84 (2012) 3125–3131.
[87] R. Vogel, A.K. Pal, S. Jambhrunkar, P. Patel, S.S. Thakur, E. Reátegui, H.S. Parekh, P. Saá, A. Stassinopoulos, M.F. Broom, High-resolution single particle zeta potential characterisation of biological nanoparticles using tunable resistive pulse sensing, Scientific Reports (1) (2017) 1–13.
[88] J.C. Vickerman, D. Briggs, ToF-SIMS: Materials Analysis by Mass Spectrometry, IM Publications, 2013.
[89] V.R. Deline, W. Katz, C.A. Evans Jr, P. Williams, Mechanism of the SIMS matrix effect, Applied Physics Letters 33 (1978) 832–835.
[90] Y. Pei, D.J.H. Cant, R. Havelund, M. Stewart, K. Mingard, M.P. Seah, C. Minelli, A.G. Shard, Argon cluster sputtering reveals internal chemical distribution in submicron polymeric particles, Journal of Physical Chemistry C 124 (2020) 23752–23763.
[91] L. Yang, M.P. Seah, I.S. Gilmore, R.J.H. Morris, M.G. Dowsett, L. Boarino, K. Sparnacci, M. Laus, Depth profiling and melting of nanoparticles in secondary ion mass spectrometry (SIMS), Journal of Physical Chemistry C 117 (2013) 16042–16052.
[92] A. Gulin, A. Shakhov, A. Vasin, A. Astafiev, O. Antonova, S. Kochev, Y. Kabachii, A. Golub, V. Nadtochenko, ToF-SIMS depth profiling of nanoparticles: chemical structure of core-shell quantum dots, Applied Surface Science 481 (2019) 144–150.

[93] A.G.H.R. Shard, M.P. Seah, S.J. Spencer, I.S. Gilmore, N. Winograd, D. Mao, T. Miyayama, E. Niehuis, D. Rading, R. Moellers, Argon cluster ion beams for organic depth profiling: results from a VAMAS interlaboratory study, Analytical Chemistry 18 (2012) 7865–7873.
[94] D. Dollimore, P. Spooner, A. Turner, The BET method of analysis of gas adsorption data and its relevance to the calculation of surface areas, Surface Technology 4 (1976) 121–160.
[95] T. Cedervall, I. Lynch, S. Lindman, T. Berggård, E. Thulin, H. Nilsson, K.A. Dawson, S. Linse, Understanding the nanoparticle–protein corona using methods to quantify exchange rates and affinities of proteins for nanoparticles, Proceedings of the National Academy of Sciences 104 (2007) 2050–2055.
[96] I. Lynch, T. Cedervall, M. Lundqvist, C. Cabaleiro-Lago, S. Linse, K.A. Dawson, The nanoparticle–protein complex as a biological entity; a complex fluids and surface science challenge for the 21st century, Advances in Colloid and Interface Science 134 (2007) 167–174.
[97] I. Lynch, K.A. Dawson, Protein–nanoparticle interactions, Nano-Enabled Medical Applications 3 (2020) 231–250.
[98] L. Vroman, A.L. Adams, G.C. Fischer, P.C. Munoz, Interaction of high molecular weight kininogen, factor XII, and fibrinogen in plasma at interfaces, Blood 55 (1980) 156–159.
[99] F. Alexis, E. Pridgen, L.K. Molnar, O.C. Farokhzad, Factors affecting the clearance and biodistribution of polymeric nanoparticles, Molecular Pharmaceutics 5 (2008) 505–515.
[100] J.V. Jokerst, T. Lobovkina, R.N. Zare, S.S. Gambhir, Nanoparticle PEGylation for imaging and therapy, Nanomedicine 6 (2011) 715–728.
[101] S.R. Meyers, M.W. Grinstaff, Biocompatible and bioactive surface modifications for prolonged in vivo efficacy, Chemical Reviews 112 (2012) 1615–1632.
[102] B.D. Ratner, A.S. Hoffman, in: Biomaterials Science, third ed., 2013, pp. 241–247. San Diego.
[103] G. Schmid, Clusters and Colloids: From Theory to Applications, John Wiley & Sons, 2008.
[104] A.J. Coury, in: A.S. Hoffman, F.J. Schoen, J.E. Lemons (Eds.), Biomaterials Science, third ed., 2013, pp. 696–715. San Diego, CA.
[105] A. Sikora, A.G. Shard, C. Minelli, Size and ζ-potential measurement of silica nanoparticles in serum using tunable resistive pulse sensing, Langmuir 32 (2016) 2216–2224.
[106] F. Caputo, J. Clogston, L. Calzolai, M. Rösslein, A. Prina-Mello, Measuring particle size distribution of nanoparticle enabled medicinal products, the joint view of EUNCL and NCI-NCL. A step by step approach combining orthogonal measurements with increasing complexity, Journal of Controlled Release 299 (2019) 31–43.
[107] D. Tsikritsis, E.J. Legge, N.A. Belsey, Practical considerations for quantitative and reproducible measurements with stimulated Raman scattering microscopy, Analyst 147 (2022) 4642–4656.
[108] Y. Yang, B. Chu, J. Cheng, J. Tang, B. Song, H. Wang, Y. He, Bacteria eat nanoprobes for aggregation-enhanced imaging and killing diverse microorganisms, Nature Communications 13 (2022) 1–15.
[109] X. Zhao, L.R. Hilliard, S.J. Mechery, Y. Wang, R.P. Bagwe, S. Jin, W. Tan, A rapid bioassay for single bacterial cell quantitation using bioconjugated nanoparticles, Proceedings of the National Academy of Sciences 101 (2004) 15027–15032.

[110] ISO/IEC Guide 21-1:2005 Regional or national adoption of International Standards and other International Deliverables. Part 1: Adoption of International Standards.
[111] http://www.vamas.org/.
[112] D.L. Kaiser, K. Chalfin, Standards from ASTM international technical committee E 56 on nanotechnology, in: Metrology and Standardization of Nanotechnology: Protocols and Industrial Innovations, 2017, pp. 269–278.

Navigating the nanoscale: Principles of body navigation

Saed Abassi[1], Anjaneyulu Dirisala[2], Daniel Gonzalez-Carter[3], West Kristian Paraiso[4], Junjie Li[5] and Theofilus A. Tockary[2]

[1]Center for Nanomedicine at the Wilmer Eye Institute, The Johns Hopkins University School of Medicine, Baltimore, MD, United States; [2]Innovation Center of NanoMedicine, Kawasaki Institute of Industrial Promotion, Kawasaki, Japan; [3]Institute for Bioengineering of Catalonia (IBEC), Barcelona Institute for Science and Technology (BIST), Barcelona, Spain; [4]Department of Basic Sciences, Faculty of Medicine and Health Sciences, Universitat Internacional de Catalunya, Barcelona, Spain; [5]Institute for Materials Chemistry and Engineering, Kyushu University, Fukuoka, Japan

1. Introduction

Drug Delivery System (DDS) can be defined as any pharmacologically active or inactive material that is used to assist the performance of the main active ingredient, aiming to enhance its pharmacokinetics and/or pharmacodynamics. The optimal DDS should maximise the therapeutic efficacy and minimise the side effects of a drug. Utilisation of DDS in pharmaceutical development has a long history, which evolved from its use as an additive excipient in pharmaceutical formulation to a more sophisticated smart nano-system that is indispensable in the efficacy of some new drug formulations. DDS science started as pharmaceutical formulation approach to enhance the performance of already existing drug products. On a macroscopic level, for example, surface coating of tablets enabled controlled drug released in a desirable manner. In recent years, DDS have benefited from the application of nanotechnology to create supramolecular nanoassemblies with therapeutic payloads to act as nanoDDS capable of providing innovative solutions to common and rare diseases. NanoDDS have instigated a paradigm shift in therapeutic intervention, with many in clinical use, and a more significant number steadily progressing in the pipeline. NanoDDS can bring many

Nanotechnology Tools for Infection Control. https://doi.org/10.1016/B978-0-12-823994-0.00002-5

physical and pharmacological advantages over standard formulations, such as improved solubility and bioavailability, reduced toxicity and increased target-tissue selectivity. With proper tuning of physicochemical characteristics, such as composition, size, shape, charge and surface modifications, nanoDDS can also accurately navigate organ and cellular barriers, acting as versatile platforms to deliver theranostic agents to their targets.

Various classes of nanoDDS have emerged during the last few decades, such as liposomes, polymeric nanoparticles (NPs) and micelles, inorganic NPs and many others. NanoDDS can be used to deliver already existing therapeutic agents such as anticancer drugs. Recently, the use of nanoDDS has become indispensable in the delivery of newer generations of therapeutics such as nucleic acid therapies. Onpattro is the first targeted RNA interference therapeutic for rare genetic diseases transthyretin amyloidosis, which was enabled by the use of lipid NPs for specific liver parenchymal cell targeting, and subsequent control of intracellular distribution.

In general terms, in order to properly navigate the body and reach its desired site of action, nanoDDS need to overcome a series of biological barriers in a hierarchical order (Fig. 5.1): firstly, nanoDDS should protect the drug payload from metabolic

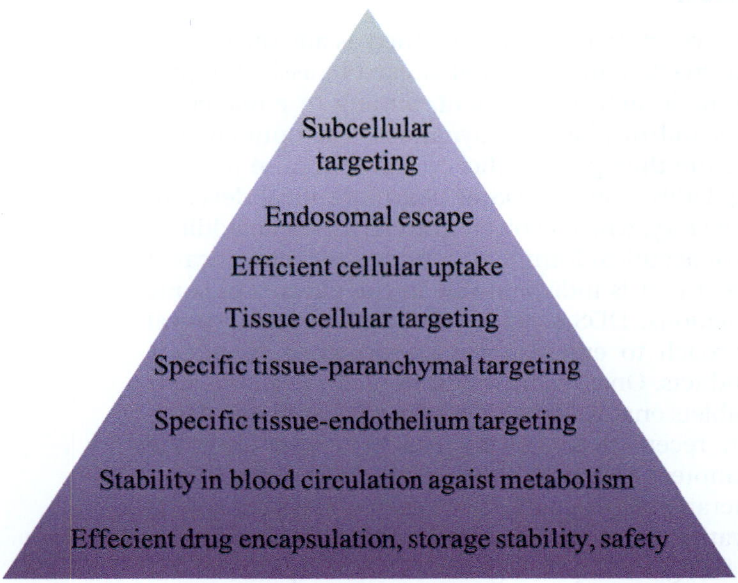

Figure 5.1 Hierarchal order of barriers a nanoDDS needs to navigate to maximise drug efficacy and minimise its toxicity.

degradation and immune recognition (clearance) in the blood circulation for a sufficient period of time. In other words, the nanoDDS should provide stealth properties to the drug payload to allow it to navigate through the body until it reaches its tissue target. Incorporation of hydrophilic polymers such as polyethylene glycol (PEG) represents the gold standard for achieving stealth protection of the nanoDDS. Other strategies involve the use of biomimetic approaches such as the masking of nanoDDS using plasma membranes derived from blood cells.

Secondly, once the nanoDDS has achieved stealth properties and prolonged blood circulation, it would need to be internalised by, and in some instances penetrate across, specific vascular endothelium barriers to reach its desired site of action. In some therapeutic indications, the pathophysiology arises from dysfunctional endothelium, and targeting the endothelium itself can result in satisfactory therapeutic outcomes. For instance, targeting of liver sinusoidal endothelial cells (LSEC) to provide cytoprotection in hepatic ischemia/reperfusion injury would be clinically beneficial. Similarly, targeting and ablating the endothelium is a promising strategy to cut the nutritional supply in disease tissues such as the adipose tissue in morbid obesity or tumour mass in cancers. However, in most instances, the drug payload would need to cross into the parenchyma of the organ to reach its site of action. In some cases, utilisation of anatomical differences between health and diseases tissues can be utilised to mediate the targeting of nanoDDS to the parenchyma. Solid tumours are characterised by leaky vasculature and impaired lymphatic drainage system, a process known as the enhanced retention and permeation (EPR) effect. The same phenomenon was also observed in inflammatory tissues. A significant body of work has been focussed on targeting nanoDDS based on the EPR effect. In another therapeutic indication, the delivery of lipid NPs into liver parenchyma has been reported to occur through passing through fenestration on LSECs, a pathway that natural lipoproteins such as chylomicrons follow for their metabolism in the liver. However, difference in anatomical features does not account for many diseases and thus fails to provide a mechanism of drug targeting in many tissues. In contrast, in tissues such as the brain, the anatomy of the vasculature is strictly orchestrated to prevent entry of foreign substances. Delivering drugs into brain parenchyma is a substantial challenge due to the presence of blood–brain barrier (BBB). Crossing the BBB by exploiting its own transcytosis mechanisms [e.g. employing the transferrin receptor (TfR)-1 transporter] is one of the most studied strategies to achieve significant drug accumulation in the brain.

Thirdly, after crossing the endothelium and arriving at the parenchyma, the nanoDDS has one of two main modes of drug delivery: either to release the drug in the vicinity of disease or target cells or to deliver the drug inside the target cell following internalisation. A combination of both pathways is also expected to take place in most of cases, as it is difficult to exclusively target one pathway and exclude the other. Environment-responsive strategies have been utilised to enable time and spatial-triggered drug release. The stimuli can be external such as in the case of ultrasound or near infrared light, or internal such as body temperature, pH levels and ion concentrations. Within the classes of internal stimuli, extracellular stimulus entails drug release outside the cell, followed by drug entry in the free form. Intracellular stimuli include release in the endosomal/lysosomal acidic compartment, or cytosolic drug release in response to reducing agents such as glutathione.

Finally, depending on the pharmacological mechanism of drug action, subcellular targeting is also needed. In some cases, biphasic pharmacodynamics are observed using some drugs due to their action on different subcellular targets in the same cell. In this case, delivering the drug to its specific target is beneficial. In other cases, such as in the case of plasmid DNA (DNA), the drug/payload needs to enter the nucleus in order to initiate the process of protein expression. A nanoDDS that increases the efficiency of nuclear targeting is usually beneficial for pDNA delivery. Additionally, organelle targeting provides an interesting tool to control organelle-specific diseases, such as mitochondrial diseases.

2. Modulating nanoparticle pharmacodynamics: Avoiding liver and RES clearance

Prolonging the systemic retention of nanomedicines increases their accumulation at desired sites by promoting their interaction with blood-vessel targets.

Hence, the targeting efficiency of nanomedicines is highly correlated with their blood circulation profile. However, most nanomedicines are rapidly eliminated from the circulation by the reticulothendothelial system (RES) organs/cells, notably the liver, which is capable of clearing 30%–99% of the injected dose (ID) of NPs [1–4]. Therefore, strategies to reduce liver uptake to redirect nanomedicines to the intended organ will be key for successful clinical translation. In this section, we will first discuss our current understanding of how the microenvironment of the liver facilitates elimination of nanome from the bloodstream. Secondly, we will discuss various strategies to modulate the liver microenvironment to improve the delivery of nanomedicines to the target sites.

2.1 The liver architecture and location of scavenger RE cells within the liver affect their interaction with nanomedicines

The liver the largest RES organ in the body, is a highly connected complex network of closely interrelated cells, consisting of parenchymal hepatocytes (60%–70% of total cell number or ~90% of the total liver mass) [5] and non-parenchymal cells (NPC) including liver sinusoidal endothelial cells (LSECs), Kupffer cells (KCs), fat-storing stellate cells (Ito cells), pit cells (natural killer cells), and cholangiocytes.

LSEC constitute ~50% of the total NPC number and volume and are characterised by the presence of fenestrae and lack of a basement membrane underneath the endothelium. In addition, LSECs are particularly aggressive pinocytic cells, thereby removing ('scavenging') soluble macromolecules, colloidal waste, cellular debris, and pathogens from the blood. These structural and phenotypic features make the liver microvasculature the most permeable of all endothelium in the body.

The KCs are liver-resident macrophages that are anatomically juxtaposed on top of the LSECs. The strategic position of KCs at the luminal side within the sinusoids permits them to perform as sentinel cells to monitor the blood percolating through the sinusoids to recognise, capture and metabolise foreign bodies including NPs [6]. Together, the KCs and LSECs serve as the main 'scavenger sinusoidal wall' to remove NPs from the blood. In addition to the inherent physiological scavenging functions, the reduced blood flow rate within the liver sinusoids (1000 times slower than systemic circulation in blood vessels) promotes uptake of NPs [7].

To avoid unwanted clearance by the liver scavenger sinusoidal wall, various nanomedicines engineering designs and strategies have been explored, particularly modulating their physicochemical properties [8–10]. For instance, stealth shielding by nonionic hydrophilic polymers, e.g. PEG [11–13] and other polymers such as poly(2-oxazoline)s [14,15], polysarcosines [16], polyglycerols, polysaccharides, and zwitterionic polymers such as polybetaines [17]. This stealth shielding prevents the adsorption of opsonic proteins, thereby avoiding the nonspecific sequestration by liver scavenger RE cells. The prolonged systemic retention due to stealth shielding can increase nanomedicines accumulation at the disease site 10 to 100-fold compared to free drugs [18–21]. However, this stealth shielding strategy often has several limitations. First, stealth coating deteriorates the targeted delivery either by decreasing the internalisation efficiency ('stealth dilemma') [22,23], or efficiency of targeting by hiding the ligand within the own bulky shell polymer strands. Second, polymers used for stealth coating may cause immune responses, leading to accelerated blood clearance on repeated injections based due to immune recognition of NP polymer coating [24,25]. Third, stealth coating may be incompatible with NPs whose functionality relies on their surface characteristics, such as surface catalysis [26,27]. Fourth, depending on nanomedicines formulation and their cargo contents, it is often difficult to obtain sufficient stealth coating without compromising functionalities. Besides stealth coating, biomimetic approaches such as wrapping the nanomedicines within natural cell membranes (cellular camouflage) [28,29] and noncovalent attachment of nanomedicines as 'backpacks' on circulating blood cells (cellular hitchhiking) [30,31] or dysopsonins such as albumin have been explored [32,33]. Moreover, nanomedicines clearance can also be evaded by conjugating 'self-markers' such as CD47, which help to avoid nanomedicines phagocytosis by macrophages [34,35].

Though effective, strategies involving nanomedicines design and surface engineering cannot completely avoid unwanted liver uptake depending on the type of nanomedicines formulation and its cargo contents. Moreover, it is still ambiguous whether efficient biomimicry can be implemented for arbitrary nanomedicines without adversely altering their prime functionalities [36]. Therefore, a combination of other strategies that do not impose restrictions on the nanomedicines surface will greatly improve the delivery efficiency. As such, the biological environment of RE organs/cells can also be regulated to inhibit nanomedicines elimination. In particular, pretreatment strategies to manipulate the liver environment to reduce the recognition and thereby phagocytic capture of nanomedicines is a promising option [37,38]. Such priming strategies could modulate the structure or function of liver RE cells in ways that favour the reduced sequestration of nanomedicines through the 'don't see and scavenge me' mechanisms. A variety of mechanisms of liver RE cell blockade have been proposed including (i) depletion of opsonic proteins prior to the administration of nanomedicines, (ii) dysopsonin corona formation around the surface of nanomedicines before in vivo application, (iii) transient depletion (and/or deactivation/inhibition) of RE cells, (iv) pharmacological inhibition of endocytosis, (v) physical saturation of phagocytic cell activity by scavenger receptor ligands, decoy particles, or antibody-sensitised blood cells prior to nanomedicines treatment and (vi) transient and selective stealth coating of the scavenger sinusoidal wall.

2.2 Preconditioning adjuvant strategies of the liver microenvironment to reduce nanomedicines clearance mechanisms

2.2.1 Depletion of opsonic proteins

Immediately after intravenous injection, nanomedicines come into direct contact with protein-enriched blood, where proteins form a coating layer ('protein corona') around the nanomedicines surface. This protein corona affects the NP's original size, charge and aggregation, conferring a new 'biological identity' which may promote the recognition and uptake by RE cells [39]. The protein corona consists of either opsonins or dysopsonins, which promote or inhibit phagocytosis, respectively [39–41]. Therefore, depletion of opsonins using decoy materials before NPs administration could be used to prolong the blood circulation. For instance, preinjection of gelatinised triolein lipid emulsion temporarily depleted available opsonins and blocked RE uptake, resulting in a reduced elimination rate of the second dose of colloid [42–44]. Empty viral capsids have also been used as decoys to deplete the preexisting neutralising antibodies, leading to increased gene transduction efficiency after systemic delivery [45]. Moreover, transient degradation of preexisting circulating antibodies using IgG-degrading enzymes before adeno-associated virus (AAV) introduction has also been developed to improve AAV transduction efficiency [46–48].

2.2.2 Dysopsonin corona formation

Dysopsonins have the opposite effect to above-described opsonins [49]. Examples of dysopsonins are albumin, lipoproteins, apolipoproteins (Apos) B100, E, A4 and C3. Coating of dysopsonins around NPs either before (precoating) or after (post-coating) injection into the body helps evade phagocyte capture [50]. For example, precoating of albumin corona around various NPs [51–53] provided protective effects against the adsorption of other plasma proteins and suppressed the complement activation, thus resulting in a substantial reduction in the liver disposition and prolonged systemic retention. In addition to precoating, real-time in-situ cloaking of NPs in blood vessels with the body own dysopsonins has been exploited to induce a stealth effect. For example, in-situ ApoE and clusterin adsorption onto PEG–PLGA NPs at low PEG density-induced stealth effect, prevented the uptake by RE cells, and thus resulted in prolonged circulation, irrespective of size [54]. Insertion of the albumin-binding domain into adenoviral capsid hexon binds the albumin of the bloodstream, shielding the virus against not only macrophage recognition but also preexisting neutralising antibodies [55]. Even relatively exotic strategies, such as molecular imprinting, have been exploited to achieve a stealth effect. In-situ cloaking of molecularly imprinted nanogels through the formation of albumin corona immediately after injection provided efficient stealth properties [56]. In the ever-evolving landscape of nanotechnology, molecular imprinting has emerged as a groundbreaking strategy to design NPs with exquisite precision for drug delivery applications [57–63]. Molecularly imprinting represent a sophisticated approach where the selective recognition of target molecules is achieved through the creation of tailor-made binding sites within the material matrix. This process mimics the specificity and affinity found in biological systems, allowing for a level of precision targeting that was previously elusive. At the heart of molecular imprinting lies a synthetic process that involves the co-polymerisation of functional monomers and cross-linkers in the presence of a template molecule – the target of interest. As the polymerisation progresses, the template is removed, leaving behind cavities that mirror the size, shape, and chemical functionality of the original drug. These molecularly imprinted sites serve as lock-and-key binding sites within the NPs, ensuring a highly selective and specific interaction with the target molecule. The unique properties of molecularly imprinted NPs also extend beyond targeting, encompassing controlled release kinetics. The well-defined binding sites within MIP NPs allow for the precise regulation of drug release, offering a sustained and controlled delivery profile. Moreover, the size and surface properties of MIP NPs can be fine-tuned to optimise their interaction with biological interfaces, facilitating efficient transport across cellular membranes and enhancing overall bioavailability [64–70].

2.2.3 Transient depletion of RE cells

Transient systemic reduction of liver RE cells has been examined by employing inactivating agents such as clodronate [71], propamidine [72], gadolinium chloride ($GdCl_3$) [73], λ-carrageenan [74,75], dextran sulphate (500-kDa) [76] and methyl palmitate [77,78]. The most commonly used method is the liposome-mediated delivery of clodronate. The clodronate liposomes are readily phagocytosed by the macrophages and the liposomal phospholipid bilayer is digested by phospholipases of lysophagosomes. The released clodronate is then metabolised to an analog of ATP which competitively inhibits ADP/ATP translocase and thus suppresses mitochondrial oxygen consumption, ultimately inducing macrophage apoptosis [79,80]. Clodronate transiently depletes the number of KCs in the liver, with the cells reappearing within 10 days post-administration [79,81]. Depleting KCs by clodronate liposomes substantially increased the tumour delivery efficiency of various NPs and nanomedicines [71,82,83] and significantly enhanced transgene expression of adenoviral gene vector in liver hepatocytes [84,85]. However, complete depletion of KCs by frequent and large intravenous dosing has been shown to be toxic [86]. $GdCl_3$ not only suppresses the phagocytic activity as a result of calcium transport inhibition across the cell membrane by the Gd(III) ion but also eliminates the KCs [87]. $GdCl_3$ pretreatment prevented quantum dot capture by KCs, which further translated to improved blood circulation and tumour accumulation [30]. However, $GdCl_3$-induced KC elimination increased cytokine release including TNF-α and interleukin-1 [88]. Complete or partial depletion of macrophages may disturb the integrity of the innate immune system and could possibly result in increased susceptibility to pathogenic infections, thus clinically may not be a viable strategy [89].

2.2.4 Pharmacological inhibition of endocytosis

Pharmacological/chemical inhibitors to block endocytic pathways may be employed to suppress the uptake of nanomedicines by phagocytes. For example, chloroquine, an FDA-approved antimalarial drug, specifically inhibits the expression of phosphatidylinositol-binding clathrin assembly lymphoid-myeloid leukemia (PICALM) protein, which binds to clathrin, phosphoinositol and adaptor protein complex 2 to assist the formation of endocytic pits. Therefore, depleting PICLAM inhibits clathrin-mediated internalisation, which is one of major endocytic pathways of nanomedicines elimination. A clinically relevant dose of chloroquine pretreatment in mice led to 28.5% and 22% reduction in the liver accumulation of intravenously injected liposome (soft) and discoidal silicon (hard) NPs, respectively, which consequently resulted in 2-fold and 1.5-fold increase accumulation to the tumour and lung, respectively [90]. Chloroquine-induced macrophage-preconditioning strategy is simple, widely applicable and, due to its long history of clinical use, could be easily implementable in clinical settings to augment site-specific delivery of nanomedicines [91]. However, the systemic distribution of chloroquine might also impede the RES-mediated clearance of pathogens and cellular debris. Furthermore, chloroquine pretreatment potentially suppresses the uptake and slow-release drug reservoir behaviour of nanotheranostics by tumour-associated macrophages, thus decreasing the intratumoural accumulation in certain types of tumours [92–94]. Furthermore, preferential uptake of exosomes by clathrin heavy chain 1 (Cltc)-mediated endocytosis in the liver and spleen compromised the delivery efficiency to the targeted organs. Prior knock-down of the Cltc specifically in the liver and spleen macrophages using exosomes encapsulated siRNA against Cltc substantially boost the delivery efficiency of therapeutic exosomes targeted to the heart [95]. However, simultaneous inhibition of other endocytic pathways could further improve the delivery efficacy as some of the exosomes are still taken up by macrophages even after suppressing Ctlc protein.

2.2.5 Preinduced physical saturation of phagocytic cell activity

Saturating the capacity of RE cells to engulf and eliminate foreign particulates from the bloodstream may be exploited to enhance nanomedicines delivery to target sites. To this purpose, various strategies have been adopted to saturate the availability of NPs recognition sites on RE cells, including (a) predosing large doses of scavenger receptor (SR) ligands, (b) overloading liver RES with decoy nano- and micron-sized particles (RES blockade) and (c) overloading liver RES by body's own intact blood cells (RES cytoblockade).

2.2.5.1 Scavenger receptor (SR) ligands

RE cells can also largely rely on opsonin-independent recognition of wide variety of NPs via SRs [96]. Therefore, saturating the SRs with their ligands could lessen the nonspecific recognition sites of nanomedicines on RE cells. One such approach is preadministration of SR ligands such as fucoidan [97], polyinosinic acid (poly-I) [98], λ-carrageenan [74,75], and dextran sulphate (DS) [99]. Preemptive administration of poly-I reduced the sequestration of adenoviral gene vectors by KCs, augmenting the transgene expression in the liver, spleen and heart by 5- to 15-fold [98]. Fucoidan preadministration prolonged the circulatory half-life of ferucarbotran SPIONs and concomitantly increased tumour accumulation [97]. However, scavenger receptor saturation by ligands has limited clinical use due to (i) induction of systemic inflammation [100,101], and anticoagulation properties [102], (ii) scavenger receptors are recycling receptors which constantly requires the large amount of ligand to suppress their function [103], and (iii) scavenger receptor saturation inhibit only opsonin-independent endocytosis despite the fact that the phagocytes has diverse clearance pathways including opsonin-dependent clearance.

2.2.5.2 RES blockade

The scavenging and clearance function of RE cells may be overloaded/saturated by injecting large doses of decoy blocker particles (empty particles containing no drug cargo), thereby decreasing the uptake of subsequently injected NPs by the RE cells. The decoy particles can be either NPs such as polymer-albumin NPs [104,105], liposomes [106–111], and small unilamellar vesicles [109] or micron-sized particles such as fat emulsions [112], colloidal carbon [113], and latex beads [107]. Predosing of liposomes into tumour-bearing mice successfully decreased the liver and spleen uptake and thereby increase the tumour accumulation of subsequently gold nanorods [110] and SPIONs and TAXOL [111]. Alternatively, suppressing the liver RES function by pretreatment with liposomes led to enhanced accumulation of second dosed test liposome to the spleen in healthy mice ('spillover to spleen') [114–116]. Prior administration of small-size (150 nm) nanoprimer (a liposome composed 50:50 M ratio of 1,2-dipalmitoyl-*sn*-glycero-3-phosphoethanolamine-*N*-(succinyl) and cholesterol) physically saturates liver cells to lower liver accumulation, and thereby increase anti-tumour efficacy of sequentially injected anti-cancer NPs [117]. In addition to retargeting from the liver to other organs, cell-specific retargeting within the liver can also be modulated by liver RE cell saturation. For example, a saturation of liver RE cells by predosing phosphatidylcholine liposome or intralipid reduced the elimination of adenoviral gene vectors by scavenger wall, concurrently enhancing hepatocyte transduction [118]. Moreover, prior administration of liposomal nanoprimers larger in size compared to the fenestrae of the liver sinusoids dramatically decreased the endocytic activity of KCs and LSECs without interacting with hepatocytes, thereby increasing the bioavailability of the lipid NPs of mRNA or siRNA to the hepatocytes [117]. The efficacy of decoy particle-based blockading strategies could be determined by the administered dose (particle number [119] or mass [110,117,120], size [120], ζ-potential [110], surface coating [120] and material composition [114]). For instance, cholesterol-free liposomes were more effective in suppressing the liver RES function than the cholesterol-rich liposomes [114]. Also, the time interval between the first dose of blocker particle and the second dose of the theragnostic particle [110] could modulate the RES blockade efficiency. Furthermore, the RES blockade efficiency could be influenced by the type of disease model (tumour-bearing, liposaccharide-inflamed, and healthy) and genetical strain (Balb/c, C57B1/6, and CD-1) of animals [120].

Considering the total number of clearance sites and SRs of the sinusoidal wall, the uptake by the liver should be decreased once the number of NP exceeds the number of effective receptors and clearance sites available on the sinusoidal wall. Towards this understanding, a recent study revealed that an NP dose above one trillion particles in mice (equals to a threshold of 1.5 quadrillion particles in humans) surpasses the number of effective receptors and clearance sites, therefore, overwhelm the kinetic limit of RE cell uptake rate. An NP dose above this threshold nonlinearly suppressed liver elimination, resulted in prolonged systemic retention, and increased NP tumour delivery of Caelyx/Doxil (increased the delivery efficiency up to 12% ID/g tumour and delivery to 93% of tumour cells) [119].

Overwhelming the RES by decoy particles is a simple and general strategy with broad applicability and versatility. However, this strategy has several limitations which might inhibit its adaptation to clinical practice. First, full saturation of RE cell function requires an extremely large dose [112], which ultimately raises dose-related toxicity considerations. Second, the efficiency of RES blockade is dependent on mouse strain and type of tumour or inflammation [120], thus various physicochemical characteristics must be thoroughly investigated in order to maximise the delivery efficiency. Third, prolonged retention of decoy blocker particles for months after administration because of their slow and limited excretion out of the body not only induce chronic toxicity risks but also interfere with therapeutic responses [121,122].

2.2.5.3 RES cytoblockade

The principle of RES cytoblockade exploits the natural function of RE cells to remove senescent or damaged blood cells [36], therefore employs the organism's own blood cells to achieve blockage, as opposed to the exogenous blockading agents employed by RE blockade strategies. Pre-administering allogeneic anti-red blood cell (RBC) antibodies into the circulation selectively marks RBCs for sequestration by the RE cells. As a result, RE cells are overwhelmed by endocytic uptake capacity, reducing the elimination of subsequently injected nanomedicines. RES cytoblockade significantly reduced the liver accumulation of different types of nano- and micro-particles of varying size, surface coverings and ligands, consequently increasing circulation half-life and accumulation efficiency to the target organs. Most importantly, RES cytoblockade substantially inhibited tumour growth using magnetically guided doxorubicin-magnetite-encapsulated liposome and clinically approved Caelyx in mice bearing melanoma tumour. RES cytoblockade has several advantages. First, it uses a substantially lower dose (two to three orders of magnitude) of anti-RBC antibody compared to lipid emulsion RES blockade [112], potentially avoiding dose-related toxicities. Second, the anti-RBC antibodies have been widely used clinically for decades [123]. However, the application of anti-RBC antibodies is related to the increased risk of intravascular haemolysis. Furthermore, RBC sensitisation by anti-RBC antibodies may induce alloimmunisation [124] and tolerance induction [125]. Hence, the potential risks and side effects of RES erythroblockade should be carefully investigated.

2.2.6 Transient and selective stealth coating of the scavenger sinusoidal wall

The principle of stealth coating of the liver's scavenger sinusoidal wall is based on charge interactions between positively charged peptide segment of PEG-*block*-oligopeptide and negatively charged glycosaminoglycans (GAGs) and anionic binding pockets of SRs, which are abundantly expressed on sinusoidal extracellular matrix. Cells of the scavenger sinusoidal wall use diverse clearance pathways to eliminate the nanomedicines from the bloodstream by recognition through several nonspecific receptors [3,4]. In such cases, receptor saturation strategies may not be ideal because they suppress only specific pathways of clearance, despite the fact that the liver uses numerous clearance pathways. To circumvent this issue, stealth coating of the scavenger sinusoidal wall was developed by using PEGylated oligopeptides to inhibit all the clearance pathways of the scavenger wall by the steric repulsion of PEG. However, the most important clinical considerations are (i) the coating should be selective to liver scavenger wall because coating to other vessel walls of the body would not only result in adverse toxicity but also decrease the delivery amount to the parenchyma of the target tissue, and (ii) the coating is recommended be transient because long-term coating might impair the normal scavenger functions of the liver sinusoids such as removal of damaged cells and pathogens. Taking these clinical considerations into account, the oligo(L-lysine) attaching two-armed PEG

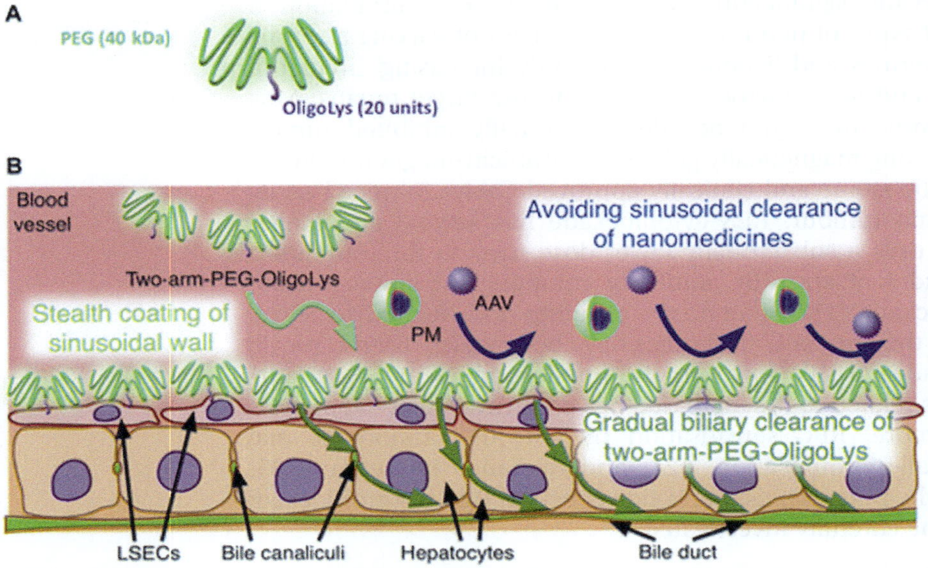

Figure 5.2 In situ stealth coating of liver scavenger sinusoidal wall using two-arm-PEG—OligoLys. (A) OligoLys was conjugated to a Y-shaped PEG (each arm is 40-kDa, thus total M_w is 80-kDa) at its carboxyl end (two-arm-PEG—OligoLys). (B) Schematic illustration of in situ stealth coating of liver scavenger wall. Two-arm-PEG—OligoLys selectively coat the liver scavenger wall to prevent the sequestration of nanomedicines, such as polyplex micelle (PM) and AAV, to the wall via stealth property of PEG. Two-arm-PEG—OligoLys is gradually cleared to the bile to avoid prolonged disturbance of normal physiological functions of the liver sinusoids. Reproduced with permission from Dirisala et al. [37].

(two-arm-PEG—OligoLys) was developed for anchoring PEG to the liver scavenger wall (Fig. 5.2). The PEGylation of OligoLys prevents the nonspecific binding of OligoLys to the extra-hepatic endothelium, presumably via the steric hindrance of PEG, while with preserved anchoring capacity to liver scavenger wall due to high binding affinity of oligocations to the anionic GAGs and SRs, which can intrinsically recognise cations. Furthermore, two-arm-PEG—OligoLys was removed from the sinusoidal wall and excreted to the bile within 6 hours, posing no toxicity issues, while one-arm-PEG—OligoLys persisted at the sinusoidal wall. The coating successfully prevented the sinusoidal recognition and capture of both viral and nonviral gene delivery agents, representatives of nature-derived and artificially engineered nanomedicines, highlighting its broad applicability. As a result of suppressed sinusoidal capture, the viral and nonviral nanomedicines are eventually redirected from the liver to their intrinsic target organs, thus substantially improving their gene transfer efficiency. Unlike decoy nano and microparticles, PEG coating does not need any prior formation of particles. The PEG coating with two-arm-PEG–OligoLys could be clinically safe as this agent was excreted to the bile within hours and elicited negligible haemolysis and acute toxicity markers [126,127]. Besides clinical safety, two-arm-PEG–Oligocation is easy to scale up through good manufacturing practices, and production is potentially cost-effective. Encouragingly, two-armed PEG-*block*-oligo(L-Ornithine) has already entered into human clinical trials for delivering siRNA.

3. Brain targeting: Crossing the blood–brain barrier

3.1 The blood–brain barrier

Successfully treating brain infections and other diseases and disorders (e.g. Alzheimer's or tumours) is severely hindered by the presence of the blood–brain barrier (BBB), a protective cellular barrier composed primarily by the specialised endothelial cells lining the brain microvasculature. The close interaction of brain endothelial cells (BECs) with astrocytes, pericytes and neurons results in BEC possessing a highly impermeable phenotype. Transport of molecules in between BEC (i.e. paracellular transport) is highly restricted by the presence of protein complexes termed tight-junctions which 'seal off' cell-to-cell contact points. These cellular connections are composed of inter-cellular proteins, such as occludin and the claudin family, which bring adjacent cellular membranes closely against each other; and intracellular proteins, such as zona occludens-1, which tether occludin and claudins to the actin cytoskeleton, thereby providing stability.

In addition, the transport of molecules through the BEC (i.e. transcellular transport) is also highly restricted. Unlike peripheral endothelial cells, the formation of endocytic vesicles within BEC is highly restricted by their particular lipid composition [128]. This lack of pinocytic activity leads to a low level of endocytic vesicles transporting cargo through the BEC, thereby preventing entry into the brain parenchyma.

3.2 Current strategies to achieve nanoparticle brain targeting

The high impermeability of brain endothelial cells, both to paracellular and transcellular transport, leads to extremely low accumulation levels of therapeutics in the brain. Hence, penetrating the BBB is one of the most challenging and pressing medical issues today. While the BBB is highly impermeable, the brain does possess endogenous protein transport systems to shuttle molecules which are crucial for the brain's homoeostasis, such as glucose and the iron-carrying protein transferrin. Therefore, exploiting such systems would allow for efficient delivery of therapies into the brain. Nanotechnology holds great potential to achieve such efficient therapeutic brain delivery by creating specialised nano-vehicles capable of protecting therapeutic cargo and directing it across the BBB. To achieve this, a wide range of NPs have been functionalised with ligands for transporter proteins (i.e. channel transporters such as the glucose transporter (Glut)-1, and endocytic receptor transporters such as Transferrin Receptor (TfR)-1) which have relatively high expression levels at the BBB, with the aim of exploiting the intrinsic transport mechanism of the protein targets to induce the NPs to 'piggy-back' on the ligand's BBB transcytosis [129–132].

3.2.1 Nanoparticle functionalisation targeting channel-transporter proteins

A widely targeted channel transporter for BBB nanoparticle penetration has been Glut-1, which is highly expressed on brain endothelial cells [133–135]. Glut-1 transports glucose into the cell by undergoing a conformational shift following glucose binding which results in free glucose moving through a 0.8–2.5 nm wide channel spanning the cell membrane [136–138]. Following intracellular glucose release, Glut-1 reverts to its original conformation, thereby allowing continued transport of glucose by the membrane embedded transporter without endocytosis [139–141].

Several classes of NPs have been functionalised with glucose and glucose analogues to target Glut-1as a brain delivery mechanism. Glucose-modified liposomes (diameter c.100 nm) penetrate the BBB to a higher extent than control liposomes both in vitro and in vivo [142,143]. Similarly, gold NPs with a core size of 4 nm have been shown to be able to cross an in vitro BBB model and enter astrocytes [144].

Recently, Anraku et al. have shown glucose-decorated polymeric nano-micelles (30 nm diameter) specifically enter the brain under conditions designed to increase luminal Glut-1 localisation [145].

Similarly to Glut-1, the L-Type amino acid transporter protein (LAT-1) is highly overexpressed at the BBB [146]. LAT-1 is structured in a cylindrical trans-membrane helix conformation with a ligand binding cavity of 1 nm diameter which transports large, neutral amino acids and neurotransmitters (e.g. L-DOPA) into the brain as a sodium-independent antiporter [147–149]. Hence, upon ligand binding, LAT-1 undergoes a conformational change to transport amino acids in and out of the cell, allowing ligand transportation to occur continuously in membrane integrated LAT-1 [150–153].

LAT-1 targeting has been examined for several nanoparticle configurations. For instance, amino acid-functionalisation of solid lipid NPs and liposomes (diameter c. 160 and 80 nm, respectively) enhanced their brain uptake in rodents [154,155]. Similarly, regarding 'hard' nanomaterials, gold NPs with a core size of c. 90 nm functionalised with the LAT-1 targeting ligand L-DOPA have a higher rate of in vitro BBB transportation compared to AuNP functionalised with a non-targeting ligand [156].

A third type of transporter exploited for BBB targeting is the choline transporter (ChT). Choline is a precursor for the neurotransmitter acetyl choline, therefore is efficiently transported into the brain. The exact identity of the BBB ChT remains unclarified, with two proteins suggested as the most likely candidates: sodium-independent choline transporter like protein type 1 (CTL1/SLC44A1) and the sodium-dependent choline transporter type 1 (CHT1/SLC5A7) [157]. Both proteins belong to the solute carrier (SLC) transporter superfamily, therefore, consisting of 12 transmembrane helices conforming a central ligand binding cavity similarly to the Glut-1 and LAT-1 transporters [152,158]. Hence, choline transportation occurs through the membrane-embedded protein along a cavity of a few nanometres in diameter.

ChT targeting has been applied to various nanoparticle systems. Li et al. have shown that poly-L-lysine dendrigrafts (c. 90 nm diameter) functionalised with choline analogues have an increase in brain penetration which, when coupled to EGFP encoding DNA, translates into higher GFP brain expression. Furthermore, the increase in dendrigraft penetration provides beneficial therapeutic effect against brain tumours when the dendrigrafts are coupled to apoptosis-promoting DNA and chemotherapeutics [159,160].

Using a related targeting strategy, Wu et al. recently demonstrated polymeric nanocapsules (30 nm diameter) containing a single protein cargo are efficiently transported across the BBB both in vitro and in vivo when decorated with a choline analogue [161].

In addition to the choline transporter, interaction with the nicotinic acetyl choline receptor (nAChR) has been employed as a brain-targeting strategy. Unlike the SLC transporters, nAChR is an ionotropic receptor, therefore binding of its ligand induces opening of the central channel to allow an ion influx. The transporter is formed by a cylindrical channel with an estimated diameter of 0.8–2 nm [162,163].

Targeting nAChR has mainly been achieved through functionalisation of NPs with RVG29, a 29 amino acid peptide derived from the rabies virus which specifically binds to nAChR to induce uptake independently from the nAChR ionotropic properties [164,165]. RVG29 functionalisation of polyamidoamine dendrimers complexed with DNA results in higher nanoparticle endocytosis by brain endothelial cells, translating into enhanced brain penetration. Furthermore, the NPs are able to functionally deliver a reporter gene to the brain parenchyma [166]. Similarly, RVG29 decorated polymeric poly(ethylene glycol)-*block*-poly(lactide-*co*-glycolide) (PEG-*b*-PLGA) NPs (c.170 nm radius) are able to efficiently transport the non-brain permeable iron chelator deferoxamine into the brain of a Parkinson's disease (PD) mouse model, successfully improving PD-related motor dysfunction [167].

3.2.2 Nanoparticle functionalisation targeting endocytic receptors

A second class of transporters targeted for brain-specific nanoparticle delivery are receptors capable of endocytic intracellular transport following ligand conjugation. In general terms, internalisation of ligands targeting such receptors relies on clusters of transmembrane receptors localised in clathrin-coated pits recruiting accessory and scaffold proteins (e.g. AP-2, FCHO1, dynamin, CLASPs) to build the endocytic machinery necessary for driving cell membrane bending, actin cytoskeleton rearrangement and vesicle fission [168].

The most widely targeted endocytic receptor is the receptor for the iron-carrying protein transferrin (TfR). NPs have been functionalised with TfR ligands (both transferrin analogues and anti-TfR antibodies) to induce brain-targeted transcytosis. Experiments indicate brain penetration is dependent on ligand functionalisation number and receptor affinity, reflecting an optimal balance between the extent of cellular internalisation (endocytosis rate) and ability to dissociate from the internalised target (exocytosis rate).

Similarly to TfR, the leptin receptor ObR has been targeted for nanoparticle brain entry. Leptin is synthesised in the periphery following caloric intake to terminate feeding. Therefore, it is required to be transported efficiently into the brain to relay its satiety signals. Leptin is thought to cross the BBB mediated by BBB-expressed ObR through receptor-mediated endocytosis [169], though the exact role of ObR in BBB transcytosis is debated [170]. PLGA NPs (c. 200 nm diameter) functionalised with leptin-derived peptides spanning the amino acid sequence responsible for BBB transcytosis show enhanced brain penetration over non-functionalised NPs [171].

The low-density lipoprotein (LDL) receptor-related protein 1 (LRP-1) transporter has also been targeted as a brain-delivery strategy. LRP-1 conforms a single transmembrane spanning protein capable of transporting lipoproteins and other ligands across the BBB through receptor-mediated transcytosis. A wide range of NPs, such as amphiphilic polymersomes [172,173], liposomes [174] and gold NPs [175] functionalised with peptides targeting LRP-1 have been shown to have increased brain penetration both in vitro and in vivo, demonstrating the capacity of targeting this transporter to promote brain delivery.

3.3 Nanoparticle avidity as a modulator of transcytosis

Although functionalising NP with ligands targeting BBB transporter proteins might induce NP internalisation into BEC, several studies have shown that actual escape into the brain parenchyma (i.e. full transcytosis) is a much more nuanced processed, highly depending on the multivalency of nanoparticle decoration. For instance, the transport of polymeric nanomicelles across the BBB by exploiting Glut-1 binding has been shown to have an optimal degree of glucose decoration on the nanoparticle surface [145]. A similar effect of ligand number has been seen in gold NPs targeting TfR1 [176], as well as polymeric NP decorated with anti-ICAM antibodies [177]. These studies demonstrate that at low ligand density, NPs fail to significantly engage their cell surface targets, resulting in low BEC endocytosis and hence low brain entry. However, at high ligand density, the NP–receptor interaction becomes too high for efficient NP release from the endocytic vesicle, again resulting in low brain entry due to intracellular entrapment. Only at an intermediate ligand decoration is efficient brain entry seen, indicating NP avidity must be carefully modulated for successful brain parenchymal delivery. Interestingly, NP formulation may be engineered to modulate NP avidity intracellularly and hence be able to separate high-avidity NP from their receptors within the endosome, thereby promote brain entry. Such approach has been examined by Clark et al., who demonstrated that addition of an acid-cleavable bond between gold NPs and their anti-TfR1 ligands promotes release of the NP from TfR1 during endosome acidification, thereby promoting parenchymal brain entry in mice [178].

In addition to simply modulating the extent of endocytic release, NP avidity has been shown to be able to modulate the actual intracellular trafficking mechanisms employed by brain endothelial cells. For instance, the avidity of polymeric NPs towards LRP-1 (by modulating the number of decorating angiopep-2 ligands) is able to control whether NP are endocytosed and trafficked in discrete vesicular packages leading to intracellular trapping and lysosomal degradation (at high avidity) or whether the NPs are incorporated into continuous endocytic tubular structures which transport the NPs efficiently across the cell for transcytotic release into the brain parenchyma (moderate avidity) [179]. The effect of avidity was demonstrated to rely on whether the NP-induced endosome interaction with membrane curvature stabilising proteins (e.g. syndapin-2), which promoted the consolidation of transcellular tubules for efficient transcytosis.

This effect has also been seen with antibodies targeting TfR1 [180], where monovalent (and hence low affinity) antibodies were able to be trafficked in tubular structures across BEC, while bivalent (high affinity) antibodies had impaired tubular trafficking and were ultimately trafficked for degradation. Interestingly, transcytosis of bivalent antibodies could be improved by forcing endocytic tubulation, hinting at possible intervention mechanisms to improve brain delivery of NP.

3.4 Generating brain-specific targets

While the current brain targeting strategies binding transporter proteins overexpressed at the BBB have demonstrated their ability to increase NP delivery into the brain, they also suffer from specificity limitations, as the target proteins are also significantly expressed in the peripheral vasculature. A possible strategy to overcome this limitation is to exploit the BBB phenotype to generate brain-specific targets. As such, the lower endocytic rate of brain endothelial cells compared to peripheral endothelial cells may be exploited to promote retention of molecular labels specifically on the surface of the brain vasculature [128]. The feasibility of such an approach has been recently examined by employing a biotinylated anti-PECAM1 antibody to generate biotin targets specifically in the brain vasculature [181]. The authors demonstrated that the uptake of avidin-decorated NPs was increased in the lung, heart, pancreas and brain of mice if the NP were injected a short time-interval (15 minutes) after injection of biotinylated anti-PECAM1 antibody, corresponding to biotin targets having been generated on the vasculature of all these organs. However, if the NPs were injected a long time-interval (8 hours) after injection of biotinylated anti-PECAM1 antibody, uptake of NP was only increased in the brain, indicating the biotin targets had been removed (endocytosed) from all peripheral organs and only remained on the surface of brain endothelial cells. Generating the required brain-specific targets for NP delivery is expected to improve clinical translation by not only decreasing detrimental peripheral NP uptake increase but also by avoiding interfering with protein transport systems which are crucial for proper brain homoeostasis. For instance, the disruption of brain iron uptake by TfR is known to lead to cognitive dysfunction and promote neurodegeneration [182].

3.5 Delivering NPs to treat brain infections

Functionalising therapy-loaded NPs with ligands against transporter proteins expressed on BEC has been employed to transport therapies against CNS-related infections across the BBB, although the majority of the research developed relates to viral infections. For instance, Prabhakar et al. encapsulated the antiretroviral Indinavir within lipid emulsions functionalised with transferrin protein to promote binding of TfR-1 to increase penetration across the BBB as a strategy to treat HIV CNS infection [183]. The authors demonstrated their nanoformulation significantly increased brain penetration within 15 minutes following intravenous injection compared to free drug. Similarly, Gong et al. successfully delivered the anti-retroviral elvitegravir across an in vitro BBB model by encapsulating it within PLGA NPs coated with the surfactant poloxamer-188, which in turn allows binding of Apo-E for recognition of the LDL receptor present in BEC [184,185]. Their nanoformulation strategy significantly decreased HIV-1 viral load in macrophages following BBB crossing compared to administration of free elvitegravir. In addition, Surnar et al. have developed PLGA-PEG-triphenylphosphonium (PLGA-PEG-TPP) polymeric NPs capable of increased interaction with BEC to deliver various antiretroviral therapies in combination with neuroprotectant antioxidants and anti-inflammatory agents as a synergistic strategy to reduce the HIV viral burden in the brain and reduce neuronal damage by glial cells [186].

Targeted NPs have also been used to treat other types of CNS infections. Zhang et al. have recently demonstrated exosome NPs functionalised with the rabies-derived glycoprotein RVG are capable of delivering siRNA across the BBB to prevent Zika virus infection in foetal mouse brains [187].

4. Brain targeting: Delivery, targeting and efflux within the brain parenchyma

4.1 Components of the brain parenchyma

Upon entry into the brain tissue following vascular extravasation, NPs undergo distribution and elimination processes which involve diffusion, extracellular fluid (ECF) and cerebrospinal fluid (CSF) bulk flow, metabolism and clearance. NPs decorated with ligands on their surface may also bind to specific binding sites (e.g. target proteins expressed on the surface of different brain cells) and non-specific binding sites (e.g. extra-cellular matrix (ECM) components). The cells comprising the brain parenchyma account for 80% of brain tissue volume and can be classified into neurons, glial cells and pericytes [188]. Neurons are cells which are electrically excitable, processing and transmitting information to other cells through intercellular synapses [189]. The typical anatomy of a neuron shows a single axon and multiple dendrites, which trigger the flow of information in the CNS [190]. Glial cells, comprised of astrocytes, oligodendrocytes and microglia, provide support and protection to the neurons [188]. Among them, astrocytes are most abundant in the CNS. Astrocytes regulate neurotransmitter and electrolyte balance, thereby supporting neuronal function. They envelope the BBB and possess protrusions that wrap the blood vessels and synapses of the neurons, providing a connection between vasculature and neuronal circuits [191]. The contact between the astrocytic end-feet and the abluminal part of the CNS microvessels augment endothelial cell tight junctions, increasing BBB integrity [192]. Oligodendrocytes are cells that myelinate axonal fibres. They are diverse in terms of morphology and location, with some types functioning in the regulation of neuronal excitability and metabolic support of axons [193]. Microglia are the main immune cells in the CNS and are the first to respond in case of any pathological intrusions. They survey the brain environment, phagocytose particles, and release cytokines. Thus, they are highly motile to provide constant monitoring and response [194]. Pericytes border the abluminal side of the CNS endothelial cells and regulate endothelial cell proliferation, migration, differentiation, vascular branching and survival, as well as regulating the blood-flow of capillaries [195]. Pericytes are key players in BBB maintenance, where they are crucial in the formation of gap junctions, peg-and-socket junctions [196].

In addition to the different brain cells, the brain parenchyma is composed of the ECF, which comprises about 20% of the parenchyma [197], surrounding the cells and circulating throughout the tissue. Paracellular transport of endogenous and exogenous molecules between brain parenchymal cells occurs mainly through the ECF [197]. Since the BBB prohibits entry of proteins and most large molecules into the brain, the ECF composition is comparable to that of the plasma but with less protein concentration [198].

Separate from the ECF, the CSF encompasses the brain and flows between the brain ventricles, sub-arachnoid space and the spinal cord [198]. It is important in providing protection to the brain against injury, as well as in clearance of waste. It also balances changes in blood volume in the brain throughout the cardiac cycle [199]. The epithelial cells of the choroid plexus in the brain ventricles are the major producers of the CSF [199]. The CSF is a clear fluid with a low protein concentration, similarly to the ECF [198].

4.2 Movement of fluids in the brain

Homoeostasis within the brain parenchyma is maintained through recycling and clearance of the brain ECF [200]. The cellular layers that separate the brain ECF and the CSF in the brain ventricles and in the sub-arachnoid space are permeable enough to allow free fluid circulation between the two fluids [201]. The brain capillary endothelial wall secretes fluid resulting from passive water transport across the BBB, producing brain ECF [200]. Bulk flow of this fluid is driven by hydrostatic pressure [201] or cerebral arterial pulsation [202] and is led in the direction of the CSF in the brain ventricles and sub-arachnoid space where the CSF acts as sink or drained across the capillary and arterial walls, into the lymphatic system [203].

The relevance of brain ECF bulk flow as a mechanism of fluid transport as opposed to diffusion is under dispute [201]. Fluid transport from the para-arterial to para-venous space that is regulated by the glial cells is referred to as the glymphatic system [204]. The term 'glymphatic' is derived from its association with glial cells and its similarity to the lymphatic system-dependent waste clearance in the periphery [205,206]. This system helps brain fluids maintain stable environments for neuronal function while quickly removing neuronal and glial waste [204]. Integral to this mechanism is the exchange of fluid between the ECF and CSF, where the CSF enters the ECF from the arteries, while the ECF leaves through the veins. This exchange depends on aquaporin-4 (AQP4) channels at the astrocytic end-feet, which are facilitators of water transport across barriers [205]. Transport within the ECF is dominated by diffusion, as shown by mathematical simulation of brain transport which considered glymphatic clearance [207]. However, there is evidence that brain ECF bulk flow is important in certain neurological conditions like epilepsy [200].

4.3 Movement of NPs within the brain fluids

Drugs and NPs that enter the brain parenchyma encounter a heterogeneous tissue environment comprised of cellular bodies, cell processes, ECM and ECF [208]. Diffusion of NPs in the ECF is hampered by obstructions like brain cells which determine the geometry and width of the narrow channels of the extracellular space (ECS) [209]. The ECS is small, measuring merely tens of nanometres, which is narrow compared to the diameter of the brain capillaries and is about 5%–36% (19% average) of healthy brain volume [210]. The effective diffusion is additionally lowered by dead-space microdomains, which are characterised as voids within the ECF in which NPs can be trapped momentarily, increasing residence time. These were discovered in diseased rat brain [211]. Aside from the geometrical factors, the ECF contains various binding sites that reduce movement of molecules. For example, when drug molecules bind to ECM proteins, their diffusion is hindered. Because of all these, effective diffusion of a drug in brain ECF is much lower than in water [198]. NPs can also be affected by viscous drag because of the finite ECS width and pores in the brain ECM [208]. NP PEGylation has enabled further understanding of the brain ECS. When surface PEG density is sufficiently high, 114-nm NPs can diffuse effectively in human, rat and mouse brains [212]. This has since been confirmed in further studies, and now ECS widths are perceived to be 80–220 nm in diameter while pores are around 100 nm [213–215]. Increased PEG surface density is also shown to restrain cellular uptake of NPs [216], which removes another impediment for diffusion.

NP surface coatings can also interact with the ECM. The brain ECM is primarily composed of anionic glycosaminoglycans that can be suspended or wrapped around cells. ECM chemical composition can alter ECS width and geometry, as demonstrated by differing NP diffusion in hyaluronidase-treated brain [214]. By nature of their anionic charge, glycosaminoglycans can either repel negatively charged substances or attract those with positive charge, which can trigger divergence from normal diffusion [217]. Colloidal stability is also an important consideration for NP diffusion in the brain parenchyma. Assuming that particles remain stable in the brain microenvironment, size and surface charge can be good predictors of particle diffusion. However, NP interactions with the changing concentrations of ions in the brain ECF can impact its colloidal stability [218]. For example, calcium ion concentration and pH are known to show spatial and temporal variations in the brain [219,220]. NPs whose surfaces display a carboxylate functional group are mostly negatively charged in higher pH, and may interact with Ca^{2+}, producing aggregates [218,221], which decrease their diffusion capabilities. Assessing NP stability in media that mimic the brain microenvironment is therefore essential.

Depending on the administration route, ECF bulk flow may also be an important mechanism of drug distribution in the brain [222]. Convection-enhanced delivery (CED) employs bulk flow produced by a pressure gradient instead of a concentration gradient. Diffusion depends on a concentration gradient and follows Fick's law:

$$J = -D\nabla C$$

where $D =$ tissue diffusivity and $\nabla C =$ concentration gradient, which says that molar flux is proportional to the concentration gradient multiplied by tissue diffusivity, which in turn is determined by molecular weight. Large-molecule drugs will consequently have longer diffusion times and will require higher concentrations to propel movement in the ECF. Bulk flow on the other hand relies on pressure gradient for distribution and is governed by Darcy's law:

$$v = -K\nabla p$$

where $K =$ hydraulic conductivity and $\nabla p =$ pressure gradient, which affirms that velocity of the molecule is directly proportional to the hydraulic conductivity and the pressure gradient [223,224].

By maintaining this pressure gradient from the cannula tip to the surrounding brain tissues, CED is able to deliver small and large molecules, including NPs, in clinically relevant significant volumes [225]. The CED-induced positive pressure directs flow through the tissue through convection until a limit, which depends on infusion volume and rate, is reached. Beyond this, diffusion will become the dominant mechanism. Velocity of flow is therefore most critical factor in drug transport near the cannula tip, but as the drug molecule travels along the parenchyma, size becomes increasingly significant. CED benefits large molecule drugs the most, including antibodies and NPs, and hence large-molecule therapeutics is where it finds most of its application [226].

5. Tumour targeting: Peripheral cancers

5.1 EPR effect

The vasculature is distributed throughout the body to transport nutrients and remove waste, as well as being a highly controlled and dynamic interphase between the blood and tissue [227]. Unfortunately, the vasculature also behaves as a sturdy palisade to block the entry of blood-borne nanotherapeutics into tissues [228]. Nanotherapeutics could passively enter through fenestrated vasculature and accumulate in inflamed or tumoral tissue with slow clearance – a phenomenon known as enhanced permeability and retention (EPR) effect [229]. However, the pores distribute randomly and the size ranges widely (e.g. 0.3–4.7 μm for MCa-IV mouse mammary carcinomas), leading to nonuniform leakiness of nanotherapeutics into the tissue parenchyma that directly affect the therapeutic efficacy [230,231]. To improve the therapeutic index, the vascular permeability in different tumour types (e.g. hypopermeable and hyperpermeable tumours) should be considered as a paramount parameter to customise the nanotherapeutics aimed at treating cancer [232,233]. In addition, irregular branching pattern and poor vascularisation in hypoxic regions will also result in an uneven distribution [234,235]. A relatively high interstitial fluid pressure (IFP) due to impaired lymphatic drainage and vasculature compression decreases blood perfusion in tumour sites [236]. In addition, the heterogeneity of vasculature among individuals further complicates the situation [237]. Therefore, only a limited amount of nanotherapeutics could manage overcome the vasculature barriers simply by virtue of the inherent vascular leakiness. Worthy of note, currently the research has primarily focussed on early phase accumulation, but rarely sheds light on NPs retention after accumulation, which is critical to improve the bioavailability of therapeutics.

5.2 Smart nanotherapeutics

Besides vasculature abnormality, solid tumours display a distinct pathophysiological microenvironment, including acidity, redox status, hypoxia and protein (e.g. protease, cytokines/chemokines, growth factor and receptor) expression. Building on these pathophysiological features, tremendous efforts have been invested in developing smart nanotherapeutics capable of navigating the diseased site to advance the in vivo functionality (e.g. specific targeting, tissue distribution, intracellular trafficking

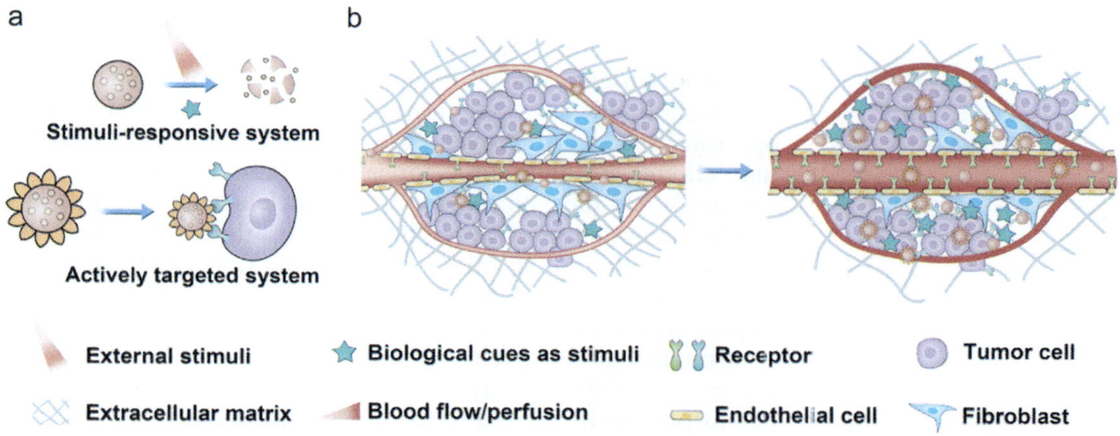

Figure 5.3 Schematic illustration of (A) stimuli-responsive and/or actively targeted nanotherapeutics based on vasculature characteristics (paracellular leakiness) and microenvironment (e.g. pH gradient, redox status changes, enzyme concentration and receptor expression) or available exogenous stimuli (e.g. light), (B) tumour microenvironment-reprogramming strategies for rejuvenating nanotherapeutics via improving accumulation and responsiveness based on enhancing vascular permeability/tissue perfusion, upregulating receptor concentration, or upregulating concentration of environment cues as the stimuli. Adapted with permission from Li and Kataoka [242].

and drug release) [238–241]. In this section, we will discuss the related strategies of smart nanotherapeutics (Fig. 5.3) [242].

5.2.1 Microenvironment-responsive nanotherapeutics

The pH of the tissue microenvironment has been extensively exploited to trigger the function of nanotherapeutics through sophisticated chemistry-based design (e.g. cleavage and protonation of effector units). Most nanotherapeutics could traffic into acidic endosomes/lysosomes through endocytosis, concurrently facilitating designing pH-responsive nanotherapeutics for intracellular delivery. For example, pH-cleavable maleic acid amide derivatives-based charge-conversion delivery system was proved to be capable of regenerating positive charges to enhance endosomal escape of protein and gene cargos [243–246]. Further fine-tuning of chemical structure (e.g. 2,3-dimethylmaleic amide) enable the cleavage by extracellular acidity to enhance tissue penetration and cellular uptake [247–250]. Cationic polymers bearing protonatable groups (e.g. secondary and tertiary amines) could exert ‘proton sponge’ effect to enhance opportunities for endosomal escape reaching the drug target [251]. Particularly, for gene delivery, it is vital to break the endosomal trapping before degradation of nucleic acid can take place, thus jeopardising the transfection success. For instance, poly(amino acids)-based polycations possessing repeating aminoethylene units were widely utilised to deliver nucleic acids, in which a delicate odd–even effect of aminoethylene units – related to pH buffering capacity – on transfection efficiency was discovered [252,253]. Interestingly, the opposite trend of odd–even effect for mRNA and pDNA implies that chemical tuning of cytoplasmic stability and endosomal escape should have consideration for nucleic acid type. mRNA is highly susceptible to cleavage by nucleases, therefore stability is a primary limitation of mRNA translation. Conversely, pDNA is more stable than mRNA, making endosomal escape the limiting step of pDNA transfection.

Intracellular drug release could be triggered by endosomal acidity in acid-labile polymeric prodrug system, such as PEG-*b*-poly(aspartate hydrazone doxorubicin/epirubicin) [254–257]. In particular, phase I clinical trials have already validated the safety of epirubicin-conjugated micelles (NC-6300). Given the 'PEG dilemma', pH-cleavable PEGylation has been adopted as a strategy to enhance endosomal escape [258].

Besides assisting drug delivery, pH could serve as a target for imaging purposes. For example, tumour extracellular acidity-induced sharp dissociation of fluorophore-conjugated tertiary amine-based ionisable polymeric micelles, which de-quenched fluorescence to a large extent, was exploited to amplify the imaging signal [259,260]. Particularly, this nanoprobe bound with indocyanine green (ICG) has entered clinical trials for surgical navigation in resection procedures [261]. Similarly, extracellular acidity-induced sharp ionisation of piperidine-functionalised block polymer remarkably improved the membrane permeability of glucose oxidase (GOD)-loaded therapeutic vesicular nanoreactors [262]. Consequently, the nanoreactors could be selectively activated at the acidic sites to catalyse glucose oxidation for amplifying oxidative stress to promote a cytotoxic effect.

Redox metabolism may also be exploited in the design of redox-responsive nanotherapeutics. Intracellular antioxidants (e.g. glutathione) can break disulfide bonds. Thus, a disulfide linker has been reversibly incorporated into nanotherapeutics, such as gene-loaded polyplex micelles and drug-conjugated NPs, to not only stabilise their structure but in addition to achieve cytosolic release of the therapeutic load [263–268]. It should be mentioned that, besides disulfide crosslinking of nanocarriers, therapeutics themselves could alternatively be bridged by thiol bonds. For example, for gene-loaded polyplex micelles, increasing the charge of nucleic acid by disulfide bridging strengthened and stabilised electrostatic interactions [269,270]. Disulfide-bridged cleavable PEGylation was also used to enhance endosomal escape facilitating intracellular trafficking of therapeutics [271–273]. High oxidative stress in certain disease sites suggests that nanocarrier integrated with ROS-cleavable units (e.g. boronic ester and thioketal groups) has the potential to selectively deliver the therapeutics [262,274,275]. To improve the sensitivity of nanotherapeutics, reduction and ROS dual-responsive systems have also been proposed [276].

ATP, the major biological energy currency, is available to trigger the intracellular release of therapeutics (e.g. siRNA, pDNA and chemotherapy drug) by competitive exchange with units in nanocarrier (e.g. boronic ester linkage) [277–280]. Additionally, it is reasonable to incorporate multitype supramolecular forces to stabilise nanotherapeutics. For example, hydrophobic interaction has often been utilised to increase the stability of gene-loaded polyplex micelles. In one example, the mixtures of PEG-*b*-poly[*N*-[*N*-(2-aminoethyl)-2-aminoethyl]aspartamide] [PAsp(DET)] and poly(*N*-isopropylacrylamide)-*b*-PAsp(DET) copolymers condensed pDNA at 25°C, followed by incubation at 37°C that allowed poly(*N*-isopropylacrylamide) with lower critical solution temperature (LCST) below physiological temperature to form hydrophobic intermediate layers between PEG shells and pDNA cores [281]. The hydrophobic poly(*N*-isopropylacrylamide) layers not only compensated the instability of polyplex micelles from counterion dissociation but also inhibited nuclease digestion due to steric hindrance, improving transfection efficiency of pDNA encoding an anti-angiogenic protein to remarkably suppress malignant growth in H22-bearing mice. The effect of hydrophobic layer was similarly observed using a triblock copolymer composed of poly(2-ethyl-2-oxazoline) (PEtOx) as hydrophilic segments, poly(2-n-propyl-2-oxazoline) (PnPrOx) as thermoresponsive segments, and poly(L-lysine) (PLys) as polycation segments [282].

Enzymes such as cathepsins and matrix metalloproteinases (MMPs) have been implicated in tumour progression and could serve as a trigger for enhancing therapeutics delivery and specific tissue imaging. Some polymeric systems already entered clinical trials. For example, Kopecek et al. pioneered poly[*N*-(2-hydroxypropyl) methacrylamide]–GlyPheLeuGly (GPLG)–Doxorubicin, a first example of clinically investigated polymeric prodrug conjugate, in which lysosomal cathepsins could cleave the peptidyl linker of GPLG to release doxorubicin [283].

5.2.2 Externally triggerable nanotherapeutics

An alternative to microenvironment-responsive nanotherapeutics is using external energy (e.g. light, magnetic field and ultrasound) to interact with tissue-retained nanotherapeutics to activate functionality, that may partly reduce the effect of micro-environment heterogeneity [284].

Light illumination changes the physico-chemical properties of the nanocarriers, such as photocleavage/photoisomerisation reaction and photodynamic/photothermal effect, thus improving in vivo therapeutics bioavailability. For example, physical techniques [e.g. photochemical internalisation (PCI)] could markedly promote intracellular delivery [285]. A tri-layered gene-loaded polyplex micelle featured with the compartmentalisation of pDNA and photosensitiser, that avoided photochemical damage to gene, was developed to safely induce PCI effect for endosomal escape [286]. In another example, a multistage system was proposed for deep delivery of a photosensitiser to enhance photodynamic therapy based on ROS-cleavable size-shrinkable polymersomes under near-infrared light irradiation [287]. In clinical settings, lyso-thermosensitive liposomal doxorubicin (ThermoDox) is an example of the release of doxorubicin under the treatment of radiofrequency (RF) thermal ablation [288]. For implementing external energy-triggered nanotherapeutics, the common disadvantages include invasive procedures (e.g. the usage of RF needle electrodes), cumbersome optimisation of irradiation (e.g. time point, period, location and intensity) and initiation of only transient effects. Although polymeric nanotherapeutics are quite rare in clinical practice, it will be interesting and promising to see the synergy between external trigger and distinct advantage of polymeric nanotherapeutics (e.g. structural versatility and ease of functionalisation). Specifically, the better stability of drug-conjugated polymeric nanotherapeutics would be anticipated to enable precise activation. The above-mentioned NC-6300 was already utilised as a sonosensitiser for improving the efficacy of sonodynamic therapy based on high-intensity focussed ultrasound to treat canine cancer and small-scale clinical trials in human patients were also initiated [289].

5.2.3 Actively targeted nanotherapeutics

Actively targeted nanotherapeutics refers to surface functionalisation of therapy-loaded nanocarriers with affinity ligands, allowing engagement of receptors to induce prolonged tissue retention and increased cellular uptake, consequently improving therapeutics bioavailability [290]. Small molecules, antibodies, peptides and aptamers have been widely utilised as ligands to target tumour parenchyma and vasculature [290]. A unique advantage of active targeting is improving the efficiency of targeting lesions with poor EPR effect, e.g. micrometastases that are significantly responsible for cancer recurrence [291,292]. In addition, vasculature-targeting strategies provide the possibility to bypass the EPR effect, showing the potential to inhibit malignant growth [293].

Apart from retention and uptake, transcytosis as a distinct function of vasculature-targeted nanotherapeutics using specific ligands (e.g. RGD motif, glucose, glutathione and Angiopep-2) could improve tissue accumulation and distribution [242]. Notably, glutathione liposomal doxorubicin and paclitaxel-Angiopep-2 conjugates, which engage glutathione transporter and LRP-1 transport systems, respectively, have entered clinical trials [294,295]. However, for some ligands, such as cell-penetrating peptides and positively charged moieties, rapid off-target effects inevitably overshadow their utility. To balance the specificity versus non-specificity dilemma, various triggerable strategies were adopted to activate non-specific ligands in situ [296–299]. Until now, though, no clear clinical benefits have been demonstrated for actively targeted nanotherapeutics. The results for the first clinically tested actively targeted nanotherapeutic, BIND-014, were not a striking and conclusive success [300].

5.3 Microenvironment heterogeneity

Targeting using smart nanotherapeutics is based on exploiting the distinct microenvironment surrounding the specific tissues, which is inevitably restricted by its heterogeneity. In brief, (i) the microenvironment fluctuates over the course of disease progression. (ii) The regional distribution characteristics of microenvironment requires customised nanotherapeutics to be delivered into a specific destination, but it is always difficult to control in a complex biological environment. (iii) Tissue-specific delivery and activation was also compounded by slight differences of microenvironment between normal and malignant tissue, given over 90% nanotherapeutics will distribute into normal tissue eventually risking off-target activity. (iv) Inter-individual diversity further poses additional challenges.

5.4 Microenvironment-reprogramming strategies for rejuvenating nanotherapeutics

In light of the microenvironment heterogeneity, implementing smart nanotherapeutics necessitates extra efforts to guarantee desirable functionality by improving specific tissue accumulation and responsiveness of nanotherapeutics.

5.4.1 Amplification of tissue accumulation

The appealing trials for amplifying accumulation focus on enhancing vascular permeability/tissue perfusion for passively targeted nanotherapeutics and upregulating receptors for actively targeted nanotherapeutics.

Vascular normalisation through modulation of vascular endothelial growth factor (VEGF) signalling, developed by Jain et al., could restore tissue vasculature functionality, and therefore improve the perfusion [301]. Given synchronously reducing vascular pore size, unsurprisingly, vascular normalisation would profoundly promote accumulation of nanomedicines with small size (<60 nm) [302,303]. The widely used therapeutics to normalise vasculature are small molecules, always being accompanied by unsatisfactory pharmacokinetics, pharmacodynamics and toxicokinetics [304]. As a consequence, nanotherapeutic delivery platforms have been proposed to deal with these issues for vascular normalisation, such as nitric oxide (NO)-donor molecule-loaded lipid-PLGA hybrid NPs [305]. In addition, vascular promotion could improve the delivery of small-molecule chemotherapeutics, but the effect on nanotherapeutics remains unclear [306]. Besides vascular normalisation/promotion, reducing the malignant tissue stroma relieves solid stress and decompresses the vasculature, thereby improving the accumulation and diffusion/penetration of nanotherapeutics. For instance, losartan, an angiotensin-II receptor antagonist, induced reduction of collagen, hyaluronan and stromal fibroblasts, facilitating the accumulation of NPs of 12 nm, 60 nm and 125 nm in diameter [307]. Dexamethasone, a glucocorticoid medication, has been demonstrated to reduce IFP, tissue stiffness and solid stress, thereby increasing the accumulation and penetration of DACHPt-loaded micelles in the target breast tissue [308]. Modulating TGF-β signalling has shown benefits in amplifying accumulation by decreasing pericyte or ECM and improving tissue perfusion [309–311]. Furthermore, enzymatic degradation of ECM by hydrolases (e.g. hyaluronidase) has also been attempted [312]. Importantly, these strategies to reverse poor delivery of nanotherapeutics would remarkably increase the therapeutic index in the case of cancer tissues characterised by remarkable desmoplasia (e.g. pancreatic and breast) [313].

Physically improving vascular permeability based on radiotherapy, photodynamic therapy, hyperthermia and focussed ultrasound is also feasible [314]. For instance, super-enhanced permeability and retention effects were reported due to massive depletion of perivascular cells using near-infrared photoimmunotherapy [315]. Hyperthermia could increase blood flow/perfusion and vascular permeability [316]. Beyond the direct effect on vascular permeability, radiation therapy and photosensitisation could prime the tissue microenvironment for nanotherapeutics delivery via activating macrophage-mediated vascular bursts and neutrophil infiltration, respectively [317,318]. Worthy of note, physical effects could be strengthened through nanotherapeutic delivery of sensitisers (e.g. photosensitiser, radiosensitiser, photothermal agent and sonosensitiser).

A potential pitfall of increasing vascular permeability is providing easier access to the main blood flow to malignant cells [319]. Thus, a vital prerequisite to safely implement pharmacological and physical methods for amplifying the nanotherapeutics accumulation is optimising the therapeutic window (e.g. doses and dosing schedules).

The issues of active targeting differ from the major bottleneck of passive targeting (tissue permeability/perfusion) in that heterogeneous receptor expression may further affect the efficacy [320]. Consequently, the solutions of increasing receptor numbers have been proposed. Most trials focussed on externally inducing a rise in stress and inflammatory biomarkers [321]. For example, coagulation cascade induced by photothermal effect or truncated tissue factor protein could increase the accumulation of liposomes decorated with coagulation-targeting peptides by 40-fold [322]. Hyperthermia or vascular disrupting agents could upregulate stress-related proteins (e.g. p32 and heat shock protein) as ligands to recruit actively targeted nanotherapeutics [323–325]. Similarly, neoantigen generation (e.g. P-selectin, CAM and $\alpha_{2b}\beta_3$) from radiotherapy within vasculature and parenchyma can be profitably utilised in drug delivery and imaging [326–328]. It should be clinically practicable to combine radiotherapy with actively targeted nanotherapeutics given >50% cancer patients would receive radiotherapy [329]. Alternatively, although expensive, ad hoc gene transfer could be exploited to upregulate expression of receptors [330,331]. Besides the genetic approach, attractively, metabolic glycoengineering through hijacking biosynthetic machinery has been applied for labelling of malignant cell surfaces with chemical groups that functionally serve as receptor [332]. For instance, azide-tagged tissues were capable of recruiting more (nano)therapeutics through bioorthogonal click reactions [333,334].

5.4.2 Amplification of the responsiveness of nanotherapeutics

A biological basis for stimuli-responsive nanotherapeutics is represented by a biological microenvironment that can trigger a desirable functionality (e.g. drug release) to a large extent. However, it might not always realistically occur, given our current superficial understanding of complex nano-bio interactions and of the microenvironment itself. To our mind, drug release/production is a decisive factor of therapeutic index. Unfortunately, so far, there is an extreme lack of in vivo evaluation, although release profiles are well demonstrated in vitro. Despite noticeable improvement in target tissue accumulation of nanotherapeutics compared with free agents, unignorable issues – inefficient drug release or prodrug transformation – may contribute to non-functional accumulation, as evidenced by some examples, including NK102, CRLX101 and liposomal formulations consisting of doxorubicin, cisplatin or CPT-11 [335–341]. For instance, NK102, SN-38–conjugated polymeric micelle, could release SN-38 by slow hydrolysis, only producing less than 1% free SN-38 in HT-29 tumour 24 hours post administration [335]. Although externally triggerable nanotherapeutics could partially resolve this issue, limitations as described above exist. Ultrasensitive systems may remarkably improve drug release and prodrug transformation, but at the cost of risking off-target activation and with undoubtedly more complex design and manufacturing difficulties [342,343]. Therefore, new strategies to amplify the responsiveness of nanotherapeutics are needed, such as artificially upregulating microenvironmental factors as the stimuli.

In fact, enzyme/prodrug therapy (EPT) is well documented in pre-clinical and clinical studies to improve small-molecule prodrug transformation by therapeutically introducing exogenous enzymes [344–346]. It deserves to be mentioned, though, that the enzymatic activation of a prodrug primarily depends on accessibility of substrate (e.g. scissile bond) by the active site, implying more consideration is required for using this strategy to amplify the responsiveness of nanotherapeutics, because the nanocarrier itself (e.g. hydrophobic core) will constitute the barrier to the ultimate enzymatic activation [347]. Instead of enzyme, upregulating small biochemicals should be profitably applicable. For example, several GOD-loaded polymeric prodrug-based nanoreactors were proposed to specifically catalyse glucose oxidation at the target site for producing ROS, not only inducing cytotoxic activity through oxidative stress but also improving ROS-responsive polymeric prodrug transformation [348–350]. Systematic evaluation of drug release kinetics in blood, liver and malignant tissue demonstrated that prodrug transformation preferentially occurred in the latter one, which essentially differs from small-molecule prodrug with normal tissues (e.g. blood and liver) as drug factory [349]. In addition, enzyme-free counterparts of the drug nanoreactors exhibited low activation efficiency, signifying that the tissue intrinsic ROS level is insufficient for prodrug transformation. This strategy is further capable of weakening the effect of the above-mentioned barriers for nanotherapeutics because released small-molecule drugs could more easily flood the entire target tissue and always exhibit stronger toxicity.

These investigations strongly argue that the responsiveness – including but not limited to drug release – of nanotherapeutics should be considered as a critical determinant of therapeutic index. There is clearly an urgent need to bridge in vivo responsiveness to the functionality of nanotherapeutics. We envision that the strategies to amplify the responsiveness of nanotherapeutics should be practicable in clinical settings, being an area of increasing attention.

6. Immune system targeting

6.1 Targeting immune system organs and their associated immune cells using NPs

Immune system organs may be classified as primary or secondary lymphoid organs if they generate special immune cells called lymphocytes or if they serve as collection sites to pool lymphocytes together with other immune cells, respectively. Lymphoid organs participate in the regulation of immune responses, homoeostasis and maintenance of a diverse repertoire of immune functions [351]. Primary lymphoid organs comprise the bone marrow and the thymus, while secondary lymphoid organs consist of the spleen, lymph nodes and certain tissues of the body [351]. All of these organs are important targets for NPs-mediated therapeutic modulation of immune function [352], such as vaccinations [353], immunotherapy [353], cancer treatment [354] and treatment of autoimmune diseases [355].

Among the immune cells targeted by NPs for immunomodulation are macrophages, dendritic cells, T-cells, B-cells and natural killer cells (NK cells) [356–358]. Some of these cells participate solely in forming innate immunity, others may solely participate in adaptive immunity, and there are a few others such as dendritic cells that may be involved in both. In targeting the immune system at this cellular level, cellular uptake mechanism has to be considered as it may influence response of these cells towards NPs and ultimately towards its cargo. In general, immune cells have the option of performing phagocytosis to engulf NPs in addition to receptor-mediated endocytosis. This character has been exploited in targeting the immune systems using NPs.

A unique characteristic of immune system therapeutic targeting is that the main goal is more often not to kill or to supply a surrogate component missing in a healthy cell. More commonly the goal is for the NPs to participate in driving or altering cell priming so that a desired effector cell is produced. In dendritic cells, for example, NPs may be used to drive maturation, cytokine release, and modulation of the immune response. T-cells are targeted to increase, or decrease their activity, promote T-cell expansion and improve T-cells infiltration to a diseased site. B-cells may be targeted to elicit tolerogenic responses towards non-diseased cells. The opportunities that come with targeting immune cells with NPs are vast yet complicated as NPs are used to alter certain cells to subsequently interact with another.

Targeting the immune system using NPs has been performed through various injection routes, such as intravenous (i.v.), subcutaneous (s.c.) or intramuscular (i.m) injections, and also direct injection to the diseased site. These broad options are available because the target site for immune system targeting is accessible through either the lymphatic drainage or blood circulation depending on the targeted immune organs and types of NPs. Noting the complexity of how the immune system works, though, selected delivery routes matter more than they do for other targets because they may affect the quality of response in addition to quantity [359]. Therefore, it is crucial to select the proper administration routes based on the intended goal of the study.

6.2 Targeting immune cells for vaccination

Historically, vaccination has been associated more closely with prevention of infectious diseases. For this purpose, NPs may serve as a platform to load antigens with or without adjuvant. The main targets for NPs are the lymph nodes, and administration is commonly achieved through s.c. or i.m local administration routes [360]. The i.v. route is less preferable because an outburst of the antigenic cargo may not produce the desired effect. When injected through s.c. and i.m. routes, the NPs may either work locally at the injected site to interact with resident antigen-presenting cells (APC), or with APC at the lymph node, the most important being the dendritic cells. NPs here are expected to unload their cargo to be processed by dendritic cells for presentation on the major histocompatibility complex (MHC) type I and II. If adjuvant is also included in the nanoparticle formulation, the nanoparticle may also be used to elicit cytokine release that may help with dendritic cells maturation and elicit priming of the immune cells to ultimately cause the desired effect of adaptive immunity.

More recently, vaccination has been expanded to include vaccination against cancers. The effort came as a result of improved understanding that cancers have defective proteins called tumour-associated antigens within their surface that may serve as targets for cancer recognition. For this application, there is the additional option of administrating NPs through the bloodstream for more potent effect. In addition to the above, the target organ for this approach may include the spleen and thymus as administration by the route is a systemic one.

Similar to the strategy for vaccination against infectious diseases, NPs can be decorated with ligands to enhance interaction with dendritic cells. For instance, Ossendorp et al. utilised PLGA-NP-vaccines to encapsulate ovalbumin antigen together with the adjuvants Pam3Csk4 (TLR2L) and Poly(I:C) (TLR3L) and to target DC via CD40, a tumour necrosis factor-receptor family cell-surface receptor highly expressed on DC [361]. They used a ligand to CD40, namely murine αCD40-mAb FGK45 to promote a CD40/CD40L ligation that has been reported to have role in the maturation of DC into APC and in $CD8^+$ T cell priming. Using this strategy, the study reported robust priming of Ag-specific $CD8^+$ T cells with the capacity to suppress tumour and prolong survival. A different strategy was employed by Kim et al. by using injectable dual-scale mesoporous silica vaccine consisting of mesoporous silica microrods (MSRs) coupled with mesoporous silica NPs (MSNs) [362], where DC-recruiting chemokine was loaded in the mesopores of MSRs to lead dendritic cells into the scaffold to bring it closer to MSNs that were co-loaded with an antigen and Toll-like receptor 9 agonist. This strategy leads to the generation of antigen-presenting activated DCs, larger number of antigen-specific T cells, and ultimately was able to inhibit melanoma model tumour in mice.

References

[1] E.C. Dreaden, L.A. Austin, M.A. Mackey, M.A. El-Sayed, Size matters: gold nanoparticles in targeted cancer drug delivery, Therapeutic Delivery 3 (4) (2012) 457–478, https://doi.org/10.4155/tde.12.21.

[2] Y.N. Zhang, W. Poon, A.J. Tavares, I.D. McGilvray, W.C.W. Chan, Nanoparticle-liver interactions: cellular uptake and hepatobiliary elimination, Journal of Controlled Release 240 (2016) 332–348, https://doi.org/10.1016/j.jconrel.2016.01.020.

[3] F. Campbell, F.L. Bos, S. Sieber, G. Arias-Alpizar, B.E. Koch, J. Huwyler, A. Kros, J. Bussmann, Directing nanoparticle biodistribution through evasion and exploitation of stab2-dependent nanoparticle uptake, ACS Nano 12 (3) (2018) 2138–2150, https://doi.org/10.1021/acsnano.7b06995.

[4] B. Yin, K.H.K. Li, L.W.C. Ho, C.K.W. Chan, C.H.J. Choi, Toward understanding in vivo sequestration of nanoparticles at the molecular level, ACS Nano 12 (3) (2018) 2088–2093, https://doi.org/10.1021/acsnano.8b00141.
[5] B.Z. Stanger, Cellular homeostasis and repair in the mammalian liver, Annual Review of Physiology 77 (2015) 179–200, https://doi.org/10.1146/annurev-physiol-021113-170255.
[6] C.I. Colino, J.M. Lanao, C. Gutierrez-Millan, Targeting of hepatic macrophages by therapeutic nanoparticles, Frontiers in Immunology 11 (2020) 218, https://doi.org/10.3389/fimmu.2020.00218.
[7] K.M. Tsoi, S.A. MacParland, X.Z. Ma, V.N. Spetzler, J. Echeverri, B. Ouyang, S.M. Fadel, E.A. Sykes, N. Goldaracena, J.M. Kaths, et al., Mechanism of hard-nanomaterial clearance by the liver, Nature Materials 15 (11) (2016) 1212–1221, https://doi.org/10.1038/nmat4718.
[8] Z. Fan, P. Zhu, Y. Zhu, K. Wu, C.Y. Li, H. Cheng, Engineering long-circulating nanomaterial delivery systems, Current Opinion in Biotechnology 66 (2020) 131–139, https://doi.org/10.1016/j.copbio.2020.07.006.
[9] J. Wolfram, M. Ferrari, Clinical cancer nanomedicine, Nano Today 25 (2019) 85–98, https://doi.org/10.1016/j.nantod.2019.02.005.
[10] E. Blanco, H. Shen, M. Ferrari, Principles of nanoparticle design for overcoming biological barriers to drug delivery, Nature Biotechnology 33 (9) (2015) 941–951, https://doi.org/10.1038/nbt.3330.
[11] K. Kataoka, A. Harada, Y. Nagasaki, Block copolymer micelles for drug delivery: design, characterization and biological significance, Advanced Drug Delivery Reviews 47 (1) (2001) 113–131, https://doi.org/10.1016/s0169-409x(00)00124-1.
[12] D.E. Owens 3rd, N.A. Peppas, Opsonization, biodistribution, and pharmacokinetics of polymeric nanoparticles, International Journal of Pharmacy 307 (1) (2006) 93–102, https://doi.org/10.1016/j.ijpharm.2005.10.010.
[13] M.L. Immordino, F. Dosio, L. Cattel, Stealth liposomes: review of the basic science, rationale, and clinical applications, existing and potential, International Journal of Nanomedicine 1 (3) (2006) 297–315.
[14] T. Lorson, M.M. Lubtow, E. Wegener, M.S. Haider, S. Borova, D. Nahm, R. Jordan, M. Sokolski-Papkov, A.V. Kabanov, R. Luxenhofer, Poly(2-oxazoline)s based biomaterials: a comprehensive and critical update, Biomaterials 178 (2018) 204–280, https://doi.org/10.1016/j.biomaterials.2018.05.022.
[15] N. Adams, U.S. Schubert, Poly(2-oxazolines) in biological and biomedical application contexts, Advanced Drug Delivery Reviews 59 (15) (2007) 1504–1520, https://doi.org/10.1016/j.addr.2007.08.018.
[16] A. Birke, J. Ling, M. Barz, Polysarcosine-containing copolymers: synthesis, characterization, self-assembly, and applications, Progress in Polymer Science 81 (2018) 163–208, https://doi.org/10.1016/j.progpolymsci.2018.01.002.
[17] Z. Amoozgar, Y. Yeo, Recent advances in stealth coating of nanoparticle drug delivery systems, Wiley Interdisciplinary Reviews Nanomedicine Nanobiotechnology 4 (2) (2012) 219–233, https://doi.org/10.1002/wnan.1157.
[18] E.A. Forssen, D.M. Coulter, R.T. Proffitt, Selective in vivo localization of daunorubicin small unilamellar vesicles in solid tumors, Cancer Research 52 (12) (1992) 3255–3261.

[19] J. Merian, R. De Souza, Y. Dou, S.N. Ekdawi, F. Ravenelle, C. Allen, Development of a liposome formulation for improved biodistribution and tumor accumulation of pentamidine for oncology applications, International Journal of Pharmacy 488 (1–2) (2015) 154–164, https://doi.org/10.1016/j.ijpharm.2015.04.060.
[20] Y. Chau, N.M. Dang, F.E. Tan, R. Langer, Investigation of targeting mechanism of new dextran-peptide-methotrexate conjugates using biodistribution study in matrix-metalloproteinase-overexpressing tumor xenograft model, Journal of Pharmaceutical Sciences 95 (3) (2006) 542–551, https://doi.org/10.1002/jps.20548.
[21] R. Suzuki, T. Takizawa, Y. Kuwata, M. Mutoh, N. Ishiguro, N. Utoguchi, A. Shinohara, M. Eriguchi, H. Yanagie, K. Maruyama, Effective anti-tumor activity of oxaliplatin encapsulated in transferrin-PEG-liposome, International Journal of Pharmacy 346 (1–2) (2008) 143–150, https://doi.org/10.1016/j.ijpharm.2007.06.010.
[22] R.-L. Hong, C.-J. Huang, Y.-L. Tseng, V.F. Pang, S.-T. Chen, J.-J. Liu, F.-H. Chang, Direct comparison of liposomal doxorubicin with or without polyethylene glycol coating in C-26 tumor-bearing mice: is surface coating with polyethylene glycol Beneficial?1, Clinical Cancer Research 5 (11) (1999) 3645–3652. (Accessed 2 January 2024).
[23] H. Hatakeyama, H. Akita, H. Harashima, The polyethyleneglycol dilemma: advantage and disadvantage of PEGylation of liposomes for systemic genes and nucleic acids delivery to tumors, Biological and Pharmaceutical Bulletin 36 (6) (2013) 892–899, https://doi.org/10.1248/bpb.b13-00059.
[24] A.S. Abu Lila, H. Kiwada, T. Ishida, The accelerated blood clearance (ABC) phenomenon: clinical challenge and approaches to manage, Journal of Controlled Release 172 (1) (2013) 38–47, https://doi.org/10.1016/j.jconrel.2013.07.026.
[25] P. Grenier, I.M.d.O. Viana, E.M. Lima, N. Bertrand, Anti-polyethylene glycol antibodies alter the protein corona deposited on nanoparticles and the physiological pathways regulating their fate in vivo, Journal of Controlled Release 287 (2018) 121–131, https://doi.org/10.1016/j.jconrel.2018.08.022.
[26] H. Lin, Y. Chen, J. Shi, Nanoparticle-triggered in situ catalytic chemical reactions for tumour-specific therapy, Chemical Society Reviews 47 (6) (2018) 1938–1958, https://doi.org/10.1039/C7CS00471K.
[27] V.R. Cherkasov, E.N. Mochalova, A.V. Babenyshev, A.V. Vasilyeva, P.I. Nikitin, M.P. Nikitin, Nanoparticle beacons: supersensitive smart materials with on/off-switchable affinity to biomedical targets, ACS Nano 14 (2) (2020) 1792–1803, https://doi.org/10.1021/acsnano.9b07569.
[28] C.-M.J. Hu, L. Zhang, S. Aryal, C. Cheung, R.H. Fang, L. Zhang, Erythrocyte membrane-camouflaged polymeric nanoparticles as a biomimetic delivery platform, Proceedings of the National Academy of Sciences 108 (27) (2011) 10980–10985, https://doi.org/10.1073/pnas.1106634108. (Accessed 1 February 2024).
[29] R. Molinaro, C. Corbo, J.O. Martinez, F. Taraballi, M. Evangelopoulos, S. Minardi, I.K. Yazdi, P. Zhao, E. De Rosa, M.B. Sherman, et al., Biomimetic proteolipid vesicles for targeting inflamed tissues, Nature Materials 15 (9) (2016) 1037–1046, https://doi.org/10.1038/nmat4644.
[30] A.C. Anselmo, V. Gupta, B.J. Zern, D. Pan, M. Zakrewsky, V. Muzykantov, S. Mitragotri, Delivering nanoparticles to lungs while avoiding liver and spleen through adsorption on red blood cells, ACS Nano 7 (12) (2013) 11129–11137, https://doi.org/10.1021/nn404853z.

[31] I.V. Zelepukin, A.V. Yaremenko, V.O. Shipunova, A.V. Babenyshev, I.V. Balalaeva, P.I. Nikitin, S.M. Deyev, M.P. Nikitin, Nanoparticle-based drug delivery via RBC-hitchhiking for the inhibition of lung metastases growth, Nanoscale 11 (4) (2019) 1636–1646, https://doi.org/10.1039/C8NR07730D.

[32] A. Paix, A. Folkmann, D.H. Goldman, H. Kulaga, M.J. Grzelak, D. Rasoloson, S. Paidemarry, R. Green, R.R. Reed, G. Seydoux, Precision genome editing using synthesis-dependent repair of Cas9-induced DNA breaks, Proceedings of the National Academy of Sciences 114 (50) (2017) E10745–E10754, https://doi.org/10.1073/pnas.1711979114. (Accessed 1 February 2024).

[33] L. Feng, F. Amber, Y. Xing, H. Leaf, Dysopsonin activity of serum DNA-binding proteins favorable for gene delivery, Journal of Pharmacology and Experimental Therapeutics 332 (2) (2010) 500, https://doi.org/10.1124/jpet.109.159541.

[34] P.L. Rodriguez, T. Harada, D.A. Christian, D.A. Pantano, R.K. Tsai, D.E. Discher, Minimal "self" peptides that inhibit phagocytic clearance and enhance delivery of nanoparticles, Science 339 (6122) (2013) 971–975, https://doi.org/10.1126/science.1229568. (Accessed 1 February 2024).

[35] Y.-C. Hsu, M. Acuña, S.M. Tahara, C.-A. Peng, Reduced phagocytosis of colloidal carriers using soluble CD47, Pharmaceutical Research 20 (10) (2003) 1539–1542, https://doi.org/10.1023/A:1026114713035.

[36] M.P. Nikitin, I.V. Zelepukin, V.O. Shipunova, I.L. Sokolov, S.M. Deyev, P.I. Nikitin, Enhancement of the blood-circulation time and performance of nanomedicines via the forced clearance of erythrocytes, Nature Biomedical Engineering 4 (7) (2020) 717–731, https://doi.org/10.1038/s41551-020-0581-2.

[37] A. Dirisala, S. Uchida, K. Toh, J. Li, S. Osawa, T.A. Tockary, X. Liu, S. Abbasi, K. Hayashi, Y. Mochida, et al., Transient stealth coating of liver sinusoidal wall by anchoring two-armed PEG for retargeting nanomedicines, Science Advances 6 (26) (2020) eabb8133, https://doi.org/10.1126/sciadv.abb8133. (Accessed 1 February 2024).

[38] A. Khalid, S. Persano, H. Shen, Y. Zhao, E. Blanco, M. Ferrari, J. Wolfram, Strategies for improving drug delivery: nanocarriers and microenvironmental priming, Expert Opinion on Drug Delivery 14 (7) (2017) 865–877, https://doi.org/10.1080/17425247.2017.1243527.

[39] S. Tenzer, D. Docter, J. Kuharev, A. Musyanovych, V. Fetz, R. Hecht, F. Schlenk, D. Fischer, K. Kiouptsi, C. Reinhardt, et al., Rapid formation of plasma protein corona critically affects nanoparticle pathophysiology, Nature Nanotechnology 8 (10) (2013) 772–781, https://doi.org/10.1038/nnano.2013.181.

[40] S. Ritz, S. Schöttler, N. Kotman, G. Baier, A. Musyanovych, J. Kuharev, K. Landfester, H. Schild, O. Jahn, S. Tenzer, et al., Protein corona of nanoparticles: distinct proteins regulate the cellular uptake, Biomacromolecules 16 (4) (2015) 1311–1321, https://doi.org/10.1021/acs.biomac.5b00108.

[41] H.H. Gustafson, D. Holt-Casper, D.W. Grainger, H. Ghandehari, Nanoparticle uptake: the phagocyte problem, Nano Today 10 (4) (2015) 487–510, https://doi.org/10.1016/j.nantod.2015.06.006.

[42] C.R. Jenkin, D. Rowley, The role of opsoins in the clearance of living and inert particles by cells of the reticuloendothelial system, Journal of Experimental Medicine 114 (3) (1961) 363–374, https://doi.org/10.1084/jem.114.3.363. (Accessed 2 January 2024).

[43] J.C. Pisano, J.T. Patterson, N.R. Di Luzio, Reticuloendothelial blockade: effect of puromycin on opsonin-dependent recovery, Science 162 (3853) (1968) 565–567, https://doi.org/10.1126/science.162.3853.565. (Accessed 1 February 2024).
[44] T.M. Saba, N.R. Di Luzio, Reticuloendothelial blockade and recovery as a function of opsonic activity, American Journal of Physiology-Legacy Content 216 (1) (1969) 197–205, https://doi.org/10.1152/ajplegacy.1969.216.1.197. (Accessed 1 February 2024).
[45] F. Mingozzi, X.M. Anguela, G. Pavani, Y. Chen, R.J. Davidson, D.J. Hui, M. Yazicioglu, L. Elkouby, C.J. Hinderer, A. Faella, et al., Overcoming preexisting humoral immunity to AAV using capsid decoys, Science Translational Medicine 5 (194) (2013), https://doi.org/10.1126/scitranslmed.3005795. (Accessed 1 February 2024).
[46] Z.C. Elmore, D.K. Oh, K.E. Simon, M.M. Fanous, A. Asokan, Rescuing AAV gene transfer from neutralizing antibodies with an IgG-degrading enzyme, JCI Insight 5 (19) (2020), https://doi.org/10.1172/jci.insight.139881.
[47] C. Leborgne, E. Barbon, J.M. Alexander, H. Hanby, S. Delignat, D.M. Cohen, F. Collaud, S. Muraleetharan, D. Lupo, J. Silverberg, et al., IgG-cleaving endopeptidase enables in vivo gene therapy in the presence of anti-AAV neutralizing antibodies, Nature Medicine 26 (7) (2020) 1096–1101, https://doi.org/10.1038/s41591-020-0911-7.
[48] S.C. Jordan, T. Lorant, J. Choi, C. Kjellman, L. Winstedt, M. Bengtsson, X. Zhang, T. Eich, M. Toyoda, B.-M. Eriksson, et al., IgG endopeptidase in highly sensitized patients undergoing transplantation, New England Journal of Medicine 377 (5) (2017) 442–453, https://doi.org/10.1056/NEJMoa1612567. (Accessed 1 February 2024).
[49] G. Berrecoso, J. Crecente-Campo, M.J. Alonso, Unveiling the pitfalls of the protein corona of polymeric drug nanocarriers, Drug Delivery and Translational Research 10 (3) (2020) 730–750, https://doi.org/10.1007/s13346-020-00745-0.
[50] E. Papini, R. Tavano, F. Mancin, Opsonins and dysopsonins of nanoparticles: facts, concepts, and methodological guidelines, Frontiers in Immunology 11 (2020) Review, https://doi.org/10.3389/fimmu.2020.567365.
[51] Q. Peng, S. Zhang, Q. Yang, T. Zhang, X.-Q. Wei, L. Jiang, C.-L. Zhang, Q.-M. Chen, Z.-R. Zhang, Y.-F. Lin, Preformed albumin corona, a protective coating for nanoparticles based drug delivery system, Biomaterials 34 (33) (2013) 8521–8530, https://doi.org/10.1016/j.biomaterials.2013.07.102.
[52] A. Vila, A. Sánchez, M. Tobío, P. Calvo, M.J. Alonso, Design of biodegradable particles for protein delivery, Journal of Controlled Release 78 (1) (2002) 15–24, https://doi.org/10.1016/S0168-3659(01)00486-2.
[53] K. Furumoto, J.-I. Yokoe, K.-i. Ogawara, S. Amano, M. Takaguchi, K. Higaki, T. Kai, T. Kimura, Effect of coupling of albumin onto surface of PEG liposome on its in vivo disposition, International Journal of Pharmaceutics 329 (1) (2007) 110–116, https://doi.org/10.1016/j.ijpharm.2006.08.026.
[54] N. Bertrand, P. Grenier, M. Mahmoudi, E.M. Lima, E.A. Appel, F. Dormont, J.-M. Lim, R. Karnik, R. Langer, O.C. Farokhzad, Mechanistic understanding of in vivo protein corona formation on polymeric nanoparticles and impact on pharmacokinetics, Nature Communications 8 (1) (2017) 777, https://doi.org/10.1038/s41467-017-00600-w.

[55] L.A. Rojas, G.N. Condezo, R. Moreno, C.A. Fajardo, M. Arias-Badia, C. San Martín, R. Alemany, Albumin-binding adenoviruses circumvent pre-existing neutralizing antibodies upon systemic delivery, Journal of Controlled Release 237 (2016) 78–88, https://doi.org/10.1016/j.jconrel.2016.07.004.
[56] T. Takeuchi, Y. Kitayama, R. Sasao, T. Yamada, K. Toh, Y. Matsumoto, K. Kataoka, Molecularly imprinted nanogels acquire stealth in situ by cloaking themselves with native dysopsonic proteins, Angewandte Chemie International Edition 56 (25) (2017) 7088–7092, https://doi.org/10.1002/anie.201700647. (Accessed 1 February 2024).
[57] A. Poma, A.P.F. Turner, S.A. Piletsky, Advances in the manufacture of MIP nanoparticles, Trends in Biotechnology 28 (12) (2010) 629–637, https://doi.org/10.1016/j.tibtech.2010.08.006.
[58] A. Poma, A. Guerreiro, M.J. Whitcombe, E.V. Piletska, A.P.F. Turner, S.A. Piletsky, Solid-phase synthesis of molecularly imprinted polymer nanoparticles with a reusable Template–"Plastic antibodies", Advanced Functional Materials 23 (22) (2013) 2821–2827, https://doi.org/10.1002/adfm.201202397. (Accessed 1 February 2021).
[59] A. Poma, M. Whitcombe, S. Piletsky, Plastic antibodies, in: S.A. Piletsky, M.J. Whitcombe (Eds.), Designing Receptors for the Next Generation of Biosensors, Springer Berlin Heidelberg, 2013, pp. 105–129.
[60] S. Subrahmanyam, A. Guerreiro, A. Poma, E. Moczko, E. Piletska, S. Piletsky, Optimisation of experimental conditions for synthesis of high affinity MIP nanoparticles, European Polymer Journal 49 (1) (2013) 100–105, https://doi.org/10.1016/j.eurpolymj.2012.09.022.
[61] A. Poma, A. Guerreiro, S. Caygill, E. Moczko, S. Piletsky, Automatic reactor for solid-phase synthesis of molecularly imprinted polymeric nanoparticles (MIP NPs) in water, RSC Advances 4 (8) (2014) 4203–4206, https://doi.org/10.1039/c3ra46838k.
[62] R. Liu, A. Poma, Advances in molecularly imprinted polymers as drug delivery systems, Molecules 26 (2021).
[63] X. Ma, J.C. Knowles, A. Poma, Biodegradable and sustainable synthetic antibodies—a perspective, Pharmaceutics 15 (2023).
[64] E. Moczko, A. Poma, A. Guerreiro, I. Perez de Vargas Sansalvador, S. Caygill, F. Canfarotta, M.J. Whitcombe, S. Piletsky, Surface-modified multifunctional MIP nanoparticles, Nanoscale 5 (9) (2013) 3733–3741, https://doi.org/10.1039/C3NR00354J.
[65] A. Guerreiro, A. Poma, K. Karim, E. Moczko, J. Takarada, I.P. de Vargas-Sansalvador, N. Turner, E. Piletska, C.S. de Magalhães, N. Glazova, et al., Influence of surface-imprinted nanoparticles on trypsin activity, Advanced Healthcare Materials 3 (9) (2014) 1426–1429, https://doi.org/10.1002/adhm.201300634.
[66] K. Muzyka, K. Karim, A. Guerreiro, A. Poma, S. Piletsky, Optimisation of the synthesis of vancomycin-selective molecularly imprinted polymer nanoparticles using automatic photoreactor, Nanoscale Research Letters 9 (1) (2014) 154, https://doi.org/10.1186/1556-276x-9-154.
[67] A. Poma, H. Brahmbhatt, J.K. Watts, N.W. Turner, Nucleoside-tailored molecularly imprinted polymeric nanoparticles (MIP NPs), Macromolecules 47 (18) (2014) 6322–6330, https://doi.org/10.1021/ma501530c.
[68] A. Poma, H. Brahmbhatt, H.M. Pendergraff, J.K. Watts, N.W. Turner, Generation of novel hybrid aptamer-molecularly imprinted polymeric

nanoparticles, Advanced Materials 27 (4) (2015) 750–758, https://doi.org/10.1002/adma.201404235.
[69] H. Brahmbhatt, A. Poma, H.M. Pendergraff, J.K. Watts, N.W. Turner, Improvement of DNA recognition through molecular imprinting: hybrid oligomer imprinted polymeric nanoparticles (oligoMIP NPs), Biomaterials Science 4 (2) (2016) 281–287, https://doi.org/10.1039/C5BM00341E.
[70] T.S. Bedwell, N. Anjum, Y. Ma, J. Czulak, A. Poma, E. Piletska, M.J. Whitcombe, S.A. Piletsky, New protocol for optimisation of polymer composition for imprinting of peptides and proteins, RSC Advances 9 (48) (2019) 27849–27855, https://doi.org/10.1039/C9RA05009D.
[71] Y. Ohara, T. Oda, K. Yamada, S. Hashimoto, Y. Akashi, R. Miyamoto, A. Kobayashi, K. Fukunaga, R. Sasaki, N. Ohkohchi, Effective delivery of chemotherapeutic nanoparticles by depleting host Kupffer cells, International Journal of Cancer 131 (10) (2012) 2402–2410, https://doi.org/10.1002/ijc.27502. (Accessed 1 February 2024).
[72] N. Van Rooijen, A. Sanders, Kupffer cell depletion by liposome-delivered drugs: comparative activity of intracellular clodronate, propamidine, and ethylenediaminetetraacetic acid, Hepatology 23 (5) (1996) 1239–1243, https://doi.org/10.1002/hep.510230544. (Accessed 1 February 2024).
[73] P. Diagaradjane, A. Deorukhkar, J.G. Gelovani, D.M. Maru, S. Krishnan, Gadolinium chloride augments tumor-specific imaging of targeted quantum dots in vivo, ACS Nano 4 (7) (2010) 4131–4141, https://doi.org/10.1021/nn901919w.
[74] E.F. Fowler, A.W. Thomson, Effect of carrageenan on activity of the mononuclear phagocyte system in the mouse, British Journal of Experimental Pathology 59 (2) (1978) 213–219.
[75] I.B. Magaña, R.B. Yendluri, P. Adhikari, G.P. Goodrich, J.A. Schwartz, E.A. Sherer, D.P. O'Neal, Suppression of the reticuloendothelial system using λ-carrageenan to prolong the circulation of gold nanoparticles, Therapeutic Delivery 6 (7) (2015) 777–783, https://doi.org/10.4155/tde.15.33. (Accessed 1 February 2024).
[76] D. Gemsa, M. Seitz, W. Kramer, G. Till, K. Resch, The effects of phagocytosis, dextran sulfate, and cell damage on PGE1 sensitivity and PGE1 production of macrophages, The Journal of Immunology 120 (4) (1978) 1187–1194, https://doi.org/10.4049/jimmunol.120.4.1187. (Accessed 2 January 2024).
[77] P. Cai, B.S. Kaphalia, G.A.S. Ansari, Methyl palmitate: inhibitor of phagocytosis in primary rat Kupffer cells, Toxicology 210 (2) (2005) 197–204, https://doi.org/10.1016/j.tox.2005.02.001.
[78] S. Sarkar, M.F. Khan, B.S. Kaphalia, G.A.S. Ansari, Methyl palmitate inhibits lipopolysaccharide-stimulated phagocytic activity of rat peritoneal macrophages, Journal of Biochemical and Molecular Toxicology 20 (6) (2006) 302–308, https://doi.org/10.1002/jbt.20150. (Accessed 1 February 2024).
[79] N.V. Rooijen, A. Sanders, Liposome mediated depletion of macrophages: mechanism of action, preparation of liposomes and applications, Journal of Immunological Methods 174 (1) (1994) 83–93, https://doi.org/10.1016/0022-1759(94)90012-4.
[80] N. van Rooijen, Liposomes for targeting of antigens and drugs: immunoadjuvant activity and liposome-mediated depletion of macrophages, Journal of Drug Targeting 16 (7–8) (2008) 529–534, https://doi.org/10.1080/10611860802228426.

[81] R. van, A. Sanders, Elimination, blocking, and activation of macrophages: three of a kind? Journal of Leukocyte Biology 62 (6) (1997) 702–709, https://doi.org/10.1002/jlb.62.6.702. (Accessed 1 February 2024).
[82] D. Simberg, T. Duza, J.H. Park, M. Essler, J. Pilch, L. Zhang, A.M. Derfus, M. Yang, R.M. Hoffman, S. Bhatia, et al., Biomimetic amplification of nanoparticle homing to tumors, Proceedings of the National Academy of Sciences 104 (3) (2007) 932–936, https://doi.org/10.1073/pnas.0610298104. (Accessed 1 February 2024).
[83] A.J. Tavares, W. Poon, Y.-N. Zhang, Q. Dai, R. Besla, D. Ding, B. Ouyang, A. Li, J. Chen, G. Zheng, et al., Effect of removing Kupffer cells on nanoparticle tumor delivery, Proceedings of the National Academy of Sciences 114 (51) (2017) E10871–E10880, https://doi.org/10.1073/pnas.1713390114. (Accessed 1 February 2024).
[84] G. Schiedner, S. Hertel, M. Johnston, V. Dries, N. van Rooijen, S. Kochanek, Selective depletion or blockade of Kupffer cells leads to enhanced and prolonged hepatic transgene expression using high-capacity adenoviral vectors, Molecular Therapy 7 (1) (2003) 35–43, https://doi.org/10.1016/S1525-0016(02)00017-5. (Accessed 1 February 2024).
[85] G. Wolff, S. Worgall, N. van Rooijen, W.R. Song, B.G. Harvey, R.G. Crystal, Enhancement of in vivo adenovirus-mediated gene transfer and expression by prior depletion of tissue macrophages in the target organ, Journal of Virology 71 (1) (1997) 624–629, https://doi.org/10.1128/jvi.71.1.624-629.1997.
[86] Z. Li, X. Xu, X. Feng, P.M. Murphy, The macrophage-depleting agent clodronate promotes durable hematopoietic chimerism and donor-specific skin allograft tolerance in mice, Scientific Reports 6 (1) (2016) 22143, https://doi.org/10.1038/srep22143.
[87] M.J. Hardonk, F.W.J. Dijkhuis, C.E. Hulstaert, J. Koudstaal, Heterogeneity of rat liver and spleen macrophages in gadolinium chloride–induced elimination and repopulation, Journal of Leukocyte Biology 52 (3) (1992) 296–302, https://doi.org/10.1002/jlb.52.3.296. (Accessed 2 January 2024).
[88] D. Rüttinger, B. Vollmar, G.A. Wanner, K. Messmer, <em>In vivo</em> assessment of hepatic alterations following gadolinium chloride-induced Kupffer cell blockade, Journal of Hepatology 25 (6) (1996) 960–967, https://doi.org/10.1016/S0168-8278(96)80302-3. (Accessed 1 February 2024).
[89] A. Spencer, S. Wilson, E. Harpur, Gadolinium chloride toxicity in the mouse, Human & Experimental Toxicology 17 (11) (1998) 633–637, https://doi.org/10.1177/096032719801701108. (Accessed 1 February 2024).
[90] J. Wolfram, S. Nizzero, H. Liu, F. Li, G. Zhang, Z. Li, H. Shen, E. Blanco, M. Ferrari, A chloroquine-induced macrophage-preconditioning strategy for improved nanodelivery, Scientific Reports 7 (1) (2017) 13738, https://doi.org/10.1038/s41598-017-14221-2.
[91] J. Pelt, S. Busatto, M. Ferrari, E.A. Thompson, K. Mody, J. Wolfram, Chloroquine and nanoparticle drug delivery: a promising combination, Pharmacology & Therapeutics 191 (2018) 43–49, https://doi.org/10.1016/j.pharmthera.2018.06.007.
[92] R. Noy, J.W. Pollard, Tumor-associated macrophages: from mechanisms to therapy, Immunity 41 (1) (2014) 49–61, https://doi.org/10.1016/j.immuni.2014.06.010. (Accessed 1 February 2024).
[93] M.A. Miller, Y.-R. Zheng, S. Gadde, C. Pfirschke, H. Zope, C. Engblom, R.H. Kohler, Y. Iwamoto, K.S. Yang, B. Askevold, et al., Tumour-associated

macrophages act as a slow-release reservoir of nano-therapeutic Pt(IV) pro-drug, Nature Communications 6 (1) (2015) 8692, https://doi.org/10.1038/ncomms9692.
[94] T. Tanei, F. Leonard, X. Liu, J.F. Alexander, Y. Saito, M. Ferrari, B. Godin, K. Yokoi, Redirecting transport of nanoparticle albumin-bound paclitaxel to macrophages enhances therapeutic efficacy against liver metastases, Cancer Research 76 (2) (2016) 429–439, https://doi.org/10.1158/0008-5472.CAN-15-1576. (Accessed 2 January 2024).
[95] Z. Wan, L. Zhao, F. Lu, X. Gao, Y. Dong, Y. Zhao, M. Wei, G. Yang, C. Xing, L. Liu, Mononuclear phagocyte system blockade improves therapeutic exosome delivery to the myocardium, Theranostics 10 (1) (2020) 218–230, https://doi.org/10.7150/thno.38198.
[96] D. Simberg, Iron oxide nanoparticles and the mechanisms of immune recognition of nanomedicines, Nanomedicine 11 (7) (2016) 741–743, https://doi.org/10.2217/nnm.16.30. (Accessed 1 February 2024).
[97] M.R.A. Abdollah, T.J. Carter, C. Jones, T.L. Kalber, V. Rajkumar, B. Tolner, C. Gruettner, M. Zaw-Thin, J. Baguña Torres, M. Ellis, et al., Fucoidan prolongs the circulation time of dextran-coated iron oxide nanoparticles, ACS Nano 12 (2) (2018) 1156–1169, https://doi.org/10.1021/acsnano.7b06734.
[98] H.J. Haisma, J.A.A.M. Kamps, G.K. Kamps, J.A. Plantinga, M.G. Rots, A.R. Bellu, Polyinosinic acid enhances delivery of adenovirus vectors in vivo by preventing sequestration in liver macrophages, Journal of General Virology 89 (5) (2008) 1097–1105, https://doi.org/10.1099/vir.0.83495-0.
[99] M.R.A. Abdollah, T. Kalber, B. Tolner, P. Southern, J.C. Bear, M. Robson, R.B. Pedley, I.P. Parkin, Q.A. Pankhurst, P. Mulholland, et al., Prolonging the circulatory retention of SPIONs using dextran sulfate: in vivo tracking achieved by functionalisation with near-infrared dyes, Faraday Discussions 175 (0) (2014) 41–58, https://doi.org/10.1039/C4FD00114A.
[100] H.-Y. Hsu, S.-L. Chiu, M.-H. Wen, K.-Y. Chen, K.-F. Hua, Ligands of macrophage scavenger receptor induce cytokine expression via differential modulation of protein kinase signaling pathways, Journal of Biological Chemistry 276 (31) (2001) 28719–28730, https://doi.org/10.1074/jbc.M011117200. (Accessed 1 February 2024).
[101] S. Marshall-Clarke, J.E. Downes, I.R. Haga, A.G. Bowie, P. Borrow, J.L. Pennock, R.K. Grencis, P. Rothwell, Polyinosinic acid is a ligand for toll-like receptor 3, Journal of Biological Chemistry 282 (34) (2007) 24759–24766, https://doi.org/10.1074/jbc.M700188200. (Accessed 1 February 2024).
[102] K. Walton, Experiments with dextran sulphate as an anticoagulant, Proceedings of the Royal Society of Medicine 44 (7) (1951) 563–564.
[103] J. Kzhyshkowska, A. Gratchev, S. Goerdt, Stabilin-1, a homeostatic scavenger receptor with multiple functions, Journal of Cellular and Molecular Medicine 10 (3) (2006) 635–649, https://doi.org/10.1111/j.1582-4934.2006.tb00425.x. (Accessed 1 February 2024).
[104] R.J. Allen, B. Mathew, K.G. Rice, PEG-peptide inhibition of scavenger receptor uptake of nanoparticles by the liver, Molecular Pharmaceutics 15 (9) (2018) 3881–3891, https://doi.org/10.1021/acs.molpharmaceut.8b00355.
[105] N.J. Baumhover, J.T. Duskey, S. Khargharia, C.W. White, S.T. Crowley, R.J. Allen, K.G. Rice, Structure–activity relationship of PEGylated polylysine peptides as scavenger receptor inhibitors for non-viral gene

delivery, Molecular Pharmaceutics 12 (12) (2015) 4321–4328, https://doi.org/10.1021/acs.molpharmaceut.5b00513.
[106] D. Liu, A. Mori, L. Huang, Role of liposome size and RES blockade in controlling biodistribution and tumor uptake of GM1-containing liposomes, Biochimica et Biophysica Acta (BBA) - Biomembranes 1104 (1) (1992) 95–101, https://doi.org/10.1016/0005-2736(92)90136-A.
[107] Y.J. Kao, R.L. Juliano, Interactions of liposomes with the reticuloendothelial system effects of reticuloendothelial blockade on the clearance of large unilamellar vesicles, Biochimica et Biophysica Acta (BBA) - General Subjects 677 (3) (1981) 453–461, https://doi.org/10.1016/0304-4165(81)90259-2.
[108] R.L. Souhami, H.M. Patel, B.E. Ryman, The effect of reticuloendothelial blockade on the blood clearance and tissue distribution of liposomes, Biochimica et Biophysica Acta (BBA) - General Subjects 674 (3) (1981) 354–371, https://doi.org/10.1016/0304-4165(81)90366-4.
[109] R.T. Proffitt, L.E. Williams, C.A. Presant, G.W. Tin, J.A. Uliana, R.C. Gamble, J.D. Baldeschwieler, Liposomal blockade of the reticuloendothelial system: improved tumor imaging with small unilamellar vesicles, Science 220 (4596) (1983) 502–505, https://doi.org/10.1126/science.6836294. (Accessed 1 February 2024).
[110] X. Sun, X. Yan, O. Jacobson, W. Sun, Z. Wang, X. Tong, Y. Xia, D. Ling, X. Chen, Improved tumor uptake by optimizing liposome based RES blockade strategy, Theranostics 7 (2) (2017) 319–328, https://doi.org/10.7150/thno.18078.
[111] T. Liu, H. Choi, R. Zhou, I.W. Chen, RES blockade: a strategy for boosting efficiency of nanoparticle drug, Nano Today 10 (1) (2015) 11–21, https://doi.org/10.1016/j.nantod.2014.12.003.
[112] L. Liu, T.K. Hitchens, Q. Ye, Y. Wu, B. Barbe, D.E. Prior, W.F. Li, F.-C. Yeh, L.M. Foley, D.J. Bain, et al., Decreased reticuloendothelial system clearance and increased blood half-life and immune cell labeling for nano- and micron-sized superparamagnetic iron-oxide particles upon pre-treatment with Intralipid, Biochimica et Biophysica Acta (BBA) - General Subjects 1830 (6) (2013) 3447–3453, https://doi.org/10.1016/j.bbagen.2013.01.021.
[113] I.M. Murray, The mechanism of blockade of the reticuloendothelial system, Journal of Experimental Medicine 117 (1) (1963) 139–147, https://doi.org/10.1084/jem.117.1.139. (Accessed 2 February 2024).
[114] J. Dave, H.M. Patel, Differentiation in hepatic and splenic phagocytic activity during reticuloendothelial blockade with cholesterol-free and cholesterol-rich liposomes, Biochimica et Biophysica Acta (BBA) - Molecular Cell Research 888 (2) (1986) 184–190, https://doi.org/10.1016/0167-4889(86)90020-0.
[115] R.L. Souhami, The effect of colloidal carbon on the organ distribution of sheep red cells and the immune response, Immunology 22 (4) (1972) 685–694.
[116] J.B. Bradfield, Control of spillover. The importance of kupffer-cell function in clinical medicine, The Lancet 304 (7885) (1974) 883–886, https://doi.org/10.1016/S0140-6736(74)91213-6.
[117] N.R.M. Saunders, M.S. Paolini, O.S. Fenton, L. Poul, J. Devalliere, F. Mpambani, A. Darmon, M. Bergère, O. Jibault, M. Germain, et al., A nanoprimer to improve the systemic delivery of siRNA and mRNA, Nano Letters 20 (6) (2020) 4264–4269, https://doi.org/10.1021/acs.nanolett.0c00752.

[118] J. Snoeys, G. Mertens, J. Lievens, T. van Berkel, D. Collen, E.A.L. Biessen, B. De Geest, Lipid emulsions potently increase transgene expression in hepatocytes after adenoviral transfer, Molecular Therapy 13 (1) (2006) 98–107, https://doi.org/10.1016/j.ymthe.2005.06.477.

[119] B. Ouyang, W. Poon, Y.-N. Zhang, Z.P. Lin, B.R. Kingston, A.J. Tavares, Y. Zhang, J. Chen, M.S. Valic, A.M. Syed, et al., The dose threshold for nanoparticle tumour delivery, Nature Materials 19 (12) (2020) 1362–1371, https://doi.org/10.1038/s41563-020-0755-z.

[120] A.B. Mirkasymov, I.V. Zelepukin, P.I. Nikitin, M.P. Nikitin, S.M. Deyev, In vivo blockade of mononuclear phagocyte system with solid nanoparticles: efficiency and affecting factors, Journal of Controlled Release 330 (2021) 111–118, https://doi.org/10.1016/j.jconrel.2020.12.004.

[121] M. Longmire, P.L. Choyke, H. Kobayashi, Clearance properties of nano-sized particles and molecules as imaging agents: considerations and caveats, Nanomedicine 3 (5) (2008) 703–717, https://doi.org/10.2217/17435889.3.5.703. (Accessed 2 February 2024).

[122] E. Sadauskas, G. Danscher, M. Stoltenberg, U. Vogel, A. Larsen, H. Wallin, Protracted elimination of gold nanoparticles from mouse liver, Nanomedicine: Nanotechnology, Biology and Medicine 5 (2) (2009) 162–169, https://doi.org/10.1016/j.nano.2008.11.002.

[123] A.R. Crow, A.H. Lazarus, The mechanisms of action of intravenous immunoglobulin and polyclonal anti-D immunoglobulin in the amelioration of immune thrombocytopenic purpura: what do we really know? Transfusion Medicine Reviews 22 (2) (2008) 103–116, https://doi.org/10.1016/j.tmrv.2007.12.001.

[124] A.B. Ryder, J.C. Zimring, J.E. Hendrickson, Factors influencing RBC alloimmunization: lessons learned from murine models, Transfusion Medicine and Hemotherapy 41 (6) (2014) 406–419, https://doi.org/10.1159/000368995. (Accessed 2 February 2024).

[125] S. Kontos, I.C. Kourtis, K.Y. Dane, J.A. Hubbell, Engineering antigens for in situ erythrocyte binding induces T-cell deletion, Proceedings of the National Academy of Sciences 110 (1) (2013) E60–E68, https://doi.org/10.1073/pnas.1216353110. (Accessed 2 February 2024).

[126] M. Naito, H. Chaya, K. Toh, B.S. Kim, K. Hayashi, S. Fukushima, T. Nagata, T. Yokota, K. Kataoka, K. Miyata, Structural tuning of oligonucleotides for enhanced blood circulation properties of unit polyion complexes prepared from two-branched poly(ethylene glycol)-block-poly(l-lysine), Journal of Controlled Release 330 (2021) 812–820, https://doi.org/10.1016/j.jconrel.2021.01.001.

[127] S. Watanabe, K. Hayashi, K. Toh, H.J. Kim, X. Liu, H. Chaya, S. Fukushima, K. Katsushima, Y. Kondo, S. Uchida, et al., In vivo rendezvous of small nucleic acid drugs with charge-matched block catiomers to target cancers, Nature Communications 10 (1) (2019) 1894, https://doi.org/10.1038/s41467-019-09856-w.

[128] A. Ben-Zvi, B. Lacoste, E. Kur, B.J. Andreone, Y. Mayshar, H. Yan, C. Gu, Mfsd2a is critical for the formation and function of the blood-brain barrier, Nature 509 (7501) (2014) 507–511, https://doi.org/10.1038/nature13324.

[129] B. Oller-Salvia, M. Sánchez-Navarro, E. Giralt, M. Teixidó, Blood–brain barrier shuttle peptides: an emerging paradigm for brain delivery, Chemical Society Reviews 45 (17) (2016) 4690–4707, https://doi.org/10.1039/c6cs00076b.

[130] L.I. Goulatis, E.V. Shusta, Protein engineering approaches for regulating blood–brain barrier transcytosis, Current Opinion in Structural Biology 45 (2017) 109–115, https://doi.org/10.1016/j.sbi.2016.12.005.
[131] X. Dong, Current strategies for brain drug delivery, Theranostics 8 (6) (2018) 1481–1493, https://doi.org/10.7150/thno.21254.
[132] Y. Zhou, Z. Peng, E.S. Seven, R.M. Leblanc, Crossing the blood-brain barrier with nanoparticles, Journal of Controlled Release 270 (2018) 290–303, https://doi.org/10.1016/j.jconrel.2017.12.015.
[133] I.A. Simpson, N.M. Appel, M. Hokari, J. Oki, G.D. Holman, F. Maher, E.M. Koehler-Stec, S.J. Vannucci, Q.R. Smith, Blood—brain barrier glucose transporter, Journal of Neurochemistry 72 (1) (1999) 238–247, https://doi.org/10.1046/j.1471-4159.1999.0720238.x.
[134] D. Schubert, Glucose metabolism and Alzheimer's disease, Ageing Research Reviews 4 (2) (2005) 240–257, https://doi.org/10.1016/j.arr.2005.02.003.
[135] Y. Uchida, S. Ohtsuki, Y. Katsukura, C. Ikeda, T. Suzuki, J. Kamiie, T. Terasaki, Quantitative targeted absolute proteomics of human blood–brain barrier transporters and receptors, Journal of Neurochemistry 117 (2) (2011) 333–345, https://doi.org/10.1111/j.1471-4159.2011.07208.x.
[136] J. Abramson, I. Smirnova, V. Kasho, G. Verner, H.R. Kaback, S. Iwata, Structure and mechanism of the lactose permease of *Escherichia coli*, Science 301 (5633) (2003) 610–615, https://doi.org/10.1126/science.1088196.
[137] P. Cunningham, I. Afzal-Ahmed, R.J. Naftalin, Docking studies show that D-glucose and quercetin slide through the transporter GLUT1, Journal of Biological Chemistry 281 (9) (2006) 5797–5803, https://doi.org/10.1074/jbc.m509422200.
[138] A.J. Cura, A. Carruthers, Role of monosaccharide transport proteins in carbohydrate assimilation, distribution, metabolism, and homeostasis, Comprehensive Physiology 2 (2) (2012) 863–914, https://doi.org/10.1002/cphy.c110024.
[139] M. Mueckler, B. Thorens, The SLC2 (GLUT) family of membrane transporters, Molecular Aspects of Medicine 34 (2–3) (2013) 121–138, https://doi.org/10.1016/j.mam.2012.07.001.
[140] M.-S. Park, Molecular dynamics simulations of the human glucose transporter GLUT1, PLoS One 10 (4) (2015), https://doi.org/10.1371/journal.pone.0125361.
[141] T. Galochkina, M. Ng Fuk Chong, L. Challali, S. Abbar, C. Etchebest, New insights into GluT1 mechanics during glucose transfer, Scientific Reports 9 (1) (2019) 998, https://doi.org/10.1038/s41598-018-37367-z.
[142] Y. Qin, W. Fan, H. Chen, N. Yao, W. Tang, J. Tang, W. Yuan, R. Kuai, Z. Zhang, Y. Wu, et al., In vitro and in vivo investigation of glucose-mediated brain-targeting liposomes, Journal of Drug Targeting 18 (7) (2010) 536–549, https://doi.org/10.3109/10611861003587235.
[143] F. Xie, N. Yao, Y. Qin, Q. Zhang, H. Chen, M. Yuan, J. Tang, X. Li, W. Fan, Q. Zhang, et al., Investigation of glucose-modified liposomes using polyethylene glycols with different chain lengths as the linkers for brain targeting, International Journal of Nanomedicine 7 (2012) 163–175, https://doi.org/10.2147/IJN.S23771.
[144] R. Gromnicova, H.A. Davies, P. Sreekanthreddy, I.A. Romero, T. Lund, I.M. Roitt, J.B. Phillips, D.K. Male, Glucose-coated gold nanoparticles transfer across human brain endothelium and enter astrocytes in vitro,

PLoS One 8 (12) (2013) e81043, https://doi.org/10.1371/journal.pone.0081043.
[145] Y. Anraku, H. Kuwahara, Y. Fukusato, A. Mizoguchi, T. Ishii, K. Nitta, Y. Matsumoto, K. Toh, K. Miyata, S. Uchida, et al., Glycaemic control boosts glucosylated nanocarrier crossing the BBB into the brain, Nature Communications 8 (1) (2017), https://doi.org/10.1038/s41467-017-00952-3.
[146] A. Dahlin, J. Royall, J.G. Hohmann, J. Wang, Expression profiling of the solute carrier gene family in the mouse brain, Journal of Pharmacology and Experimental Therapeutics 329 (2) (2009) 558–570, https://doi.org/10.1124/jpet.108.149831.
[147] X. Gao, F. Lu, L. Zhou, S. Dang, L. Sun, X. Li, J. Wang, Y. Shi, Structure and mechanism of an amino acid antiporter, Science 324 (5934) (2009) 1565–1568, https://doi.org/10.1126/science.1173654.
[148] P.L. Shaffer, A. Goehring, A. Shankaranarayanan, E. Gouaux, Structure and mechanism of a Na+-independent amino acid transporter, Science 325 (5943) (2009) 1010–1014, https://doi.org/10.1126/science.1176088.
[149] K.E.J. Jungnickel, J.L. Parker, S. Newstead, Structural basis for amino acid transport by the CAT family of SLC7 transporters, Nature Communications 9 (1) (2018) 550, https://doi.org/10.1038/s41467-018-03066-6.
[150] E.M. del Amo, A. Urtti, M. Yliperttula, Pharmacokinetic role of L-type amino acid transporters LAT1 and LAT2, European Journal of Pharmaceutical Sciences 35 (3) (2008) 161–174, https://doi.org/10.1016/j.ejps.2008.06.015.
[151] D. Fotiadis, Y. Kanai, M. Palacín, The SLC3 and SLC7 families of amino acid transporters, Molecular Aspects of Medicine 34 (2–3) (2013) 139–158, https://doi.org/10.1016/j.mam.2012.10.007.
[152] C. Colas, P.M.-U. Ung, A. Schlessinger, SLC transporters: structure, function, and drug discovery, Medchemcomm 7 (6) (2016) 1069–1081, https://doi.org/10.1039/C6MD00005C.
[153] D. Dickens, G.N. Chiduza, G.S.A. Wright, M. Pirmohamed, S.V. Antonyuk, S.S. Hasnain, Modulation of LAT1 (SLC7A5) transporter activity and stability by membrane cholesterol, Scientific Reports 7 (2017) 43580, https://doi.org/10.1038/srep43580.
[154] P. Kharya, A. Jain, A. Gulbake, S. Shilpi, A. Jain, P. Hurkat, S. Majumdar, S.K. Jain, Phenylalanine-coupled solid lipid nanoparticles for brain tumor targeting, Journal of Nanoparticle Research 15 (11) (2013) 2022, https://doi.org/10.1007/s11051-013-2022-6.
[155] L. Li, X. Di, S. Zhang, Q. Kan, H. Liu, T. Lu, Y. Wang, Q. Fu, J. Sun, Z. He, Large amino acid transporter 1 mediated glutamate modified docetaxel-loaded liposomes for glioma targeting, Colloids and Surfaces B: Biointerfaces 141 (2016) 260–267, https://doi.org/10.1016/j.colsurfb.2016.01.041.
[156] D.A. Gonzalez-Carter, Z.Y. Ong, C.M. McGilvery, I.E. Dunlop, D.T. Dexter, A.E. Porter, L-DOPA functionalized, multi-branched gold nanoparticles as brain-targeted nano-vehicles, Nanomedicine: Nanotechnology, Biology and Medicine 15 (1) (2019) 1–11, https://doi.org/10.1016/j.nano.2018.08.011.
[157] W.M. Pardridge, Blood–brain barrier endogenous transporters as therapeutic targets: a new model for small molecule CNS drug discovery, Expert Opinion on Therapeutic Targets 19 (8) (2015) 1059–1072, https://doi.org/10.1517/14728222.2015.1042364.

[158] E. Traiffort, S. O'Regan, M. Ruat, The choline transporter-like family SLC44: properties and roles in human diseases, Molecular Aspects of Medicine 34 (2–3) (2013) 646–654, https://doi.org/10.1016/j.mam.2012.10.011.
[159] J. Li, L. Zhou, D. Ye, S. Huang, K. Shao, R. Huang, L. Han, Y. Liu, S. Liu, L. Ye, et al., Choline-derivate-modified nanoparticles for brain-targeting gene delivery, Advanced Materials 23 (39) (2011) 4516–4520, https://doi.org/10.1002/adma.201101899.
[160] J. Li, Y. Guo, Y. Kuang, S. An, H. Ma, C. Jiang, Choline transporter-targeting and co-delivery system for glioma therapy, Biomaterials 34 (36) (2013) 9142–9148, https://doi.org/10.1016/j.biomaterials.2013.08.030.
[161] D. Wu, M. Qin, D. Xu, L. Wang, C. Liu, J. Ren, G. Zhou, C. Chen, F. Yang, Y. Li, et al., Drug delivery: a bioinspired platform for effective delivery of protein therapeutics to the central nervous system, Advanced Materials 31 (18) (2019) 1807557, https://doi.org/10.1002/adma.201970127.
[162] E.X. Albuquerque, E.F.R. Pereira, M. Alkondon, S.W. Rogers, Mammalian nicotinic acetylcholine receptors: from structure to function, Physiological Reviews 89 (1) (2009) 73–120, https://doi.org/10.1152/physrev.00015.2008.
[163] J.A. Dani, Neuronal nicotinic acetylcholine receptor structure and function and response to nicotine, International Review of Neurobiology 124 (2015) 3–19, https://doi.org/10.1016/bs.irn.2015.07.001.
[164] T.L. Lentz, T.G. Burrage, A.L. Smith, J. Crick, G.H. Tignor, Is the acetylcholine receptor a rabies virus receptor? Science 215 (4529) (1982) 182–184, https://doi.org/10.1126/science.7053569.
[165] R. Huey, S. Hawthorne, P. McCarron, The potential use of rabies virus glycoprotein-derived peptides to facilitate drug delivery into the central nervous system: a mini review, Journal of Drug Targeting 25 (5) (2016) 379–385, https://doi.org/10.1080/1061186x.2016.1223676.
[166] Y. Liu, R. Huang, L. Han, W. Ke, K. Shao, L. Ye, J. Lou, C. Jiang, Brain-targeting gene delivery and cellular internalization mechanisms for modified rabies virus glycoprotein RVG29 nanoparticles, Biomaterials 30 (25) (2009) 4195–4202, https://doi.org/10.1016/j.biomaterials.2009.02.051.
[167] L. You, J. Wang, T. Liu, Y. Zhang, X. Han, T. Wang, S. Guo, T. Dong, J. Xu, G.J. Anderson, et al., Targeted brain delivery of rabies virus glycoprotein 29-modified deferoxamine-loaded nanoparticles reverses functional deficits in parkinsonian mice, ACS Nano 12 (5) (2018) 4123–4139, https://doi.org/10.1021/acsnano.7b08172.
[168] M. Kaksonen, A. Roux, Mechanisms of clathrin-mediated endocytosis, Nature Reviews Molecular Cell Biology 19 (5) (2018) 313–326, https://doi.org/10.1038/nrm.2017.132.
[169] J. Wauman, L. Zabeau, J. Tavernier, The leptin receptor complex: heavier than expected? Frontiers in Endocrinology 8 (2017) 30, https://doi.org/10.3389/fendo.2017.00030.
[170] D. Gonzalez-Carter, A.E. Goode, R. Fiammengo, I.E. Dunlop, D.T. Dexter, A.E. Porter, Inhibition of leptin–ObR interaction does not prevent leptin translocation across a human blood–brain barrier model, Journal of Neuroendocrinology 28 (6) (2016), https://doi.org/10.1111/jne.12392.
[171] G. Tosi, L. Badiali, B. Ruozi, A.V. Vergoni, L. Bondioli, A. Ferrari, F. Rivasi, F. Forni, M.A. Vandelli, Can leptin-derived sequence-modified nanoparticles be suitable tools for brain delivery? Nanomedicine 7 (3) (2012) 365–382, https://doi.org/10.2217/nnm.11.98.
[172] X. Tian, S. Nyberg, P. S Sharp, J. Madsen, N. Daneshpour, S.P. Armes, J. Berwick, M. Azzouz, P. Shaw, N.J. Abbott, et al., LRP-1-mediated

intracellular antibody delivery to the Central Nervous System, Scientific Reports 5 (2015) 11990, https://doi.org/10.1038/srep11990.
[173] A. Joseph, C. Contini, D. Cecchin, S. Nyberg, L. Ruiz-Perez, J. Gaitzsch, G. Fullstone, X. Tian, J. Azizi, J. Preston, et al., Chemotactic synthetic vesicles: design and applications in blood-brain barrier crossing, Science Advances 3 (8) (2017), https://doi.org/10.1126/sciadv.1700362.
[174] I. Papademetriou, E. Vedula, J. Charest, T. Porter, Effect of flow on targeting and penetration of angiopep-decorated nanoparticles in a microfluidic model blood-brain barrier, PLoS One 13 (10) (2018), https://doi.org/10.1371/journal.pone.0205158.
[175] C. Velasco-Aguirre, F. Morales-Zavala, E. Salas-Huenuleo, E. Gallardo-Toledo, O. Andonie, L. Muñoz, X. Rojas, G. Acosta, M. Sánchez-Navarro, E. Giralt, et al., Improving gold nanorod delivery to the central nervous system by conjugation to the shuttle Angiopep-2, Nanomedicine 12 (20) (2017) 2503–2517, https://doi.org/10.2217/nnm-2017-0181.
[176] D.T. Wiley, P. Webster, A. Gale, M.E. Davis, Transcytosis and brain uptake of transferrin-containing nanoparticles by tuning avidity to transferrin receptor, Proceedings of the National Academy of Sciences of the U S A 110 (21) (2013) 8662–8667, https://doi.org/10.1073/pnas.1307152110.
[177] R.L. Manthe, M. Loeck, T. Bhowmick, M. Solomon, S. Muro, Intertwined mechanisms define transport of anti-ICAM nanocarriers across the endothelium and brain delivery of a therapeutic enzyme, Journal of Controlled Release 324 (2020) 181–193, https://doi.org/10.1016/j.jconrel.2020.05.009.
[178] A.J. Clark, M.E. Davis, Increased brain uptake of targeted nanoparticles by adding an acid-cleavable linkage between transferrin and the nanoparticle core, Proceedings of the National Academy of Sciences of the U S A 112 (40) (2015) 12486–12491, https://doi.org/10.1073/pnas.1517048112.
[179] X. Tian, D.M. Leite, E. Scarpa, S. Nyberg, G. Fullstone, J. Forth, D. Matias, A. Apriceno, A. Poma, A. Duro-Castano, et al., On the shuttling across the blood-brain barrier via tubule formation: mechanism and cargo avidity bias, Science Advances 6 (48) (2020) eabc4397, https://doi.org/10.1126/sciadv.abc4397.
[180] R. Villaseñor, M. Schilling, J. Sundaresan, Y. Lutz, L. Collin, Sorting tubules regulate blood-brain barrier transcytosis, Cell Reports 21 (11) (2017) 3256–3270, https://doi.org/10.1016/j.celrep.2017.11.055.
[181] D. Gonzalez-Carter, X. Liu, T.A. Tockary, A. Dirisala, K. Toh, Y. Anraku, K. Kataoka, Targeting nanoparticles to the brain by exploiting the blood-brain barrier impermeability to selectively label the brain endothelium, Proceedings of the National Academy of Sciences of the U S A 117 (32) (2020) 19141–19150, https://doi.org/10.1073/pnas.2002016117.
[182] P. Matak, A. Matak, S. Moustafa, D.K. Aryal, E.J. Benner, W. Wetsel, N.C. Andrews, Disrupted iron homeostasis causes dopaminergic neurodegeneration in mice, Proceedings of the National Academy of Sciences of the U S A 113 (13) (2016) 3428–3435, https://doi.org/10.1073/pnas.1519473113.
[183] K. Prabhakar, S.M. Afzal, P.U. Kumar, A. Rajanna, V. Kishan, Brain delivery of transferrin coupled indinavir submicron lipid emulsions—pharmacokinetics and tissue distribution, Colloids and Surfaces B: Biointerfaces 86 (2) (2011) 305–313, https://doi.org/10.1016/j.colsurfb.2011.04.013.

[184] Y. Gong, P. Chowdhury, P.K.B. Nagesh, M.A. Rahman, K. Zhi, M.M. Yallapu, S. Kumar, Novel elvitegravir nanoformulation for drug delivery across the blood-brain barrier to achieve HIV-1 suppression in the CNS macrophages, Scientific Reports 10 (1) (2020) 3835, https://doi.org/10.1038/s41598-020-60684-1.
[185] N. Hartl, F. Adams, O.M. Merkel, From adsorption to covalent bonding: apolipoprotein E functionalization of polymeric nanoparticles for drug delivery across the blood-brain barrier, Advances in Therapy 4 (1) (2020) 2000092, https://doi.org/10.1002/adtp.202000092.
[186] B. Surnar, A.S. Shah, M. Park, A.A. Kalathil, M.Z. Kamran, R. Ramirez Jaime, M. Toborek, M. Nair, N. Kolishetti, S. Dhar, Brain-accumulating nanoparticles for assisting astrocytes to reduce human immunodeficiency virus and drug abuse-induced neuroinflammation and oxidative stress, ACS Nano 15 (10) (2021) 15741–15753, https://doi.org/10.1021/acsnano.0c09553.
[187] R. Zhang, Y. Fu, M. Cheng, W. Ma, N. Zheng, Y. Wang, Z. Wu, sEVs(RVG) selectively delivers antiviral siRNA to fetus brain, inhibits ZIKV infection and mitigates ZIKV-induced microcephaly in mouse model, Molecular Therapy 30 (5) (2022) 2078–2091, https://doi.org/10.1016/j.ymthe.2021.10.009.
[188] A.D. Wong, M. Ye, A.F. Levy, J.D. Rothstein, D.E. Bergles, P.C. Searson, The blood-brain barrier: an engineering perspective, Frontiers in Neuroengineering 6 (2013) 7, https://doi.org/10.3389/fneng.2013.00007.
[189] J. Garcia-Chica, W.K. D Paraiso, S. Tanabe, D. Serra, L. Herrero, N. Casals, J. Garcia, X. Ariza, S. Quader, R. Rodriguez-Rodriguez, An overview of nanomedicines for neuron targeting, Nanomedicine 15 (16) (2020) 1617–1636, https://doi.org/10.2217/nnm-2020-0088.
[190] A.P. Barnes, F. Polleux, Establishment of axon-dendrite polarity in developing neurons, Annual Review of Neuroscience 32 (2009) 347–381, https://doi.org/10.1146/annurev.neuro.31.060407.125536.
[191] N.J. Abbott, L. Rönnbäck, E. Hansson, Astrocyte–endothelial interactions at the blood–brain barrier, Nature Reviews Neuroscience 7 (1) (2006) 41–53, https://doi.org/10.1038/nrn1824.
[192] O.C. Colgan, N.T. Collins, G. Ferguson, R.P. Murphy, Y.A. Birney, P.A. Cahill, P.M. Cummins, Influence of basolateral condition on the regulation of brain microvascular endothelial tight junction properties and barrier function, Brain Research 1193 (2008) 84–92, https://doi.org/10.1016/j.brainres.2007.11.072.
[193] C. Hayashi, N. Suzuki, Heterogeneity of oligodendrocytes and their precursor cells, in: Advances in Experimental Medicine and Biology, Springer Singapore, 2019, pp. 53–62.
[194] L.-P. Bernier, E.M. York, A. Kamyabi, H.B. Choi, N.L. Weilinger, B.A. MacVicar, Microglial metabolic flexibility supports immune surveillance of the brain parenchyma, Nature Communications 11 (1) (2020) 1559, https://doi.org/10.1038/s41467-020-15267-z.
[195] C.N. Hall, C. Reynell, B. Gesslein, N.B. Hamilton, A. Mishra, B.A. Sutherland, F.M. O'Farrell, A.M. Buchan, M. Lauritzen, D. Attwell, Capillary pericytes regulate cerebral blood flow in health and disease, Nature 508 (7494) (2014) 55–60, https://doi.org/10.1038/nature13165.
[196] A. Armulik, G. Genové, M. Mäe, M.H. Nisancioglu, E. Wallgard, C. Niaudet, L. He, J. Norlin, P. Lindblom, K. Strittmatter, et al., Pericytes regulate the blood–brain barrier, Nature 468 (7323) (2010) 557–561, https://doi.org/10.1038/nature09522.

[197] C. Nicholson, E. Syková, Extracellular space structure revealed by diffusion analysis, Trends in Neurosciences 21 (5) (1998) 207–215, https://doi.org/10.1016/s0166-2236(98)01261-2.
[198] E. Vendel, V. Rottschäfer, E C.M. de Lange, The need for mathematical modelling of spatial drug distribution within the brain, Fluids and Barriers of the CNS 16 (1) (2019) 12, https://doi.org/10.1186/s12987-019-0133-x.
[199] S.B. Hladky, M.A. Barrand, Mechanisms of fluid movement into, through and out of the brain: evaluation of the evidence, Fluids and Barriers of the CNS 11 (1) (2014) 26, https://doi.org/10.1186/2045-8118-11-26.
[200] N. Marchi, M. Banjara, D. Janigro, Blood-brain barrier, bulk flow, and interstitial clearance in epilepsy, Journal of Neuroscience Methods 260 (2016) 118–124, https://doi.org/10.1016/j.jneumeth.2015.06.011.
[201] N.J. Abbott, Evidence for bulk flow of brain interstitial fluid: significance for physiology and pathology, Neurochemistry International 45 (4) (2004) 545–552, https://doi.org/10.1016/j.neuint.2003.11.006.
[202] J.J. Iliff, M. Wang, D.M. Zeppenfeld, A. Venkataraman, B.A. Plog, Y. Liao, R. Deane, M. Nedergaard, Cerebral arterial pulsation drives paravascular CSF-interstitial fluid exchange in the murine brain, Journal of Neuroscience 33 (46) (2013) 18190–18199, https://doi.org/10.1523/JNEUROSCI.1592-13.2013.
[203] C.E. Johanson, J.A. Duncan 3rd, P.M. Klinge, T. Brinker, E.G. Stopa, G.D. Silverberg, Multiplicity of cerebrospinal fluid functions: new challenges in health and disease, Cerebrospinal Fluid Research 5 (2008) 10, https://doi.org/10.1186/1743-8454-5-10.
[204] N.J. Abbott, M.E. Pizzo, J.E. Preston, D. Janigro, R.G. Thorne, The role of brain barriers in fluid movement in the CNS: is there a 'glymphatic' system? Acta Neuropathologica 135 (3) (2018) 387–407, https://doi.org/10.1007/s00401-018-1812-4.
[205] L. Xie, H. Kang, Q. Xu, M.J. Chen, Y. Liao, M. Thiyagarajan, J. O'Donnell, D.J. Christensen, C. Nicholson, J.J. Iliff, et al., Sleep drives metabolite clearance from the adult brain, Science 342 (6156) (2013) 373–377, https://doi.org/10.1126/science.1241224.
[206] J.J. Iliff, M. Wang, Y. Liao, B.A. Plogg, W. Peng, G.A. Gundersen, H. Benveniste, G.E. Vates, R. Deane, S.A. Goldman, et al., A paravascular pathway facilitates CSF flow through the brain parenchyma and the clearance of interstitial solutes, including amyloid β, Science Translational Medicine 4 (147) (2012) https://doi.org/10.1126/scitranslmed.3003748.
[207] K.E. Holter, B. Kehlet, A. Devor, T.J. Sejnowski, A.M. Dale, S.W. Omholt, O.P. Ottersen, E.A. Nagelhus, K.-A. Mardal, K.H. Pettersen, Interstitial solute transport in 3D reconstructed neuropil occurs by diffusion rather than bulk flow, Proceedings of the National Academy of Sciences of the U S A 114 (37) (2017) 9894–9899, https://doi.org/10.1073/pnas.1706942114.
[208] H. Helmbrecht, A. Joseph, M. McKenna, M. Zhang, E. Nance, Governing transport principles for nanotherapeutic application in the brain, Current Opinion in Chemical Engineering 30 (12) (2020) 112–119, https://doi.org/10.1016/j.coche.2020.08.010.
[209] E. Syková, C. Nicholson, Diffusion in brain extracellular space, Physiological Reviews 88 (4) (2008) 1277–1340, https://doi.org/10.1152/physrev.00027.2007.
[210] J. Tønnesen, V.V.G.K. Inavalli, U.V. Nägerl, Super-esolution imaging of the extracellular space in living brain tissue, Cell 172 (5) (2018), https://doi.org/10.1016/j.cell.2018.02.007.

[211] S. Hrabetová, J. Hrabe, C. Nicholson, Dead-space microdomains hinder extracellular diffusion in rat neocortex during ischemia, Journal of Neuroscience 23 (23) (2003) 8351–8359, https://doi.org/10.1523/JNEUROSCI.23-23-08351.2003.
[212] E.A. Nance, G.F. Woodworth, K.A. Sailor, T.-Y. Shih, Q. Xu, G. Swaminathan, D. Xiang, C. Eberhart, J. Hanes, A dense poly(ethylene glycol) coating improves penetration of large polymeric nanoparticles within brain tissue, Science Translational Medicine 4 (149) (2012), https://doi.org/10.1126/scitranslmed.3003594.
[213] E. Nance, K. Timbie, G.W. Miller, J. Song, C. Louttit, A.L. Klibanov, T.-Y. Shih, G. Swaminathan, R.J. Tamargo, G.F. Woodworth, et al., Non-invasive delivery of stealth, brain-penetrating nanoparticles across the blood-brain barrier using MRI-guided focused ultrasound, Journal of Controlled Release 189 (2014) 123–132, https://doi.org/10.1016/j.jconrel.2014.06.031.
[214] A.G. Godin, J.A. Varela, Z. Gao, N. Danné, J.P. Dupuis, B. Lounis, L. Groc, L. Cognet, Single-nanotube tracking reveals the nanoscale organization of the extracellular space in the live brain, Nature Nanotechnology 12 (3) (2016) 238–243, https://doi.org/10.1038/nnano.2016.248.
[215] C. Paviolo, F.N. Soria, J.S. Ferreira, A. Lee, L. Groc, E. Bezard, L. Cognet, Nanoscale exploration of the extracellular space in the live brain by combining single carbon nanotube tracking and super-resolution imaging analysis, Methods 174 (2020) 91–99, https://doi.org/10.1016/j.ymeth.2019.03.005.
[216] C. Curtis, M. McKenna, H. Pontes, D. Toghani, A. Choe, E. Nance, Predicting in situ nanoparticle behavior using multiple particle tracking and artificial neural networks, Nanoscale 11 (46) (2019) 22515–22530, https://doi.org/10.1039/c9nr06327g.
[217] S. Hrabetová, D. Masri, L. Tao, F. Xiao, C. Nicholson, Calcium diffusion enhanced after cleavage of negatively charged components of brain extracellular matrix by chondroitinase ABC, The Journal of Physiology 587 (Pt 16) (2009) 4029–4049, https://doi.org/10.1113/jphysiol.2009.170092.
[218] C. Curtis, D. Toghani, B. Wong, E. Nance, Colloidal stability as a determinant of nanoparticle behavior in the brain, Colloids and Surfaces B: Biointerfaces 170 (2018) 673–682, https://doi.org/10.1016/j.colsurfb.2018.06.050.
[219] M.J. Berridge, Neuronal calcium signaling, Neuron 21 (1) (1998) 13–26, https://doi.org/10.1016/s0896-6273(00)80510-3.
[220] M. Chesler, Regulation and modulation of pH in the brain, Physiological Reviews 83 (4) (2003) 1183–1221, https://doi.org/10.1152/physrev.00010.2003.
[221] M. Zhang, B.P. Bishop, N.L. Thompson, K. Hildahl, B. Dang, O. Mironchuk, N. Chen, R. Aoki, V.C. Holmberg, E. Nance, Quantum dot cellular uptake and toxicity in the developing brain: implications for use as imaging probes, Nanoscale Advances 1 (9) (2019) 3424–3442, https://doi.org/10.1039/C9NA00334G.
[222] E.C.M. de Lange, M. Danhof, Considerations in the use of cerebrospinal fluid pharmacokinetics to predict brain target concentrations in the clinical setting, Clinical Pharmacokinetics 41 (10) (2002) 691–703, https://doi.org/10.2165/00003088-200241100-00001.
[223] R.R. Lonser, M. Sarntinoranont, P.F. Morrison, E.H. Oldfield, Convection-enhanced delivery to the central nervous system, Journal of Neurosurgery 122 (3) (2015) 697–706, https://doi.org/10.3171/2014.10.jns14229.

[224] A.M. Mehta, A.M. Sonabend, J.N. Bruce, Convection-enhanced delivery, Neurotherapeutics 14 (2) (2017) 358–371, https://doi.org/10.1007/s13311-017-0520-4.
[225] M.S. Fiandaca, M.S. Berger, K.S. Bankiewicz, The use of convection-enhanced delivery with liposomal toxins in neurooncology, Toxins 3 (4) (2011) 369–397, https://doi org/10.3390/toxins3040369.
[226] C.A. Stine, J.M. Munson, Convection-enhanced delivery: connection to and impact of interstitial fluid flow, Frontiers Oncology 9 (2019) 966, https://doi.org/10.3389/fonc.2019.00966.
[227] H.G. Augustin, G.Y. Koh, Organotypic vasculature: from descriptive heterogeneity to functional pathophysiology, Science 357 (6353) (2017) eaal2379, https://doi.org/10.1126/science.aal2379.
[228] M.K. Danquah, X.A. Zhang, R.I. Mahato, Extravasation of polymeric nanomedicines across tumor vasculature, Advanced Drug Delivery Reviews 63 (8) (2011) 623–639, https://doi.org/10.1016/j.addr.2010.11.005.
[229] Y. Matsumura, H. Maeda, A new concept for macromolecular therapeutics in cancer chemotherapy: mechanism of tumoritropic accumulation of proteins and the antitumor agent smancs, Cancer Research 46 (12 Pt 1) (1986) 6387–6392.
[230] H. Hashizume, P. Baluk, S. Morikawa, J.W. McLean, G. Thurston, S. Roberge, R.K. Jain, D.M. McDonald, Openings between defective endothelial cells explain tumor vessel leakiness, American Journal Of Pathology 156 (4) (2000) 1363–1380, https://doi.org/10.1016/s0002-9440(10)65006-7.
[231] S.K. Hobbs, W.L. Monsky, F. Yuan, W.G. Roberts, L. Griffith, V.P. Torchilin, R.K. Jain, Regulation of transport pathways in tumor vessels: role of tumor type and microenvironment, Proceedings of the National Academy of Sciences of the United States of America 95 (8) (1998) 4607–4612.
[232] Y. Anraku, A. Kishimura, A. Kobayashi, M. Oba, K. Kataoka, Size-controlled long-circulating PICsome as a ruler to measure critical cut-off disposition size into normal and tumor tissues, Chemical Communications 47 (21) (2011) 6054–6056, https://doi.org/10.1039/c1cc11465d.
[233] H. Cabral, Y. Matsumoto, K. Mizuno, Q. Chen, M. Murakami, M. Kimura, Y. Terada, M.R. Kano, K. Miyazono, M. Uesaka, et al., Accumulation of sub-100 nm polymeric micelles in poorly permeable tumours depends on size, Nature Nanotechnology 6 (12) (2011) 815–823, https://doi.org/10.1038/nnano.2011.166.
[234] A.I. Minchinton, I.F. Tannock, Drug penetration in solid tumours, Nature Reviews Cancer 6 (8) (2006) 583–592, https://doi.org/10.1038/nrc1893.
[235] A.S. Narang, S. Varia, Role of tumor vascular architecture in drug delivery, Advanced Drug Delivery Reviews 63 (8) (2011) 640–658, https://doi.org/10.1016/j.addr.2011.04.002.
[236] C.H. Heldin, K. Rubin, K. Pietras, A. Ostman, High interstitial fluid pressure-an obstacle in cancer therapy, Nature Reviews Cancer 4 (10) (2004) 806–813, https://doi.org/10.1038/nrc1456.
[237] K. Hida, N. Maishi, Y. Sakurai, Y. Hida, H. Harashima, Heterogeneity of tumor endothelial cells and drug delivery, Advanced Drug Delivery Reviews 99 (Pt B) (2016) 140–147, https://doi.org/10.1016/j.addr.2015.11.008.

[238] S. Mura, J. Nicolas, P. Couvreur, Stimuli-responsive nanocarriers for drug delivery, Nature Materials 12 (11) (2013) 991–1003, https://doi.org/10.1038/nmat3776.
[239] Y. Lu, A.A. Aimetti, R. Langer, Z. Gu, Bioresponsive materials, Nature Review Materials 2 (1) (2016) 16075, https://doi.org/10.1038/natrevmats.2016.75.
[240] H.S. El-Sawy, A.M. Al-Abd, T.A. Ahmed, K.M. El-Say, V.P. Torchilin, Stimuli-responsive nano-architecture drug-delivery systems to solid tumor micromilieu: past, present, and future perspectives, ACS Nano 12 (11) (2018) 10636–10664, https://doi.org/10.1021/acsnano.8b06104.
[241] P. Mi, H. Cabral, K. Kataoka, Ligand-installed nanocarriers toward precision therapy, Advances in Materials 32 (13) (2020) e1902604, https://doi.org/10.1002/adma.201902604.
[242] J. Li, K. Kataoka, Chemo-physical strategies to advance the in vivo functionality of targeted nanomedicine: the next generation, Journal of the American Chemical Society 143 (2) (2021) 538–559, https://doi.org/10.1021/jacs.0c09029.
[243] Y. Lee, S. Fukushima, Y. Bae, S. Hiki, T. Ishii, K. Kataoka, A protein nanocarrier from charge-conversion polymer in response to endosomal pH, Journal of the American Chemical Society 129 (17) (2007) 5362–5363.
[244] Y. Lee, K. Miyata, M. Oba, T. Ishii, S. Fukushima, M. Han, H. Koyama, N. Nishiyama, K. Kataoka, Charge-conversion ternary polyplex with endosome disruption moiety: a technique for efficient and safe gene delivery, Angewandte Chemie International Edition 47 (28) (2008) 5163–5166, https://doi.org/10.1002/anie.200800963.
[245] Y. Lee, T. Ishii, H.J. Kim, N. Nishiyama, Y. Hayakawa, K. Itaka, K. Kataoka, Efficient delivery of bioactive antibodies into the cytoplasm of living cells by charge-conversional polyion complex micelles, Angewandte Chemie International Edition 49 (14) (2010) 2552–2555, https://doi.org/10.1002/anie.200905264.
[246] H. Takemoto, K. Miyata, S. Hattori, T. Ishii, T. Suma, S. Uchida, N. Nishiyama, K. Kataoka, Acidic pH-responsive siRNA conjugate for reversible carrier stability and accelerated endosomal escape with reduced IFNα-associated immune response, Angewandte Chemie International Edition 52 (24) (2013) 6218–6221, https://doi.org/10.1002/anie.201300178.
[247] J. Li, Y. Han, Q. Chen, H. Shi, S. Ur Rehman, M. Siddiq, Z. Ge, S. Liu, Dual endogenous stimuli-responsive polyplex micelles as smart two-step delivery nanocarriers for deep tumor tissue penetration and combating drug resistance of cisplatin, Journal of Materials Chemistry B: Materials for Biology and Medicine 2 (13) (2014) 1813–1824, https://doi.org/10.1039/c3tb21383h.
[248] J. Li, W. Ke, H. Li, Z. Zha, Y. Han, Z. Ge, Endogenous stimuli-sensitive multistage polymeric micelleplex anticancer drug delivery system for efficient tumor penetration and cellular internalization, Advanced Healthcare Materials 4 (15) (2015) 2206–2219, https://doi.org/10.1002/adhm.201500379.
[249] C.Y. Sun, Y. Liu, J.Z. Du, Z.T. Cao, C.F. Xu, J. Wang, Facile generation of tumor-pH-labile linkage-bridged block copolymers for chemotherapeutic delivery, Angewandte Chemie International Edition 55 (3) (2016) 1010–1014, https://doi.org/10.1002/anie.201509507.
[250] J.Z. Du, H.J. Li, J. Wang, Tumor-acidity-cleavable maleic acid amide (TACMAA): a powerful tool for designing smart nanoparticles to overcome

delivery barriers in cancer nanomedicine, Accounts of Chemical Research 51 (11) (2018) 2848–2856, https://doi.org/10.1021/acs.accounts.8b00195.
[251] J.P. Behr, The proton sponge: a trick to enter cells the viruses did not exploit, Chimia 51 (1–2) (1997) 34–36.
[252] H. Uchida, K. Itaka, T. Nomoto, T. Ishii, T. Suma, M. Ikegami, K. Miyata, M. Oba, N. Nishiyama, K. Kataoka, Modulated protonation of side chain aminoethylene repeats in N-substituted polyaspartamides promotes mRNA transfection, Journal of the American Chemical Society 136 (35) (2014) 12396–12405, https://doi.org/10.1021/ja506194z.
[253] H. Uchida, K. Miyata, M. Oba, T. Ishii, T. Suma, K. Itaka, N. Nishiyama, K. Kataoka, Odd-even effect of repeating aminoethylene units in the side chain of N-substituted polyaspartamides on gene transfection profiles, Journal of the American Chemical Society 133 (39) (2011) 15524–15532, https://doi.org/10.1021/ja204466y.
[254] Y. Bae, S. Fukushima, A. Harada, K. Kataoka, Design of environment-sensitive supramolecular assemblies for intracellular drug delivery: polymeric micelles that are responsive to intracellular pH change, Angewandte Chemie International Edition 42 (38) (2003) 4640–4643, https://doi.org/10.1002/anie.200250653.
[255] H. Kinoh, Y. Miura, T. Chida, X. Liu, K. Mizuno, S. Fukushima, Y. Morodomi, N. Nishiyama, H. Cabral, K. Kataoka, Nanomedicines eradicating cancer stem-like cells in vivo by pH-triggered intracellular cooperative action of loaded drugs, ACS Nano 10 (6) (2016) 5643–5655, https://doi.org/10.1021/acsnano.6b00900.
[256] S. Quader, X. Liu, Y. Chen, P. Mi, T. Chida, T. Ishii, Y. Miura, N. Nishiyama, H. Cabral, K. Kataoka, cRGD peptide-installed epirubicin-loaded polymeric micelles for effective targeted therapy against brain tumors, Journal of Controlled Release 258 (2017) 56–66, https://doi.org/10.1016/j.jconrel.2017.04.033.
[257] T. Chida, Y. Miura, H. Cabral, T. Nomoto, K. Kataoka, N. Nishiyama, Epirubicin-loaded polymeric micelles effectively treat axillary lymph nodes metastasis of breast cancer through selective accumulation and pH-triggered drug release, Journal of Controlled Release 292 (2018) 130–140, https://doi.org/10.1016/j.jconrel.2018.10.035.
[258] M. Oishi, Y. Nagasaki, K. Itaka, N. Nishiyama, K. Kataoka, Lactosylated poly(ethylene glycol)-siRNA conjugate through acid labile β-thiopropionate linkage to construct pH-sensitive polyion complex micelles achieving enhanced gene silencing in hepatoma cells, Journal of the American Chemical Society 127 (6) (2005) 1624–1625.
[259] K. Zhou, Y. Wang, X. Huang, K. Luby-Phelps, B.D. Sumer, J. Gao, Tunable, ultrasensitive pH-responsive nanoparticles targeting specific endocytic organelles in living cells, Angewandte Chemie International Edition 50 (27) (2011) 6109–6114, https://doi.org/10.1002/anie.201100884.
[260] Y. Wang, K. Zhou, G. Huang, C. Hensley, X. Huang, X. Ma, T. Zhao, B.D. Sumer, R.J. DeBerardinis, J. Gao, A nanoparticle-based strategy for the imaging of a broad range of tumours by nonlinear amplification of microenvironment signals, Nature Materials 13 (2) (2014) 204–212, https://doi.org/10.1038/nmat3819.
[261] F.J. Voskuil, P.J. Steinkamp, T. Zhao, B. van der Vegt, M. Koller, J.J. Doff, Y. Jayalakshmi, J.P. Hartung, J. Gao, B.D. Sumer, et al., Exploiting metabolic acidosis in solid cancers using a tumor-agnostic pH-activatable nanoprobe for fluorescence-guided surgery, Nature Communications 11 (1) (2020) 3257, https://doi.org/10.1038/s41467-020-16814-4.

[262] J. Li, A. Dirisala, Z. Ge, Y. Wang, W. Yin, W. Ke, K. Toh, J. Xie, Y. Matsumoto, Y. Anraku, et al., Therapeutic vesicular nanoreactors with tumor-specific activation and self-destruction for synergistic tumor ablation, Angewandte Chemie International Edition 56 (45) (2017) 14025–14030, https://doi.org/10.1002/anie.201706964.
[263] Y. Kakizawa, A. Harada, K. Kataoka, Environment-sensitive stabilization of core-shell structured polyion complex micelle by reversible cross-linking of the core through disulfide bond, Journal of the American Chemical Society 121 (48) (1999) 11247–11248.
[264] K. Miyata, Y. Kakizawa, N. Nishiyama, A. Harada, Y. Yamasaki, H. Koyama, K. Kataoka, Block catiomer polyplexes with regulated densities of charge and disulfide cross-linking directed to enhance gene expression, Journal of the American Chemical Society 126 (8) (2004) 2355–2361.
[265] R.J. Christie, K. Miyata, Y. Matsumoto, T. Nomoto, D. Menasco, T.C. Lai, M. Pennisi, K. Osada, S. Fukushima, N. Nishiyama, et al., Effect of polymer structure on micelles formed between siRNA and cationic block copolymer comprising thiols and amidines, Biomacromolecules 12 (9) (2011) 3174–3185, https://doi.org/10.1021/bm2006714.
[266] A. Dirisala, S. Uchida, T.A. Tockary, N. Yoshinaga, J. Li, S. Osawa, L. Gorantla, S. Fukushima, K. Osada, K. Kataoka, Precise tuning of disulphide crosslinking in mRNA polyplex micelles for optimising extracellular and intracellular nuclease tolerability, Journal of Drug Targeting 27 (5–6) (2019) 670–680, https://doi.org/10.1080/1061186X.2018.1550646.
[267] X. Hu, J. Hu, J. Tian, Z. Ge, G. Zhang, K. Luo, S. Liu, Polyprodrug amphiphiles: hierarchical assemblies for shape-regulated cellular internalization, trafficking, and drug delivery, Journal of the American Chemical Society 135 (46) (2013) 17617–17629, https://doi.org/10.1021/ja409686x.
[268] H.C. Yen, H. Cabral, P. Mi, K. Toh, Y. Matsumoto, X. Liu, H. Koori, A. Kim, K. Miyazaki, Y. Miura, et al., Light-induced cytosolic activation of reduction-sensitive camptothecin-loaded polymeric micelles for spatiotemporally controlled in vivo chemotherapy, ACS Nano 8 (11) (2014) 11591–11602.
[269] H. Mok, S.H. Lee, J.W. Park, T.G. Park, Multimeric small interfering ribonucleic acid for highly efficient sequence-specific gene silencing, Nature Materials 9 (3) (2010) 272–278, https://doi.org/10.1038/nmat2626.
[270] H. Takemoto, A. Ishii, K. Miyata, M. Nakanishi, M. Oba, T. Ishii, Y. Yamasaki, N. Nishiyama, K. Kataoka, Polyion complex stability and gene silencing efficiency with a siRNA-grafted polymer delivery system, Biomaterials 31 (31) (2010) 8097–8105, https://doi.org/10.1016/j.biomaterials.2010.07.015.
[271] S. Takae, K. Miyata, M. Oba, T. Ishii, N. Nishiyama, K. Itaka, Y. Yamasaki, H. Koyama, K. Kataoka, PEG-detachable polyplex micelles based on disulfide-linked block catiomers as bioresponsive nonviral gene vectors, Journal of the American Chemical Society 130 (18) (2008) 6001–6009.
[272] T. Suma, K. Miyata, Y. Anraku, S. Watanabe, R.J. Christie, H. Takemoto, M. Shioyama, N. Gouda, T. Ishii, N. Nishiyama, et al., Smart multilayered assembly for biocompatible siRNA delivery featuring dissolvable silica, endosome-disrupting polycation, and detachable PEG, ACS Nano 6 (8) (2012) 6693–6705.

[273] J. Li, Z. Ge, S. Liu, PEG-sheddable polyplex micelles as smart gene carriers based on MMP-cleavable peptide-linked block copolymers, Chemical Communications 49 (2013) 6974–6976, https://doi.org/10.1039/c3cc43576h.
[274] M.S. Shim, Y. Xia, A reactive oxygen species (ROS)-responsive polymer for safe, efficient, and targeted gene delivery in cancer cells, Angewandte Chemie International Edition 52 (27) (2013) 6926–6929, https://doi.org/10.1002/anie.201209633.
[275] S. Kwon, H. Ko, D.G. You, K. Kataoka, J.H. Park, Nanomedicines for reactive oxygen species mediated approach: an emerging paradigm for cancer treatment, Accounts of Chemical Research 52 (7) (2019) 1771–1782, https://doi.org/10.1021/acs.accounts.9b00136.
[276] J. Wang, X. Sun, W. Mao, W. Sun, J. Tang, M. Sui, Y. Shen, Z. Gu, Tumor redox heterogeneity-responsive prodrug nanocapsules for cancer chemotherapy, Advances in Materials 25 (27) (2013) 3670–3676, https://doi.org/10.1002/adma.201300929.
[277] M. Naito, T. Ishii, A. Matsumoto, K. Miyata, Y. Miyahara, K. Kataoka, A phenylboronate-functionalized polyion complex micelle for ATP-triggered release of siRNA, Angewandte Chemie International Edition 51 (43) (2012) 10751–10755, https://doi.org/10.1002/anie.201203360.
[278] R. Mo, T. Jiang, Z. Gu, Enhanced anticancer efficacy by ATP-mediated liposomal drug delivery, Angewandte Chemie International Edition 53 (23) (2014) 5815–5820, https://doi.org/10.1002/anie.201400268.
[279] R. Mo, T. Jiang, R. DiSanto, W. Tai, Z. Gu, ATP-triggered anticancer drug delivery, Nature Communications 5 (2014) 3364, https://doi.org/10.1038/ncomms4364.
[280] N. Yoshinaga, T. Ishii, M. Naito, T. Endo, S. Uchida, H. Cabral, K. Osada, K. Kataoka, Polyplex micelles with phenylboronate/gluconamide cross-linking in the core exerting promoted gene transfection through spatiotemporal responsivity to intracellular pH and ATP concentration, Journal of the American Chemical Society 139 (51) (2017) 18567–18575, https://doi.org/10.1021/jacs.7b08816.
[281] J. Li, Q. Chen, Z. Zha, H. Li, K. Toh, A. Dirisala, Y. Matsumoto, K. Osada, K. Kataoka, Z. Ge, Ternary polyplex micelles with PEG shells and intermediate barrier to complexed DNA cores for efficient systemic gene delivery, Journal of Controlled Release 209 (2015) 77–87, https://doi.org/10.1016/j.jconrel.2015.04.024.
[282] S. Osawa, K. Osada, S. Hiki, A. Dirisala, T. Ishii, K. Kataoka, Polyplex micelles with double-protective compartments of hydrophilic shell and thermoswitchable palisade of poly(oxazoline)-based block copolymers for promoted gene transfection, Biomacromolecules 17 (1) (2016) 354–361, https://doi.org/10.1021/acs.biomac.5b01456.
[283] J. Kopecek, P. Kopeckova, HPMA copolymers: origins, early developments, present, and future, Advanced Drug Delivery Reviews 62 (2) (2010) 122–149, https://doi.org/10.1016/j.addr.2009.10.004.
[284] Y. Wang, D.S. Kohane, External triggering and triggered targeting strategies for drug delivery, Nature Review Materials 2 (6) (2017) 17020, https://doi.org/10.1038/natrevmats.2017.20.
[285] M.P. Stewart, A. Sharei, X. Ding, G. Sahay, R. Langer, K.F. Jensen, In vitro and ex vivo strategies for intracellular delivery, Nature 538 (7624) (2016) 183–192, https://doi.org/10.1038/nature19764.
[286] T. Nomoto, S. Fukushima, M. Kumagai, K. Machitani, Arnida, Y. Matsumoto, M. Oba, K. Miyata, K. Osada, N. Nishiyama, et al., Three-

layered polyplex micelle as a multifunctional nanocarrier platform for light-induced systemic gene transfer, Nature Communications 5 (2014) 3545, https://doi.org/10.1038/ncomms4545.

[287] J. Li, K. Wei, S. Zuo, Y. Xu, Z. Zha, W. Ke, H. Chen, Z. Ge, Light-triggered clustered vesicles with self-supplied oxygen and tissue penetrability for photodynamic therapy against hypoxic tumor, Advances in Functional Materials 27 (33) (2017) 1702108, https://doi.org/10.1002/adfm.201702108.

[288] Y. Dou, K. Hynynen, C. Allen, To heat or not to heat: challenges with clinical translation of thermosensitive liposomes, Journal of Controlled Release 249 (2017) 63–73, https://doi.org/10.1016/j.jconrel.2017.01.025.

[289] Y. Horise, M. Maeda, Y. Konishi, J. Okamoto, S. Ikuta, Y. Okamoto, H. Ishii, S. Yoshizawa, S. Umemura, T. Ueyama, et al., Sonodynamic therapy with anticancer micelles and high-intensity focused ultrasound in treatment of canine cancer, Frontiers in Pharmacology 10 (2019) 545, https://doi.org/10.3389/fphar.2019.00545.

[290] Z. Zhao, A. Ukidve, J. Kim, S. Mitragotri, Targeting strategies for tissue-specific drug delivery, Cell 181 (1) (2020) 151–167, https://doi.org/10.1016/j.cell.2020.02.001.

[291] S. Deshayes, H. Cabral, T. Ishii, Y. Miura, S. Kobayashi, T. Yamashita, A. Matsumoto, Y. Miyahara, N. Nishiyama, K. Kataoka, Phenylboronic acid-installed polymeric micelles for targeting sialylated epitopes in solid tumors, Journal of the American Chemical Society 135 (41) (2013) 15501–15507, https://doi.org/10.1021/ja406406h.

[292] J. Wen, D. Wu, M. Qin, C. Liu, L. Wang, D. Xu, H.V. Vinters, Y. Liu, E. Kranz, X. Guan, et al., Sustained delivery and molecular targeting of a therapeutic monoclonal antibody to metastases in the central nervous system of mice, Nature Biomedical Engineering 3 (9) (2019) 706–716, https://doi.org/10.1038/s41551-019-0434-z.

[293] E.A. Murphy, B.K. Majeti, L.A. Barnes, M. Makale, S.M. Weis, K. Lutu-Fuga, W.;A.,C.D. Wrasidlo, Nanoparticle-mediated drug delivery to tumor vasculature suppresses metastasis, Proceedings of the National Academy of Sciences of the United States of America 105 (2008) 9343–9348.

[294] P.J. Gaillard, C.C. Appeldoorn, R. Dorland, J. van Kregten, F. Manca, D.J. Vugts, B. Windhorst, G.A. van Dongen, H.E. de Vries, D. Maussang, et al., Pharmacokinetics, brain delivery, and efficacy in brain tumor-bearing mice of glutathione pegylated liposomal doxorubicin (2B3-101), PLoS One 9 (1) (2014) e82331, https://doi.org/10.1371/journal.pone.0082331.

[295] P. Kumthekar, S.C. Tang, A.J. Brenner, S. Kesari, D.E. Piccioni, C. Anders, J. Carrillo, P. Chalasani, P. Kabos, S. Puhalla, et al., ANG1005, a brain-penetrating peptide-drug conjugate, shows activity in patients with breast cancer with leptomeningeal carcinomatosis and recurrent brain metastases, Clinical Cancer Research 26 (12) (2020) 2789–2799, https://doi.org/10.1158/1078-0432.CCR-19-3258.

[296] J. Li, S. Xiao, Y. Xu, S. Zuo, Z. Zha, W. Ke, C. He, Z. Ge, Smart asymmetric vesicles with triggered availability of inner cell-penetrating shells for specific intracellular drug delivery, ACS Applied Materials & Interfaces 9 (21) (2017) 17727–17735, https://doi.org/10.1021/acsami.7b02808.

[297] E.S. Olson, T. Jiang, T.A. Aguilera, Q.T. Nguyen, L.G. Ellies, M. Scadeng, R.Y. Tsien, Activatable cell penetrating peptides linked to nanoparticles as dual probes for in vivo fluorescence and MR imaging of proteases, Proceedings of the National Academy of Sciences of the United States of America 107 (9) (2010) 4311–4316, https://doi.org/10.1073/pnas.0910283107.

[298] S.R. Macewan, A. Chilkoti, Digital switching of local arginine density in a genetically encoded self-assembled polypeptide nanoparticle controls cellular uptake, Nano Letters 12 (6) (2012) 3322–3328, https://doi.org/10.1021/nl301529p.
[299] L. Zhu, T. Wang, F. Perche, A. Taigind, V.P. Torchilin, Enhanced anticancer activity of nanopreparation containing an MMP2-sensitive PEG-drug conjugate and cell-penetrating moiety, Proceedings of the National Academy of Sciences of the United States of America 110 (42) (2013) 17047–17052, https://doi.org/10.1073/pnas.1304987110.
[300] K.A. Autio, R. Dreicer, J. Anderson, J.A. Garcia, A. Alva, L.L. Hart, M.I. Milowsky, E.M. Posadas, C.J. Ryan, R.P. Graf, et al., Safety and efficacy of BIND-014, a docetaxel nanoparticle targeting prostate-specific membrane antigen for patients with metastatic castration-resistant prostate cancer: a phase 2 clinical trial, JAMA Oncology 4 (10) (2018) 1344–1351, https://doi.org/10.1001/jamaoncol.2018.2168. (Accessed 2 February 2024).
[301] T. Stylianopoulos, L.L. Munn, R.K. Jain, Reengineering the physical microenvironment of tumors to improve drug delivery and efficacy: from mathematical modeling to bench to bedside, Trends Cancer 4 (4) (2018) 292–319, https://doi.org/10.1016/j.trecan.2018.02.005.
[302] V.P. Chauhan, T. Stylianopoulos, J.D. Martin, Z. Popovic, O. Chen, W.S. Kamoun, M.G. Bawendi, D. Fukumura, R.K. Jain, Normalization of tumour blood vessels improves the delivery of nanomedicines in a size-dependent manner, Nature Nanotechnology 7 (6) (2012) 383–388, https://doi.org/10.1038/nnano.2012.45.
[303] W. Jiang, Y. Huang, Y. An, B.Y.S. Kim, Remodeling tumor vasculature to enhance delivery of intermediate-sized nanoparticles, ACS Nano 9 (9) (2015) 8689–8696.
[304] V.P. Chauhan, I.X. Chen, R. Tong, M.R. Ng, J.D. Martin, K. Naxerova, M.W. Wu, P. Huang, Y. Boucher, D.S. Kohane, et al., Reprogramming the microenvironment with tumor-selective angiotensin blockers enhances cancer immunotherapy, Proceedings of the National Academy of Sciences of the United States of America 116 (22) (2019) 10674–10680, https://doi.org/10.1073/pnas.1819889116.
[305] Y.C. Sung, P.R. Jin, L.A. Chu, F.F. Hsu, M.R. Wang, C.C. Chang, S.J. Chiou, J.T. Qiu, D.Y. Gao, C.C. Lin, et al., Delivery of nitric oxide with a nanocarrier promotes tumour vessel normalization and potentiates anti-cancer therapies, Nature Nanotechnology 14 (12) (2019) 1160–1169, https://doi.org/10.1038/s41565-019-0570-3.
[306] P.P. Wong, F. Demircioglu, E. Ghazaly, W. Alrawashdeh, M.R. Stratford, C.L. Scudamore, B. Cereser, T. Crnogorac-Jurcevic, S. McDonald, G. Elia, et al., Dual-action combination therapy enhances angiogenesis while reducing tumor growth and spread, Cancer Cell 27 (1) (2015) 123–137, https://doi.org/10.1016/j.ccell.2014.10.015.
[307] V.P. Chauhan, J.D. Martin, H. Liu, D.A. Lacorre, S.R. Jain, S.V. Kozin, T. Stylianopoulos, A.S. Mousa, X. Han, P. Adstamongkonkul, et al., Angiotensin inhibition enhances drug delivery and potentiates chemotherapy by decompressing tumour blood vessels, Nature Communications 4 (2013) 2516, https://doi.org/10.1038/ncomms3516.
[308] J.D. Martin, M. Panagi, C. Wang, T.T. Khan, M.R. Martin, C. Voutouri, K. Toh, P. Papageorgis, F. Mpekris, C. Polydorou, et al., Dexamethasone increases cisplatin-loaded nanocarrier delivery and efficacy in metastatic

breast cancer by normalizing the tumor microenvironment, ACS Nano 13 (6) (2019) 6396–6408, https://doi.org/10.1021/acsnano.8b07865.
[309] M.R. Kano, Y. Bae, C. Iwata, Y. Morishita, M. Yashiro, M. Oka, T. Fujii, A. Komuro, K. Kiyono, M. Kaminishi, et al., Improvement of cancer-targeting therapy, using nanocarriers for intractable solid tumors by inhibition of TGF-β signaling, Proceedings of the National Academy of Sciences of the United States of America 104 (9) (2007) 3460–3465.
[310] J. Liu, S. Liao, B. Diop-Frimpong, W. Chen, S. Goel, K. Naxerova, M. Ancukiewicz, Y. Boucher, R.K. Jain, L. Xu, TGF-β blockade improves the distribution and efficacy of therapeutics in breast carcinoma by normalizing the tumor stroma, Proceedings of the National Academy of Sciences of the United States of America 109 (41) (2012) 16618–16623, https://doi.org/10.1073/pnas.1117610109.
[311] M. Panagi, C. Voutouri, F. Mpekris, P. Papageorgis, M.R. Martin, J.D. Martin, P. Demetriou, C. Pierides, C. Polydorou, A. Stylianou, et al., TGF-β inhibition combined with cytotoxic nanomedicine normalizes triple negative breast cancer microenvironment towards anti-tumor immunity, Theranostics 10 (4) (2020) 1910–1922, https://doi.org/10.7150/thno.36936.
[312] H. Zhou, Z. Fan, J. Deng, P.K. Lemons, D.C. Arhontoulis, W.B. Bowne, H. Cheng, Hyaluronidase embedded in nanocarrier PEG Shell for enhanced tumor penetration and highly efficient antitumor efficacy, Nano Letters 16 (5) (2016) 3268–3277, https://doi.org/10.1021/acs.nanolett.6b00820.
[313] T.R. Cox, The matrix in cancer, Nature Reviews Cancer 21 (4) (2021) 217–238, https://doi.org/10.1038/s41568-020-00329-7.
[314] T. Ojha, V. Pathak, Y. Shi, W.E. Hennink, C.T.W. Moonen, G. Storm, F. Kiessling, T. Lammers, Pharmacological and physical vessel modulation strategies to improve EPR-mediated drug targeting to tumors, Advanced Drug Delivery Reviews 119 (2017) 44–60, https://doi.org/10.1016/j.addr.2017.07.007.
[315] K. Sano, T. Nakajima, P.L. Choyke, H. Kobayashi, Markedly enhanced permeability and retention effects induced by photo-immunotherapy of tumors, ACS Nano 7 (1) (2013) 717–724.
[316] A.L.B. Seynhaeve, M. Amin, D. Haemmerich, G.C. van Rhoon, T.L.M. Ten Hagen, Hyperthermia and smart drug delivery systems for solid tumor therapy, Advanced Drug Delivery Reviews 163–164 (2020) 125–144, https://doi.org/10.1016/j.addr.2020.02.004.
[317] M.A. Miller, R. Chandra, M.F. Cuccarese, C. Pfirschke, C. Engblom, S. Stapleton, U. Adhikary, R.H. Kohler, J.F. Mohan, M.J. Pittet, et al., Radiation therapy primes tumors for nanotherapeutic delivery via macrophage-mediated vascular bursts, Science Translational Medicine 9 (392) (2017) eaal0225.
[318] D. Chu, X. Dong, Q. Zhao, J. Gu, Z. Wang, Photosensitization priming of tumor microenvironments improves delivery of nanotherapeutics via neutrophil infiltration, Advances in Materials 29 (27) (2017) 1701021, https://doi.org/10.1002/adma.201701021.
[319] J. Garcia-Roman, A. Zentella-Dehesa, Vascular permeability changes involved in tumor metastasis, Cancer Letters 335 (2) (2013) 259–269, https://doi.org/10.1016/j.canlet.2013.03.005.
[320] R. Pasqualini, W. Arap, D.M. McDonald, Probing the structural and molecular diversity of tumor vasculature, Trends in Molecular Medicine 8 (12) (2002) 563–571.

[321] K. Seidi, H.A. Neubauer, R. Moriggl, R. Jahanban-Esfahlan, T. Javaheri, Tumor target amplification: implications for nano drug delivery systems, Journal of Controlled Release 275 (2018) 142–161, https://doi.org/10.1016/j.jconrel.2018.02.020.

[322] G. von Maltzahn, J.H. Park, K.Y. Lin, N. Singh, C. Schwoppe, R. Mesters, W.E. Berdel, E. Ruoslahti, M.J. Sailor, S.N. Bhatia, Nanoparticles that communicate in vivo to amplify tumour targeting, Nature Materials 10 (7) (2011) 545–552, https://doi.org/10.1038/nmat3049.

[323] J.H. Park, G. von Maltzahn, M.J. Xu, V. Fogal, V.R. Kotamraju, E. Ruoslahti, S.N. Bhatia, M.J. Sailor, Cooperative nanomaterial system to sensitize, target, and treat tumors, Proceedings of the National Academy of Sciences of the United States of America 107 (3) (2010) 981–986, https://doi.org/10.1073/pnas.0909565107.

[324] A.J. Gormley, N. Larson, S. Sadekar, R. Robinson, A. Ray, H. Ghandehari, Guided delivery of polymer therapeutics using plasmonic photothermal therapy, Nano Today 7 (3) (2012) 158–167, https://doi.org/10.1016/j.nantod.2012.04.002.

[325] K.Y. Lin, E.J. Kwon, J.H. Lo, S.N. Bhatia, Drug-induced amplification of nanoparticle targeting to tumors, Nano Today 9 (5) (2014) 550–559, https://doi.org/10.1016/j.nantod.2014.09.001.

[326] D.E. Hallahan, L. Geng, A.J. Cmelak, A.B. Chakravarthy, W. Martin, C. Scarfone, A. Gonzalez, Targeting drug delivery to radiation-induced neoantigens in tumor microvasculature, Journal of Controlled Release 74 (1–3) (2001) 183–191.

[327] D. Hallahan, L. Geng, S. Qu, C. Scarfone, T. Giorgio, E. Donnelly, X. Gao, J. Clanton, Integrin-mediated targeting of drug delivery to irradiated tumor blood vessels, Cancer Cell 3 (1) (2003) 63–74.

[328] C.D. Corso, A.N. Ali, R. Diaz, Radiation-induced tumor neoantigens: imaging and therapeutic implications, American Journal of Cancer Research 1 (3) (2011) 390–412.

[329] A. Detappe, S. Kunjachan, L. Sancey, V. Motto-Ros, D. Biancur, P. Drane, R. Guieze, G.M. Makrigiorgos, O. Tillement, R. Langer, et al., Advanced multimodal nanoparticles delay tumor progression with clinical radiation therapy, Journal of Controlled Release 238 (2016) 103–113, https://doi.org/10.1016/j.jconrel.2016.07.021.

[330] D.J. Buchsbaum, B.E. Rogers, M.B. Khazaeli, M.S. Mayo, D.E. Milenic, S.V. Kashmiri, C.J. Anderson, L.L. Chappell, M.W. Brechbiel, D.T. Curiel, Targeting strategies for cancer radiotherapy, Clinical Cancer Research 5 (10 Suppl. l) (1999) 3048s–3055s.

[331] M.A. Stackhouse, D.J. Buchsbaum, S.R. Kancharla, W.E. Grizzle, C. Grimes, K. Laffoon, L.C. Pederson, D.T. Curiel, Specific membrane receptor gene expression targeted with radiolabeled peptide employing the erbB-2 and DF3 promoter elements in adenoviral vectors, Cancer Gene Therapy 6 (3) (1999) 209–219.

[332] C. Agatemor, M.J. Buettner, R. Ariss, K. Muthiah, C.T. Saeui, K.J. Yarema, Exploiting metabolic glycoengineering to advance healthcare, Nature Reviews Chemistry 3 (10) (2019) 605–620, https://doi.org/10.1038/s41570-019-0126-y.

[333] H. Koo, S. Lee, J.H. Na, S.H. Kim, S.K. Hahn, K. Choi, I.C. Kwon, S.Y. Jeong, K. Kim, Bioorthogonal copper-free click chemistry in vivo for tumor-targeted delivery of nanoparticles, Angewandte Chemie International Edition 51 (47) (2012) 11836–11840, https://doi.org/10.1002/anie.201206703.

[334] H. Wang, R. Wang, K. Cai, H. He, Y. Liu, J. Yen, Z. Wang, M. Xu, Y. Sun, X. Zhou, et al., Selective in vivo metabolic cell-labeling-mediated cancer targeting, Nature Chemical Biology 13 (4) (2017) 415–424, https://doi.org/10.1038/nchembio.2297.
[335] F. Koizumi, M. Kitagawa, T. Negishi, T. Onda, S. Matsumoto, T. Hamaguchi, Y. Matsumura, Novel SN-38-incorporating polymeric micelles, NK012, eradicate vascular endothelial growth factor-secreting bulky tumors, Cancer Research 66 (20) (2006) 10048–10056, https://doi.org/10.1158/0008-5472.CAN-06-1605.
[336] A.J. Clark, D.T. Wiley, J.E. Zuckerman, P. Webster, J. Chao, J. Lin, Y. Yen, M.E. Davis, CRLX101 nanoparticles localize in human tumors and not in adjacent, nonneoplastic tissue after intravenous dosing, Proceedings of the National Academy of Sciences of the United States of America 113 (14) (2016) 3850–3854, https://doi.org/10.1073/pnas.1603018113.
[337] A.A. Manzoor, L.H. Lindner, C.D. Landon, J.Y. Park, A.J. Simnick, M.R. Dreher, S. Das, G. Hanna, W. Park, A. Chilkoti, et al., Overcoming limitations in nanoparticle drug delivery: triggered, intravascular release to improve drug penetration into tumors, Cancer Research 72 (21) (2012) 5566–5575, https://doi.org/10.1158/0008-5472.CAN-12-1683.
[338] A.L.B. Seynhaeve, B.M. Dicheva, S. Hoving, G.A. Koning, T.L.M. Ten Hagen, Intact Doxil is taken up intracellularly and released doxorubicin sequesters in the lysosome: evaluated by in vitro/in vivo live cell imaging, Journal of Controlled Release 172 (1) (2013) 330–340, https://doi.org/10.1016/j.jconrel.2013.08.034.
[339] I. Cheong, X. Huang, C. Bettegowda, L.A. Diaz Jr., K.W. Kinzler, S. Zhou, B. Vogelstein, A bacterial protein enhances the release and efficacy of liposomal cancer drugs, Science 314 (5803) (2006) 1308–1311, https://doi.org/10.1126/science.1130651.
[340] A. Schroeder, R. Honen, K. Turjeman, A. Gabizon, J. Kost, Y. Barenholz, Ultrasound triggered release of cisplatin from liposomes in murine tumors, Journal of Controlled Release 137 (1) (2009) 63–68, https://doi.org/10.1016/j.jconrel.2009.03.007.
[341] R.M. Wadkins, C.L. Morton, J.K. Weeks, L. Oliver, M. Wierdl, M.K. Danks, P.M. Potter, Structural constraints affect the metabolism of 7-Ethyl-10-[4-(1-piperidino)-1-piperidino] carbonyloxycamptothecin (CPT-11) by carboxylesterases, Molecular Pharmacology 60 (2) (2001) 355–362.
[342] C. de Gracia Lux, S. Joshi-Barr, T. Nguyen, E. Mahmoud, E. Schopf, N. Fomina, A. Almutairi, Biocompatible polymeric nanoparticles degrade and release cargo in response to biologically relevant levels of hydrogen peroxide, Journal of the American Chemical Society 134 (38) (2012) 15758–15764, https://doi.org/10.1021/ja303372u.
[343] G. Liu, G. Zhang, J. Hu, X. Wang, M. Zhu, S. Liu, Hyperbranched self-immolative polymers (hSIPs) for programmed payload delivery and ultrasensitive detection, Journal of the American Chemical Society 137 (36) (2015) 11645–11655, https://doi.org/10.1021/jacs.5b05060.
[344] G. Xu, H.L. McLeod, Strategies for enzyme/prodrug cancer therapy, Clinical Cancer Research 7 (11) (2001) 3314–3324.
[345] Y. Anraku, A. Kishimura, M. Kamiya, S. Tanaka, T. Nomoto, K. Toh, Y. Matsumoto, S. Fukushima, D. Sueyoshi, M.R. Kano, et al., Systemically injectable enzyme-loaded polyion complex vesicles as in vivo nanoreactors functioning in tumors, Angewandte Chemie International Edition 55 (2) (2016) 560–565, https://doi.org/10.1002/anie.201508339.

[346] T.A. Tockary, W. Foo, A. Dirisala, Q. Chen, S. Uchida, S. Osawa, Y. Mochida, X. Liu, H. Kinoh, H. Cabral, et al., Single-stranded DNA-packaged polyplex micelle as adeno-associated-virus-inspired compact vector to systemically target stroma-rich pancreatic cancer, ACS Nano 13 (11) (2019) 12732–12742, https://doi.org/10.1021/acsnano.9b04676.
[347] R. Walther, J. Rautio, A.N. Zelikin, Prodrugs in medicinal chemistry and enzyme prodrug therapies, Advanced Drug Delivery Reviews 118 (2017) 65–77, https://doi.org/10.1016/j.addr.2017.06.013.
[348] J. Li, W. Ke, L. Wang, M. Huang, W. Yin, P. Zhang, Q. Chen, Z. Ge, Self-sufficing H2O2-responsive nanocarriers through tumor-specific H2O2 production for synergistic oxidation-chemotherapy, Journal of Controlled Release 225 (2016) 64–74, https://doi.org/10.1016/j.jconrel.2016.01.029.
[349] J. Li, Y. Li, Y. Wang, W. Ke, W. Chen, W. Wang, Z. Ge, Polymer prodrug-based nanoreactors activated by tumor acidity for orchestrated oxidation/chemotherapy, Nano Letters 17 (11) (2017) 6983–6990, https://doi.org/10.1021/acs.nanolett.7b03531.
[350] W. Ke, J. Li, F. Mohammed, Y. Wang, K. Tou, X. Liu, P. Wen, H. Kinoh, Y. Anraku, H. Chen, et al., Therapeutic polymersome nanoreactors with tumor-specific activable cascade reactions for cooperative cancer therapy, ACS Nano 13 (2) (2019) 2357–2369, https://doi.org/10.1021/acsnano.8b09082.
[351] T. Walzer, L. Chiossone, J. Chaix, A. Calver, C. Carozzo, L. Garrigue-Antar, Y. Jacques, M. Baratin, E. Tomasello, E. Vivier, Natural killer cell trafficking in vivo requires a dedicated sphingosine 1-phosphate receptor, Nature Immunology 8 (12) (2007) 1337–1344, https://doi.org/10.1038/ni1523.
[352] J. Du, Y.S. Zhang, D. Hobson, P. Hydbring, Nanoparticles for immune system targeting, Drug Discovery Today 22 (9) (2017) 1295–1301, https://doi.org/10.1016/j.drudis.2017.03.013.
[353] D.J. Irvine, M.C. Hanson, K. Rakhra, T. Tokatlian, Synthetic nanoparticles for vaccines and immunotherapy, Chemical Reviews 115 (19) (2015) 11109–11146, https://doi.org/10.1021/acs.chemrev.5b00109.
[354] Y. Xie, T.R. Bagby, M.S. Cohen, M.L. Forrest, Drug delivery to the lymphatic system: importance in future cancer diagnosis and therapies, Expert Opinion on Drug Delivery 6 (8) (2009) 785–792, https://doi.org/10.1517/17425240903085128.
[355] P. Serra, P. Santamaria, Nanoparticle-based approaches to immune tolerance for the treatment of autoimmune diseases, European Journal of Immunology 48 (5) (2018) 751–756, https://doi.org/10.1002/eji.201747059. (Accessed 5 February 2024).
[356] E. Ben-Akiva, S. Est Witte, R.A. Meyer, K.R. Rhodes, J.J. Green, Polymeric micro- and nanoparticles for immune modulation, Biomaterials Science 7 (1) (2019) 14–30, https://doi.org/10.1039/C8BM01285G.
[357] S.-Y. Kim, Y.-W. Noh, T.H. Kang, J.-E. Kim, S. Kim, S.H. Um, D.-B. Oh, Y.-M. Park, Y.T. Lim, Synthetic vaccine nanoparticles target to lymph node triggering enhanced innate and adaptive antitumor immunity, Biomaterials 130 (2017) 56–66, https://doi.org/10.1016/j.biomaterials.2017.03.034.
[358] T. Uto, T. Akagi, T. Hamasaki, M. Akashi, M. Baba, Modulation of innate and adaptive immunity by biodegradable nanoparticles, Immunology Letters 125 (1) (2009) 46–52, https://doi.org/10.1016/j.imlet.2009.05.008.
[359] L. Van Hoecke, K. Roose, M. Ballegeer, Z. Zhong, N.N. Sanders, S. De Koker, X. Saelens, S. Van Lint, The opposing effect of type I IFN on the

T cell response by non-modified mRNA-lipoplex vaccines is determined by the route of administration, Molecular Therapy - Nucleic Acids 22 (2020) 373–381, https://doi.org/10.1016/j.omtn.2020.09.004.
[360] S. Ols, L. Yang, E.A. Thompson, P. Pushparaj, K. Tran, F. Liang, A. Lin, B. Eriksson, G.B. Karlsson Hedestam, R.T. Wyatt, et al., Route of vaccine administration alters antigen trafficking but not innate or adaptive immunity, Cell Reports 30 (12) (2020), https://doi.org/10.1016/j.celrep.2020.02.111.
[361] R.A. Rosalia, L.J. Cruz, S. van Duikeren, A.T. Tromp, A.L. Silva, W. Jiskoot, T. de Gruijl, C. Löwik, J. Oostendorp, S.H. van der Burg, et al., CD40-targeted dendritic cell delivery of PLGA-nanoparticle vaccines induce potent anti-tumor responses, Biomaterials 40 (2015) 88–97, https://doi.org/10.1016/j.biomaterials.2014.10.053.
[362] T.L. Nguyen, B.G. Cha, Y. Choi, J. Im, J. Kim, Injectable dual-scale mesoporous silica cancer vaccine enabling efficient delivery of antigen/adjuvant-loaded nanoparticles to dendritic cells recruited in local macroporous scaffold, Biomaterials 239 (2020) 119859, https://doi.org/10.1016/j.biomaterials.2020.119859.

Further reading

[1] C.D. Arvanitis, G.B. Ferraro, R.K. Jain, The blood–brain barrier and blood–tumour barrier in brain tumours and metastases, Nature Reviews Cancer 20 (1) (2020) 26–41, https://doi.org/10.1038/s41568-019-0205-x.
[2] G.P. Cribaro, E. Saavedra-López, L. Romarate, I. Mitxitorena, L.R. Díaz, P.V. Casanova, M. Roig-Martínez, J.M. Gallego, A. Perez-Vallés, C. Barcia, Three-dimensional vascular microenvironment landscape in human glioblastoma, Acta Neuropathologica Communications 9 (1) (2021) 24, https://doi.org/10.1186/s40478-020-01115-0.

6

Intracellular fate of nanosystems, their degradation and body accumulation

Loris Rizzello[1,2]
[1]*Department of Pharmaceutical Sciences (DISFARM), University of Milan, Milan, MI, Italy;* [2]*The National Institute of Molecular Genetics (INGM), Milan, MI, Italy*

1. Introduction

The human body is characterised by several different and highly specialised compartments having a specific function that is strictly dictated by the cells composing it. Together with tissue specialisation, the human body has evolved refined ways to overcome the issue of compartmentalisation, especially in the form of signalling processes. The same problem of compartmentalisation, as well as the strategies adopted to overwhelm it, applies also at the micrometre and sub-micrometre scale. Inside each cell (independently on which tissue it belongs to) there is indeed a whole separated world where thousands of biochemical reactions and a very dynamic trafficking take place [1]. The problem of reaching specific body and cellular isolated compartments, or an intracellular organelle, is the leitmoti reach the desired molecular target without interacting with other molecules and macromolecules. In addition to pharmacologists, material scientists are nowadays starting to face the same issue since the applications of materials in the biological and medical fields, the so-called biomaterials, have significantly risen in refinement in the last decades of the 20th century [2].

The current scientific panorama shows several examples of biomaterials that are daily used in the clinic (and outside) including prothesis, coating for medical devices, contact lens, wound dressings, sutures, cosmetic implants, nerve conduits and vascular grafts [3–5]. However, the advancement of knowledge in the life sciences, combined with the progression of new

Nanotechnology Tools for Infection Control. https://doi.org/10.1016/B978-0-12-823994-0.00011-6

ways to manipulate matter, has led biomaterials to evolve into new and more sophisticated versions.

A significant stimulus for the design and development of previously unforeseen classes of biomaterials has been particularly provided by the advent of nanotechnology, which enables to finely control the properties of materials at nanoscale level [6,7]. In this framework, the two main strategies employed for the nanotechnological production of biomaterials are top-down and bottom-up approaches. The former can be referred to the possibility of tuning the physicochemical characteristics of bulk materials [8]. The final result is both (or alternatively) a nano-object (as definition with at least one dimension below 100 nm in size) and a bulk material having nano-engineered structures, such as a nanopatterned surface or a surface-patterned nanoparticles (NPs). This method requires the use of complex instruments such as the 'Dip-Pen' nano lithography, soft lithography and electron-beam writing [9–11]. The bottom-up method is based on the high control of the assembly of atoms and/or molecules, which shape themselves into more complex nanomaterials. Metal-based and/or soft polymeric NPs are few examples of nanomaterials produced by this approach [12].

Most probably, when in 1959 Richard P. Feynman, unanimously considered the theoretical father of Nanotechnology, declared his 'there is plenty of room at the bottom', he could never expect the revolutionary potentiality of his thoughts, especially in the context of applying nanotechnology to biomaterials development. As scaling down their design, in fact, biomaterials principles can be applied to engineer new ways for navigating the body. The aim will be that of crossing different biological barriers and targeting specific parts with the dual purpose to deliver therapeutic cargos more efficiently, and to gather functional information for diagnostic purposes [13]. As a consequence, there are now biomedical nanomaterials for controlling tissue and cell growth, drug delivery systems, nanoscopic carriers and various sensing devices. Moreover, biomaterials are applied to push biological control, at the single cell level, to recreate organs harvesting stem cell capability [14,15].

It is evident that a critical aspect in biomaterials design is the understanding of how the materials may control, and even tailor, biological systems and how these outputs can be, in turn, translated into new material design.

Despite the plethora of literature data available in the field of NPs for biomedical applications, there is still a high level of open issues concerning their interaction with biological molecules in situ. This is mainly due to the complexity of the biological environment, together with a lack of translational information about biological dynamics of nanomaterials. The scattered information describing the interaction between nanomaterials and biological systems hinders the chance to have established translational theories on the basic mechanisms ruling this phenomenon.

With all these premises in mind, the principal aim of this chapter is to critically address the NPs fate within the body, by means of a multidisciplinary and a comprehensive viewpoint. I will describe the long itinerary of NPs by analysing step-by-step all the fundamental stages of their trip, namely from immediately after its administration, up to the final delivery and/or clearance. To do this, I will describe all the possible interactions (both desired and random) occurring with human body components, starting from the molecular level and up to the interaction occurring with cells and tissues. Along with the biological journey and the multiple interactions, I will provide useful guidelines for designing NPs targeted to a desired outcome. I believe this review will give the readers a critical tool for understanding the analytical approach required to design active/effective nano-biomedical devices, which are represented, in this specific case, by NPs.

2. The fate of nanoparticles

2.1 Preliminary considerations on NPs toxicity

The biocompatibility of NPs is surely a critical aspect in the context of applications for the healthcare. We are asked to produce something that interact with the human body to cause a positive effect, with a consequent minimal collateral damage. The aim of this section is not to report the current knowledge on nanotoxicology, as many aspects of the mechanisms of NPs toxicity have been disclosed [16–18]. We will take the preliminary assumption that each circulating NP must be biocompatible, and clinically approved or made of generally recognised as safe (GRAS) material (i.e. its components are already used and considered safe in different clinical contexts). It is not thus surprizing why biomaterials scientists are reluctant with synthesising new materials, while they are prone to use already established clinically safe ones. Material scientists must consider opting for materials that have short life in biological milieu, and that degrade into easy to metabolise components, especially in the context of intravenous injections (like polylactide, polyglycolide) [19–22]. To this respect, it has been recently observed that the human body can perform even drastic degradation, digesting both 'unbreakable' (e.g. carbon nanotubes) or biologically inert (PEO) materials [23–25].

Nevertheless, I will focus on the open issues concerning the 'potential' toxicity of the NPs, discussing specifically which analytical approaches should be exploited, and further implemented, to address their safety. First, most of the tools used to investigate the collateral damages are not universally appropriate. NP toxicity is usually assessed using cell cytotoxicity assays, and in most cases, on immortalised cell lines as this is a quick and easy way to address critical toxicity. The standard cytotoxicity screens include the viability (by MTT), the membrane damage (by LDH), the oxidative stress (by dichlorofluorescein assay) and the cellular metabolism (measure of ATP levels) assays [26,27]. Although it is worth noticing that the majority of the cytotoxicity assays are based on the conversion of a given substrate by metabolically active cells, which is then molecularly transformed into a luminescent of colourimetric readout. While providing useful information, all these assays fall short in determining whether the cells of interest are in cryostasis because of the treatment. Together with cytotoxicity, also genotoxicity studies are nowadays performed for addressing any potential hazardous effects to genetic materials [28,29]. This latter is usually based on comet or TUNEL assays. However, it is worth mentioning that all these methods do not give a full picture of potential harm in more complex systems. Alternative approaches have been thus proposed, such as tissue engineering models recreating some of the in vivo complexity [29,30]. Another way is to go deeper inside the cellular damage, by focussing on more refined investigations like autophagy, nuclear factor kB (NF-kB) translocation, endoplasmic reticulum (ER) stress, antiviral responses or even venturing into adequate gene and protein screenings. Such methods can give important information on several aspects, especially in the viewpoint to disclose unplanned outcomes (e.g. anti-inflammatory activity, immune response, stress recovery, etc.). A further improvement could be characterised by immunological evaluations with the aim to assess possible interactions with complement proteins, and on the potential effects on immune cells, trying at the same time to embrace the more established theories of immunology (e.g. the danger model) [31,32]. Even though in vitro methods provide a basic layer of insight about the characterisation of NPs, discrepancies between in vitro and in vivo studies are too often reported demonstrating not only that traditional in vitro assays remain limited but also that in vivo experiments represent the élite choice for exploring NPs toxicity in a more comprehensive way.

Again, new developments are available, as we have now access to new animal models that facilitate high-throughput (HTP) screenings. Some examples are flatworms, slugs and zebrafish [33–35]. Particularly the latter is emerging as new non-rodent vertebrate model for assessing the use of NPs in cancer or infection treatments [36,37]. Zebrafish models are easy to handle and relatively cheap to maintain. They also allow for quite sophisticated whole body and high-resolution imaging with faster and more efficient outputs [38,39]. However, they are still physiologically simple and fall short in recapitulating the biological complexity of the human body, and medical history has taught of many cases where the collateral damage was greater than the beneficial effects (Fig. 6.1).

2.2 NPs interfacing with biological barriers: An overview on the intra-body itineraries

The human body is a highly compartmentalised system with several components creating very different local compositions. Yet, physiology teaches that there are several highly gated transport mechanisms that regulate signalling, and metabolism across the different organs. These barriers inevitably hinder nanomaterials entry and diffusion within the body, and consequently new strategies are requested to set up new design principles for nanomaterials. Biological barriers cannot really be grouped in classes and each specific class is eventually rather difficult to describe, because most of them share common pathways. However, it can be roughly categorised that there is a fine control over the presence of external molecules at molecular, cellular, tissue and organ level. This mostly depends on the specific way of administration, so that one barrier may act before another one, while some of them may be completely overcome.

For this journey to begin, NPs have to be effectively carried somehow to their target. It might not be immediate, but the journey of the NPs will be significantly affected by the introduction method, as it will interface with several different barriers. There are several administration ways, e.g. subcutaneous, sublingual and topical inoculations (ocular, cutaneous and transdermal) but the most common ones are the intravenous (IV) and intramuscular injection, together with the oral administration. Assuming an IV injection, the very first molecule to come to term is water. This is the second most common molecule in the Universe, second only to molecular hydrogen, and it is surely the most important component of life. It is well known that water

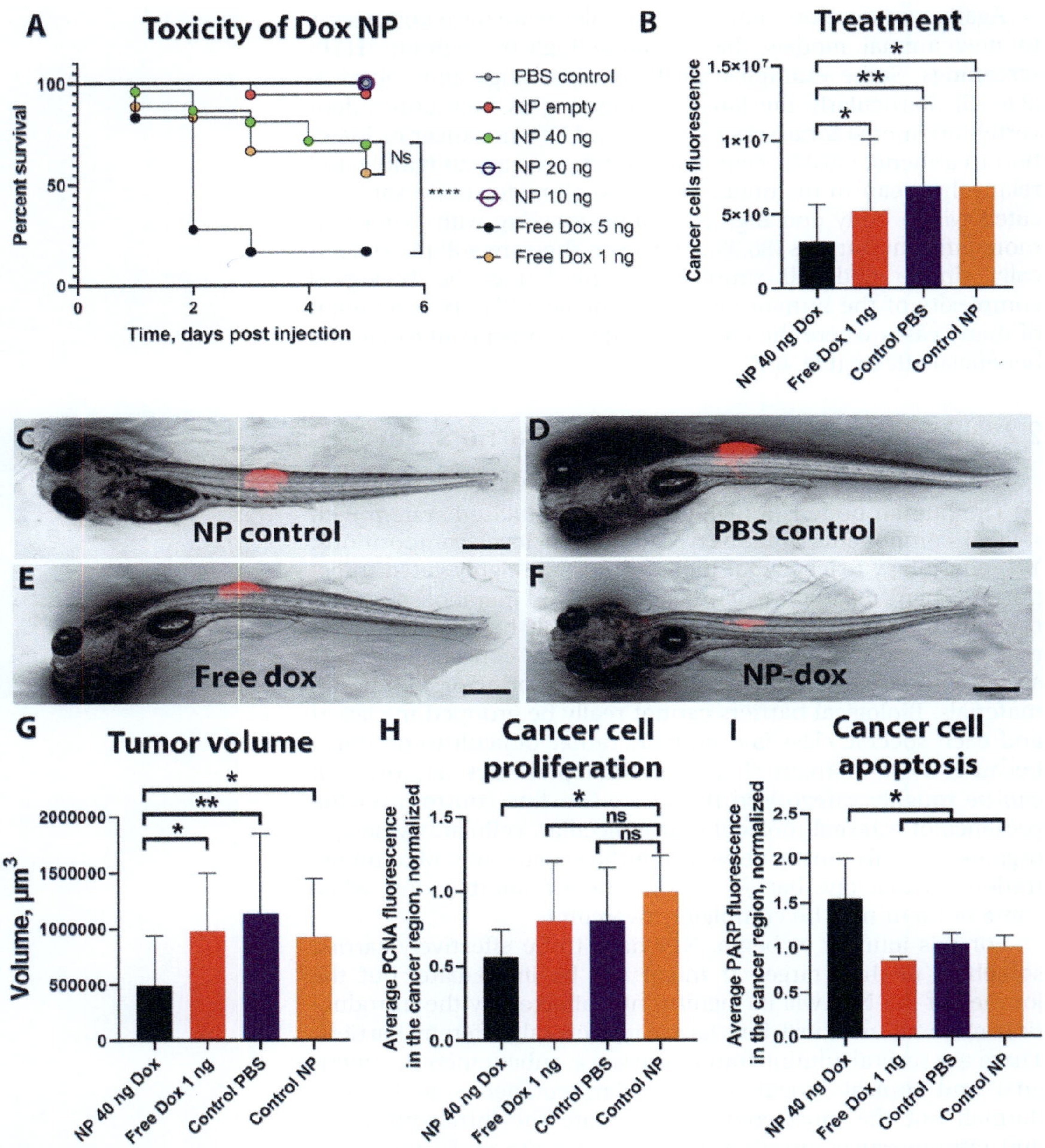

Figure 6.1 PEG-PDPA-doxorubicin toxicity and cancer therapy. (A) shows via an embryo survival graph the toxicity of PEG-PDPA-doxorubicin versus free doxorubicin. (B) shows the measurements based on fluorescence of cancer cells growth at day 7 when zebrafish received either 40 ng of doxorubicin in PEG-PDPA NP or 1 ng of free doxorubicin, or were injected with NP control (without doxorubicin) or PBS. Representative images of each group can be seen in (C), (D), (E) and (F). (G), (H) and (I) are graphs showing the quantification of tumour volume (G), cancer cell proliferation (PCNA antibody labelling, H) and cancer cell apoptosis (cPARP antibody labelling, I) of zebrafish receiving the four treatments, at 7 days after xenotransplantation.

molecules interact between each other via hydrogen bonds, forming an average of 3–3.5 bonds per molecules in the liquid state. Any guest molecule in water will induce perturbations to the water network, and they will attract or repel each other depending on how the guest can (or cannot) interact with water molecules. It goes without saying that a hypothetical hydrophobic NPs will not be able to enter the water network and it will be repelled by it (hence attract to each other's) with forces whose magnitude in some cases exceeds the attraction in the vacuum [40]. It is not indeed surprizing why most NPs are either soluble or possess a hydrophilic surface. Another important aspect is that the interaction between the NPs and water has extreme consequences in terms of interaction with other molecules, as this also occurs via hydrogen bonding perturbation. The molecular surface nature of the NPs will thus direct this interaction in one specific way. Traditionally, this approach has been adapted to the existing repertoire of theoretical models and experimental approaches created by surface scientists. However, these are often based on the simplification that surfaces are two-dimensional entities, atomically ordered, while hydrogen bonding has defined and directional bond lengths and angles. This means that, in addition to the chemical nature, the supramolecular forces can be also controlled by the three-dimensional conformation of the NPs. Within any biological fluids, and in blood in particular, the fluid phase is enriched with several other solutes including salts, small metabolites and proteins. Without going into much physicochemical details on how such complex solutions work, one important aspect to consider is that biological liquids are almost saturate in salts. This means that any electrostatic interaction is inevitably screened by this large amount of electrolyte [41]. One level up in molecular size, and the next encounter, results in dealing with proteins. The 'fouling' problem, i.e. the inevitable interaction between exogenous materials and proteins, has dominated Biomaterial Science for many decades, due to its critical impact on the final delivery of the somanaut. First described as protein 'adsorption' in the 1950 and 1960s [42,43], the concept of protein corona has rapidly evolved over the course of the recent years. At the basis of this biological phenomena there are three key concepts.

First, whatever kind of NPs will interact with plasma proteins such as albumin (HSA), apolipoproteins and immunoglobulins [44,45]. Second, these interactions will result in the formation of layers of proteins, which are classically defined as 'hard corona' and 'soft corona'. Whereby, the first comprises an inner protein layer is strongly bound onto the NPs surface, while in the second there is a dynamic exchange of proteins between the NPs surface and the environment [46,47]. There is also evidence that proteins of the 'soft corona' are covalently bound to the 'hard corona' rather than the surface of the NPs [48]. It is also worth underlining that the majority of the studies focussed on ex vivo characterisation of protein corona. However, it is now clear that although the final amount of protein present on the surface of the NPs in vivo and ex vivo are correlated, their relative abundance and variety are different. The reason for such differences lies in the absence of blood flow dynamics or interactions with cellular components outside of the body [45,49].

Third, the NPs covered by proteins will behave as a completely different nano-object because it will possess new physicochemical properties [46]. This latter event has been also found to be the main cause of dissimilar toxicity of the same batch of AuNPs incubated in two different cell culture media [50]. Concerning the nature of NPs–protein interactions, nobel metal hard NPs (e.g. gold and silver) strongly interact with cysteine-rich peptides/proteins in a quasi-covalent manner. This is because the thiol moiety is a soft ligand, with highest occupied molecular orbitals (HOMO) of high energy and will strongly bind soft cations with low unoccupied molecular orbitals (LUMO) of low energy. On the other hand, the binding between soft NPs and proteins is relatively weak, as it is mainly formed by Wan deer Waals interactions. However, this binding is highly dynamic, and it varies in conditions of health and disease. Recent work has demonstrated that the protein corona formed around nanoparticles administered in humans can be exploited as an analytic tool to investigate the circulating proteome [51].

Because of the fouling process, many efforts have been focussed on finding strategies able to avoid undesired or uncontrolled/unspecific protein adsorption. In this context, a ubiquitous approach is the use of a specific coating that comprises the appropriate physical and chemical features to interact with water more strongly than with proteins. One of the best solution is the poly(ethylene oxide) (PEO), commonly known as poly(ethylene glycol) (PEG). The anti-fouling property of PEO is the result of its chemical nature. PEO has the correct electron-acceptor character to favour water association, and to create an energy barrier that prevent protein (or any other soluble polymer) interaction [52,53]. The non-fouling character can be increased by confining PEO chains into dense brushes that create a steric repulsion hindering the protein to approach the coated NPs. Such behaviour, although yet not fully formalised, has been observed in several other polymers and surface coatings, such as phosphorylcholine [54], certain hydrophilic polysaccharides

[55] and poly-amino acids [56]. However, the PEO-based anti-fouling approach is also inevitably reductionist, so that a total biological inertness of the NPs is impossible, albeit significantly reduced. Clearly, the filp-side is that the presence of proteins on the surface of the somanaut could also prevent non-specific cellular uptake [57], and could be exploited to increase NPs targeting or reduce cytotoxicity [58].

One of the undesired effects of a NPs covered by plasma proteins could be a systemic and uncontrolled immune response. In immunological arenas, the fouling problem is often known as opsonisation. Immune-regulating proteins can opsonise (i.e. cover) the NPs surface with more or less affinity. Among these there are immunoglobulins and complement proteins (word derived from the original observation that some proteins 'complemented' together with antibodies in the bacteria lysis). Due to the high binding specificity of immunoglobulin, it is quite unlikely that NPs may be opsonised. On the other side, a complement-mediated recognition may occur. In particular, the complement consists of a pool of more than 30 serum proteins that are in the form of inactive precursor (i.e. the zymogen) within the blood stream.

In this framework, the circulating NPs are likely to interact with the complement protein C3 because it has affinity to several non-self-material, with a consequent possible activation of complement system. In particular, there are evidences that charged sulfide, lipids and cyclodextrine-modified NPs are more prone to activate the complement system comparing to their respective unmodified counterpart [48,59], while PEG coatings were found to reduce the complement activation [60]. A NPs-induced constitutive activation of C3 may indeed lead to mild and transient reactions, also known as C activation-related pseudo-allergy (CARPA) as reported for Doxil [61,62],

The protein fouling of somanaut may be thus associated with an immune response, and the way the human body recognises endogenous from exogenous material is via the use of specific immune-modulators motifs. Discher and colleagues have exemplified this approach by using NPs displaying the self-peptide extracted from the CD47 receptor. They observed that this 'don't eat me' signal on the particles prevents inflammation, inhibits microparticle phagocytosis and promotes persistent circulation of virus-like nanoparticles in vivo [63,64]. Such an immune modulator effect expands beyond the molecular level, and it is an exemplary approach on how molecular level interactions control more complex biological processes. These are examples on how synthetic strategies may be exploited to modulate a desired biological outcome that is, in this case, an immune regulation.

The design of NPs is crucial in the context of overcoming the molecular barriers of the interactions occurring at the solid–liquid interfaces. The water molecules, as well as the huge number of proteins present in the blood stream, will significantly impact both the NPs stability in situ and their final fate as a function of uncontrolled opsonisation. The final targeting efficiency may be hence strongly affected, resulting in an overall failure in the correct delivery and effectiveness.

2.3 Targeting the cellular barriers

According to the previous descriptions, circulating NPs will interact with water and plasma proteins upon intravenous injections. However, they will also contact both circulating and tissue cells, with a possible internalisation event. In this context, it might be useful to mention that all the interactions NPs have at this level certainly affect their capacity to bind the target of interest. This is in fact a crucial topic in the current biomedical research because a good targeting needs to be specific for the site of interest and this is mandatory to avoid undesired adverse effects and prevent impairing the fate of NPs when circulating within the human body. As introduced back in time by Paul Ehlrich, this specificity is related to the ability of tailor-made macromolecules eventually present onto NPs surface, known as ligands, to bind selectively receptors expressed on the cells of interest. This concept has largely been exploited and a high number of targeted strategies have been developed mainly based on the monovalent interaction between ligands and receptors [65,66]. In this unique recognition process, however, there are few chances for this interaction to be completely selective especially for ligands with high affinity for their receptors. This is mainly because most of the time receptors are not solely expressed on the cells of interest, but they are present at low densities on other tissues. In this framework, the necessity to use receptor densities as discriminating factor for cancer therapies has seen the use of multivalency as a crucial solution to address the selectivity requirements [67]. Multivalency is based on the simultaneous interactions of multiple ligands with multiple receptors originating peculiar behaviours not observable in the correspondent monovalent binding [68]. This mechanism is very well known in nature as several aspects in cell biology are regulated by multivalency, e.g. viruses and bacterial infections [69,70], DNA modifications or antibodies-mediated processes [71,72] (Fig. 6.2).

Mammen and co-workers recognised the importance of this principle in the design of constructs able to sharply respond to receptors concentration [73]. However, a uniform and comprehensive theoretical explanation behind the correlation of multivalency with selectivity was firstly proposed by Martinez-Veracoechea and Frenkel some decades later [74]. Here the authors explain that having multiple binding arrangements between ligands and receptors is a *conditio* sine *qua non* to achieve selectivity as a function of receptors number however, an on-off regime can be exclusively established when the single ligand–receptor bond is sufficiently weak.

Having this background on ligand–receptor interaction, we should move on analysing which cells the circulating NPs will interact with. The first level of interaction is likely to occur with the most abundant cells in the blood stream, namely the red blood cells (RBCs). The literature data available on the NPs-RBC interaction is not so abundant. Complex theoretical simulations, where the cells hydrodynamics was modelled with particles Brownian motions in microcirculation conditions, confirmed the crucial role of RBC in NPs dynamics [75]. Interestingly, the motion of RBC seems to enhance the dispersion of NPs, which were predicted to preferentially group at the edge of the vessel, under flowing conditions. Such phenomenon can be explained by combining the hydrodynamic interactions with a volumetric exclusion effect of the RBC [75].

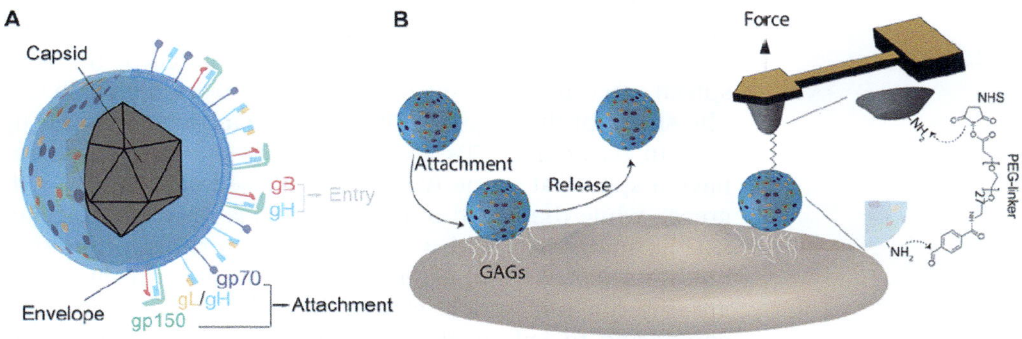

Figure 6.2 (A) Schematic model of MuHV-4 particle, showing a lipid bilayer–derived envelope (*blue*) carrying multiple glycoproteins, a subset of which are involved either in the attachment (gp70, gp150 and gL/gH) to cell surface molecules or in the entry mechanism into cells (gB and gH). (B) Schematic of HV binding to GAGs and virus release (either after attachment or after cellular infection). Before cell entry, the virus must bind to attachment factors (GAGs, HS, etc.) to concentrate virus on the cell surface before the specific binding to entry receptors. Interactions with GAG moieties will be monitored at the single-virus level using AFM, with tips derivatised with a single virion. With kind permission from Delguste et al. [69].

This is an important aspect, since RBC will affect the journey of the circulating NPs, which will probably avoid the lumen of vessel, and prefer contacting the endothelium, thus having the chance to interact with endothelial cells more efficiently. In this scenario, model human umbilical vein endothelial cell (HUVEC) were found to engulf different polystyrene NPs (in the size range of 100 nm) [76,77]. Interestingly, the NPs-cell associations were related to the quantity of protein adsorbed onto the NPs surface, rather than on the identity (i.e. the type) of a specific protein present. In particular, NPs having a bigger protein corona were up taken more efficiently by HUVEC cells, comparing to the same NPs having a small (or completely lacking) protein layer around them [77]. This would further confirm how protein corona changes the characteristics, and the final fate indeed, of nanosized circulating NPs.

During their 'trip' through the systemic circulation, the NPs are likely to interact with the reticuloendothelial system (RES), also known as mononuclear phagocyte system (MPS) [78,79]. This is a significant pool of macrophages present in the spleen, liver, bone marrow, lungs and lymph nodes. Its main role is the protection from possible invasion of microorganisms, toxins and viruses [80]. Macrophages may uptake the circulating NPs, especially those opsonised by complement proteins, thus increasing the rates of clearance and decreasing their biodistribution/bioavailability. Similarly to the NPs–protein interactions, also in this case specific strategies have been developed to avoid a RES clearance. As expected, PEG functionalisation represented the best choice [81]. However, we are still far from uncovering a general strategy for bypassing the RES clearance. There are evidences that more than 50% of the injected NPs ended in the liver and spleen after 48 hours, even though they were highly PEGylated. The shape of the NPs is an important parameter for RES uptake [82]. In particular, NPs are successfully internalised when they have a spherical shape (with a normalised curvature $\Omega \leq 45$ degrees), while the speed of phagocytosis is reversely correlated to Ω. Ellipsoidal NPs with $\Omega > 45$ degrees, on the other side, are not internalised. Moreover, NPs having a worm-like structure are internalised much slower by alveolar rat macrophages, comparing to spherical NPs. This evidence may be explained with the high dominance of low curvature (i.e. flat) regions in the 'worms' (with $\Omega = 87.5$ degrees) over the only two high curvature regions ($\Omega = 2.5$ degrees), represented by the extremities of the structure [83].

These examples highlight the complexity of the phenomena involved in the interactions occurring between NPs and the physiological components of the circulating system. It is also evident that good NPs should have a spherical shape, and an overall neutral charge, to avoid uncontrolled aggregation and/or non-specific cellular internalisation.

2.4 Cellular uptake of NPs

In the previous paragraphs I described the interactions of NPs with different biomolecules and cells, immediately after injection. Additionally, I depicted the role of circulating and resident cells in the control over the NPs delivery within the body. However, the mechanisms of NPs uptake by cells, and the specific molecular pathways involved, are also important topics to be discussed, especially in the viewpoint of the final sorting. This is a very debated and quite complex issue, where biology merges with physics, biochemistry and molecular biology. The main question is how the NPs interact with the plasma membranes, and what is the preferential uptake process.

The most accepted mechanisms of NPs entry within the cell are the phagocytosis and/or endocytosis. The former is performed by specialised/professional phagocytes, namely mast cells, macrophages, neutrophils, dendritic cells and monocytes. The process starts with an event of recognition between an extracellular ligand (usually functionalised on the surface of the NPs) and specific plasma membrane receptors present in the immune cells. Therefore, a signal cascade event leads to the local recruitment of actin filaments that, in turns, reassemble and distort the plasma membrane with a resultant formation of membrane protrusions engulfing the NPs. These plasma membranes extensions will end with the formation of the phagosome having final dimensions dictated by the specific size and shape of the NPs. The phagocytosis of NPs may be driven by the opsonisation of complement proteins. These proteins will be, in turn, recognised by their respective complement receptors on the plasma membrane of immune cells. Several reports already demonstrated that NPs may be engulfed in phagosomal vesicles having a final size of c.a. 1 um [84,85].

Unlike phagocytosis, endocytosis is not delimited to professional cells, as it is ubiquitous to almost all eukaryotes. Also, endocytosis requires the specific binding between an external molecule and its respective plasma membrane receptor. Then, the engulfment process may follow different pathways, depending on the main involved proteins, such as the Clathrin, Caveolae, RhoA, CDC42, ARF6 and Flotillin [86,87].

In addition to phagocytosis and endocytosis, macropinocytosis is another possible entry mechanism of NPs within cells. It involves the uptake of huge amount of external fluid, thanks to the extrusion of sheet-like lamellipodia from the plasma membrane. The consequent formed vesicle, named as macropinosome, has size in the range of 1–4 um. Whilst both phagocytosis and endocytosis start with a ligand–receptor binding, macropinocytosis is independent from this event.

It is worth pointing out that the physicochemical characteristics of the NPs play a pivotal role in the discrimination of the specific uptake process involved. Concerning the size, there are several evidences that smaller NPs may access the cells more efficiently comparing to bigger NPs [88–90]. However, this scenario looks slightly difficult to be categorised, mainly because of the different approaches exploited to analyse and quantify the collected data. In this context, a simple normalisation of fluorescence signal of differently sized SiO_2 NPs would suggest that the role of size is negligible for the uptake [91], a thesis supported by similar works. In this case, a combination of flow cytometry and UV-visible spectroscopy assays confirmed that the size of poly(2-methacryloyloxyethyl phosphorylcholine) (PMPC) and poly(ethylene oxide) PEO polymeric vesicles (named as polymersomes) is not a fundamental parameter for endocytosis, in human dermal fibroblast (HDF) cells [92]. On the other side, the efficacy and strength of the binding between the HDF and the NPs seem to be much more fundamental in the uptake efficiency, rather than size itself (Fig. 6.3).

In addition to size, the shape/geometry of the NPs is another parameter that can be easily tuned during the synthesis of nanomaterials. While the observations on the NPs size are contrasting, the literature data available about the effects of shape on the cellular uptake are rather concordant. In particular, spherical NPs (AuNPs) seem to be engulfed much faster than tubular structures (Au nanotubes), independent on the size and/or external functionalisation of tubes [93]. This has been very recently confirmed also by Robertson and co-workers, which explored the degree of uptake of polymeric vesicles and tubes [94]. By using flow cytometry assays, the authors discovered that the internalisation of rhodamine-labelled tubular polymersomes displays a profile having two-phase kinetics: immediately after the incubation, the tubes bind to the surface of the cells (neutrophils and FaDu cells were tested) without being engulfed; in the second step they are slowly internalised. On the other side, spherical polymersomes were rapidly internalised by the same cells [94]. Among the differently sized tubular structures, carbon nanotubes with a

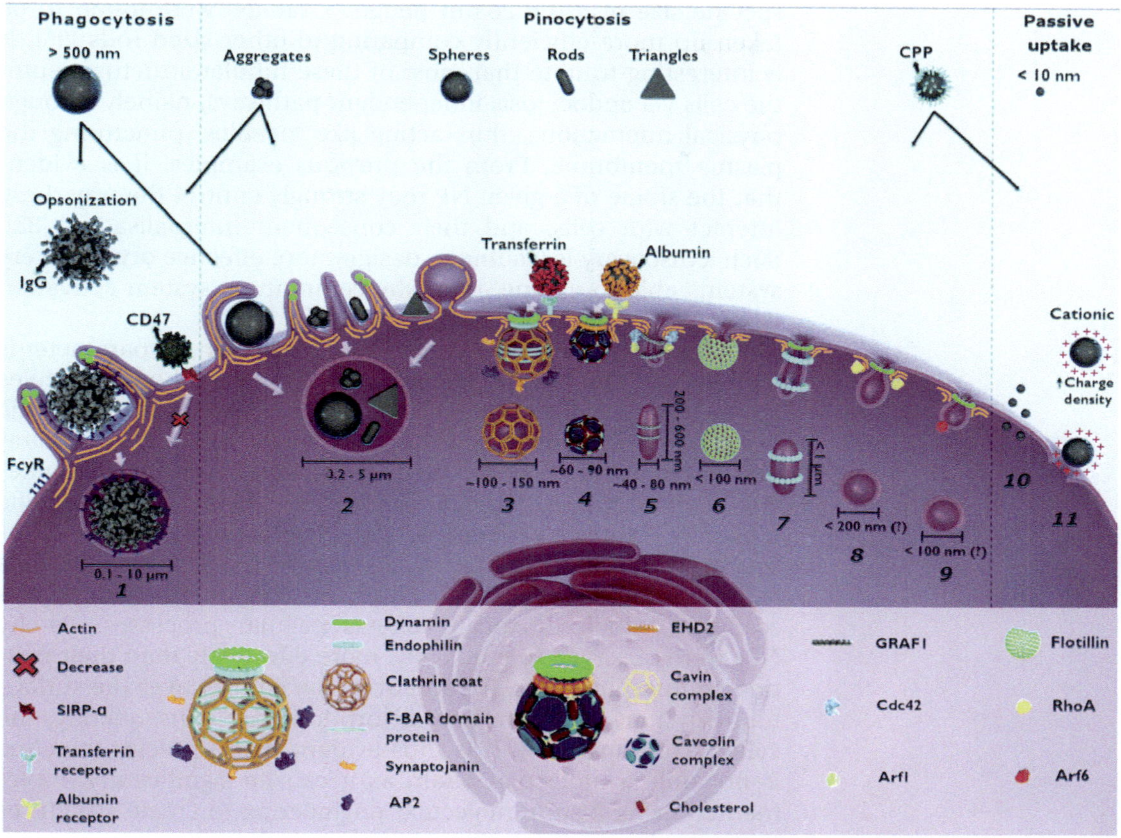

Figure 6.3 Possible entry mechanisms for nanoparticles (NPs). Large NPs (>500 nm) and aggregates enter the cell through phagocytosis [1] and macropinocytosis [2]. NP opsonisation via IgG leads to cellular recognition (FcγR) in phagocytes. Pinocytosis includes different mechanisms: Macropinocytosis [2], clathrin-mediated endocytosis [3], caveolae-dependent endocytosis [4], CLIC–GEEC [5], flotillin-assisted endocytosis [6], fast-endophilin-mediated endocytosis [7], RhoA-dependent endocytosis [8] and Arf-6-associated endocytosis [9]. As a non-selective endocytic process, macropinocytosis [2] is associated with the internalisation of different NPs. Smaller NPs (<10 nm) and cationic NPs, with high charge density, enter the cell via direct penetration [10] and pore formation [11], respectively. NPs surface functionalisation with different molecules has an impact on cellular uptake. NPs functionalised with transferrin and albumin are taken up through clathrin-mediated [3] and caveolae-dependent endocytosis [4], respectively. NPs functionalised with CPP can be internalised passively [10,11] as well as via other endocytic pathways. The functionalisation of NPs with CD47 reduces phagocytosis [1]. Flotillin-assisted endocytosis [6] and Arf-6-associated endocytosis [9] can occur both, in the presence or absence of dynamin. CPP: cell penetrating peptide. IgG: Immunoglobulin G. CD47: Cluster of differentiation 47. FcγR: Fc gamma receptor. SIRPα: Signal regulatory protein alpha. AP2: Adaptor protein 2. EHD2: Eps15-homology domain containing protein 2. GRAF1: GTPase regulator associated with focal adhesion kinase-1. CDC42: cell division cycle 42. Arf1: ADP-ribosylation factor 1. RhoA: Ras homologue family member A. Arf6: ADP-ribosylation factor 6. (?) – vesicle size still unclear. Reproduced from Ref. [90] with permission from the Royal Society of Chemistry.

specific size of 320 × 26 nm (length x radius) were found to be taken up more efficiently comparing to other sized rods [95]. It is interesting to note that most of these tubular structures enter the cells via endocytosis independent pathways, namely through physical interactions, thus acting like 'needles' puncturing the plasma membrane. From the previous examples, it is evident that the shape of a given NP may strongly control the way these interact with cells, and their consequent internalisation [82]. Such a discovery is leading to design more effective drug delivery systems able to escape, for instance, immune system activation [83].

In addition to size and shape, another important parameter is the surface topology of the NPs, which refers to how molecules and macromolecule arrange on a given interface, forming specific patterns and domains. To this respect, interface-confined separation of copolymers has been recently employed to design materials with controlled surface topology. For instance, the specific mixing of cell-inert with cell-active polymers may lead to the formation of controlled patterns. These have a size range from tens to hundreds of nanometres, either on NPs or on microporous scaffolds, which drastically affects cellular processes. Patchy NPs were observed to enter cells more effectively than their pristine counterparts [96,97]. Moreover, the control over the surface topology may affect protein adsorption and, consequently, the cellular response [98]. It is thus evident that a precise targeting is not only a molecular affair, as it can be significantly implemented using a supramolecular engineering to create structures that combine molecular recognition with mesoscopic ones.

2.5 Intracellular fate and sorting of NPs

Similarly to the uptake, also the intracellular fate of the NPs is a quite complex scenario to be depicted. This is due to the endosomal trafficking, where endocytic vesicles are shuttled to specific subcellular compartment, thanks to cytosolic motor proteins. The sorting starts with the remodelling of plasma membrane, a process regulated by a set of proteins containing the Bin/Amphiphysin/Rvs (BAR) domain. BAR proteins may act as sensor, effector and stabiliser of membrane curvature and shaping [99–101] (Fig. 6.4).

They are monomers that dimerise upon activation, and start building a complex tridimensionality displaying a positive charge on the side approaching/binding the negatively charged membrane. After membrane budding, the cleavage of the forming vesicles from the plasma membrane is regulated by dynamin, a

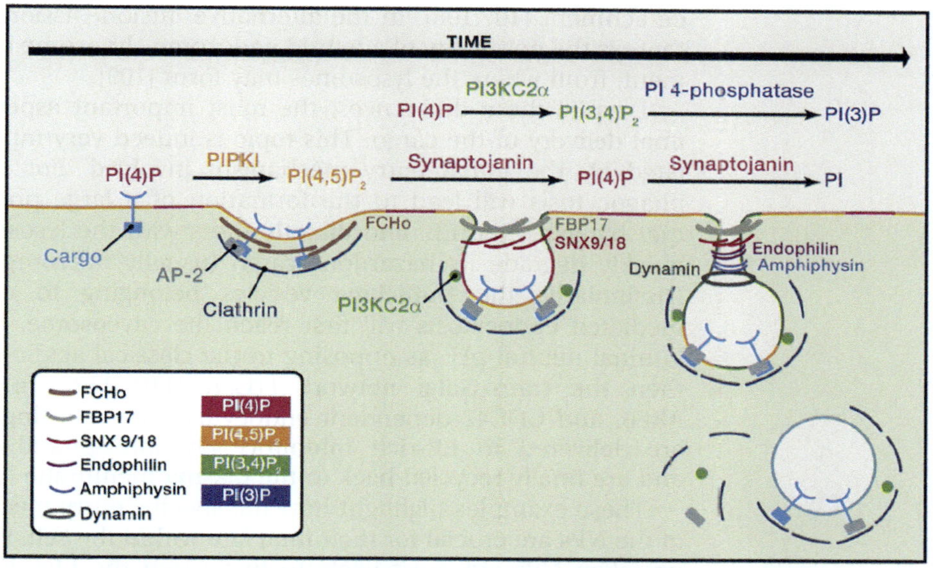

Figure 6.4 Endocytic membrane Remodelling during clathrin-mediated endocytosis.

GTPase family protein, most of the times. Experimental evidence highlighted two possible mechanisms of dynamin-mediated vesicle detachment. The 'pinch off' model suggests that dynamin tetramers assemble between the budding vesicle and the plasma membrane, forming progressively narrowing helical tubes [102,103]. In the 'helicase' mechanism, the dynamin tubules expand without changing the internal diameter [104]. Although both the two proposed model could also work together, the final result is the detachment of the vesicles, which buds from the internal side of the plasma membrane and gain access to the cytosol. The trafficking vesicles are then ready to be delivered to the respective intracellular compartments. Because of the so fast spatiotemporal dynamics of the processes involved, understanding the nature of intracellular sorting remains still a big challenge. One of the most accepted theories, for decades, was the 'maturation' process. Here, the up taken material is first delivered to the early endosome (EE), which slowly matures to a late endosome (LE), and finally to a lysosome [105,106].

However, this model looks nowadays unsatisfactory for explaining the fast process involved, especially in the viewpoint of the recycling organelles. Several recent data confirmed a possible 'kiss and run' mechanism, where endosomes and lysosomes undergo continuous cycles of temporary fusion and detachment [107,108]. In the alternative 'fusion–fission model', there is the possibility of a hybrid endosome–lysosome compartment, from where the lysosomes may form [109].

Despite these differences, the most important aspect is the final delivery of the cargo. This topic is indeed very much regulated by the initial entry mechanism involved. For example, phagocytosis will lead to the formation of a large phagosome that bypasses the EE, and directly fuses with the lysosomes, to quickly degrade its hazardous cargo (usually microorganisms). Dissimilarly, the trafficking vesicles belonging to caveolae-mediated endocytosis will first reach the caveosome, having a luminal neutral pH (as opposing to the classical acidic EE), and then the trans-Golgi network (TGN) [110–112]. In flotillin, ARF6, and CDC42-dependent endocytosis, the forming vesicles are delivered to EE-rich inhibitory glycophosphatidylinositol, and are finally recycled back to the plasma membrane [113].

These examples highlight how the specific entry mechanisms of the NPs are crucial for their final fate within the cell. However, up-taken NPs are most likely to first reach the EEs, in a time range of about 1–4 min. EEs are heterogeneous organelles having differently sized and shaped cisternae (characterised by tubes of 50–80 nm and big vesicles of c.a. 400 nm). The main role of EE is to recycle cell receptors back to the plasma membrane, and to deliver their cargo to the TGN or to the LEs, a process occurring within 10–15 min. The structure of LEs is morphologically very similar to the EEs, although they have a more acidic pH (between 5.0 and 5.5). After LEs, the final organelles are the lysosomes, which are reached in about 30 min. They are characterised by membrane whorls, and have a luminal pH of 4.5–5.0, which is kept constant, thanks to proton-pumping ATPases [114]. The main hydrolytic activity of lysosomes is due to a group of 50 different acidic hydrolyses and 25 lysosomal integral proteins [115], which act together for the degradation of both intracellular (i.e. in autophagy) and extracellular material.

It is indeed evident that, following the intracellular sorting of vesicles, most of the internalised NPs will finally reach the lysosomal compartment, resulting in their degradation that may lead to several side effects [116].

This highlights why several strategies have been adopted for the development of smart NPs able to escape the endosomal pathways, for avoiding undesired degradation. This is an important topic, especially for biomedical and drug delivery applications, where the internalised cargo must reach the intracellular target [117,118]. Particularly, scientists took inspiration from Nature in the design of NPs copying the 'escape plans' evolved by intracellular obligate and facultative bacteria/viruses. Some famous examples include NPs covered with the TAT-peptide of HIV [119,120], and the L240 or HGP peptide of the papillomavirus [121]. Because the peptides-modified NPs may be intrinsically immunogenic, other approaches focussed on synthetic polymers and lipids. These are mostly pH-sensitive molecules, so that change in the environmental pH will trigger a destabilisation of the endosomal membrane. Consequently, the cargo is released in the cytosol and ready to reach the desired intracellular target [38,118] (Fig. 6.5).

A following step in the complexity of the involved phenomena is the cytosolic navigation. Upon escaping the endosomal pathways, the NPs must 'sail' and bind to the desired targets, which could be present in the cytosol or even within the nucleus. The cell cytoplasm is a very crowded environment, full of proteins, organelles, nutrients and cytoskeletal structures. All these components will significantly impact the rheology of the NPs at cytosolic level, a parameter that will be strongly dependent on its size. In addition, any potential interaction with the cytosolic matrix may further hinder the mobility of smaller NPs, while the shape seems to be important for the navigation of bigger NPs [122].

A smart strategy for next drug development should consider the possibility of exploiting naturally available motor proteins, such as kinesin, myosin and dynein for actively directing the NPs to cytosolic targets. To this respect, Tat peptide-conjugated quantum dots (Tat-QDs) have been demonstrated to be internalised by macropynocitosis and entrapped within cytoplasmatic organelles of HeLa cells [123]. The vesicles carrying the QDs were found to be actively transported by dynein to the asymmetric perinuclear region, the microtubule organising centre (MTOC) [123].

2.6 The tissue barriers

The assembly of cells into tissues is a highly orchestrated set of biological events. Cells must be exposed to the appropriate mechanical and chemical stimuli and to the correct nutrient supply. They must be able to communicate amongst themselves, and to rearrange themselves according to the function they must perform. The ability of the NPs to go across such a complex system can be addressed by studying all the characteristics implied with its diffusion. The extravasation from the blood capillaries of the NPs is followed by interaction with highly viscous matrix present in the extracellular space. The extracellular space, or interstitium, is commonly composed of a network of collagen fibres and other molecules such as hyaluronic acid, and the nonstructural

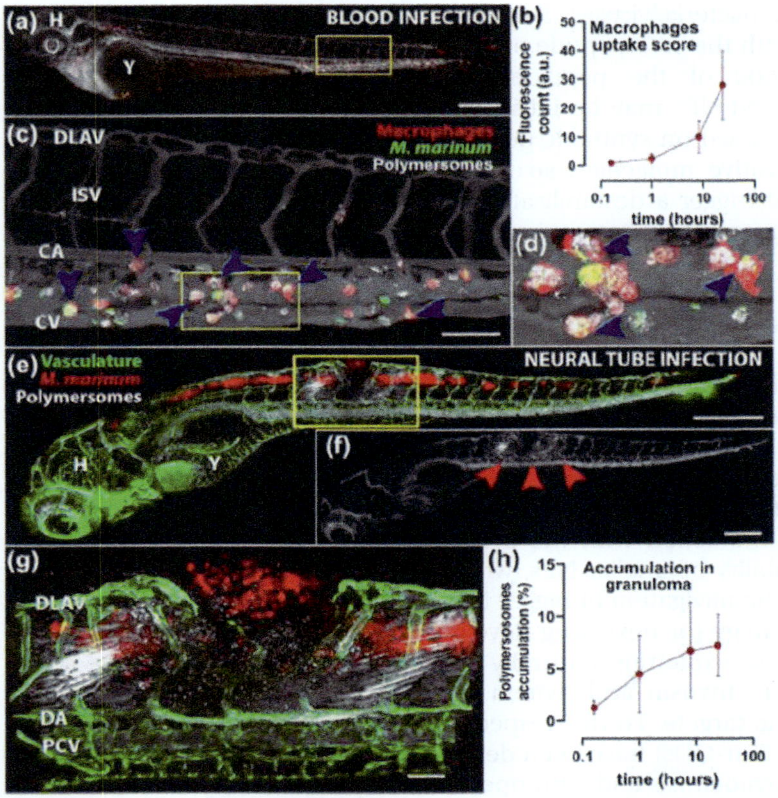

Figure 6.5 Polymersome accumulation in macrophages and granulomas in zebrafish embryos infected with *M. marinum*. (A) Zebrafish embryo fluorescently labelled with macrophages (*gray*) injected intravenously with *M. marinum* and the following day with polymersomes containing Cy5 (*white*). The image was taken 8 hours after polymersomes injection. H, head region; Y, yolk sac. (B) Quantification of polymersome uptake over time in macrophages in zebrafish larvae. (C) Enlarged area in (A) where polymersomes are detected within infected macrophages (dark gray arrows). DLAV, dorsal longitudinal anastomotic vessel. ISV, intersegmental vessel; CA, caudal artery; CV, caudal vein. (D) Enlarged area in (C) where macrophages containing *M. marinum* and polymersomes are evident (*dark gray arrows*). (E) Zebrafish embryos fluorescently labelled with endothelial cells (*white*) were injected with *M. marinum* (*light gray*) in the neural tube. Four days later, polymersomes containing Cy5 (*gray*) were injected intravenously, and the whole zebrafish was imaged 8 hours later. H, head region; Y, yolk sac. (F) The image in (E) without the signal of light gray endothelial cells and white *M. marinum* in order to better observe the selective accumulation of polymersomes (*dark gray arrows*) in the granuloma region. The *white box* in (E) is seen enlarged in (G) for observing details of polymersome accumulation in the granuloma. DLAV, dorsal longitudinal anastomotic vessel; DA, dorsal aorta; PCV, posterior cardinal vein. A graph showing accumulation over time of polymersomes in neural tube granulomas is shown in (H). Scale bars: (A) 300 μm; (C) 100 μm, (D) 25 μm, (E) 300 μm, (F) 300 μm, (G) 50 μm. Reprinted (adapted) with permission from Fenaroli et al. [118]. Copyright 2020, American Chemical Society.

proteins such as proteoglycans. Altogether, this is called extracellular matrix (ECM), which is characterised by a fluid phase consisting of water, electrolytes, nutrients and some plasma proteins. This complex and dynamic environment is where the NPs must travel through. The particles will move with Brownian random walks in between the spaces of the network structures, and it has been estimated that the fluid flows from the capillary at the low velocity of 0.1–4 m/second [124]. Thus, the movement is influenced by the matrix components [125], because of steric (collision with matrix fibres), hydrodynamic (low diffusion of water molecules due to proximity with fibres) and electrostatic interactions (for charged particles) [126,127]. The interactions with the different configuration, as well as the physicochemical properties of the ECM components, will determine the direction, speed and distance of NPs transport with a specific size and/or charge. If we take a closer look at these interactions, the electrostatic and hydrodynamic interactions are probably the most important ones.

Concerning the role played by electrostatic and hydrodynamic interactions, the diffusion in a fibrous media was the first model where the random walk of NPs was studied. In particular, it was observed that when the particle size is significantly smaller than the diameter of the fibre, the hydrodynamic interactions are negligible [128]. However, when the particle size is comparable or even larger than the fibre diameter, hydrodynamic hindrance slows down the mobility of the particle more than two-fold, and hydrodynamic interactions become crucial. Furthermore, it has been demonstrated that neutral particles might diffuse faster than cationic [126,128]. Thus, for large fibres, electrostatic repulsion might not be significant and, thus, charged particles (having charge similar to that of the fibres) will have the same diffusivity of neutral particles.

At the same time, the size of the NPs can limit the diffusion within the ECM and tissues. Nonetheless, an enhanced production of growth factors, signalling and adhesion molecules at tissue level can also further change NPs penetration within the tissue. Steric interaction can be considered negligible for small molecules, whereas they can hinder large nanoparticles movement and thus only allows for their local drug release [129]. Uniform diffusion of small NPs (64 nm in diameter) has been observed to go through neocortical extracellular space (ECS) channels. In this case, larger NPs transport may occur by different mechanisms, like entropic barriers transport or reptation. Size and the physicochemical properties play an important role for controlling the overall accumulation and penetration depth into tissues. For instance, polymeric (i.e. soft) NPs can penetrate the hard lung granuloma (the hallmark of tuberculosis infection in humans), which is one of the hardest to reach body compartment for many drugs [118].

NPs larger than 100 nm are trapped in the ECM between cells because they are not able to extravasate far beyond the blood vessel. On the other side, smaller nanoparticles (20 nm) are able to deeply penetrate within the tissues [130].

As expected, also the NPs shape is heavily involved in the tissue distribution: solubilisation, circulation time and cellular uptake are parameters that all depends on the shape of the NPs. In particular, rod-shaped or filamentous materials have been proved to better penetrate tissues comparing their spherical counterparts. Additionally, the circulation lifetime of rod-shaped micelles is 10 times longer than that of spherical micelles.

The surface chemistry of the NPs also dictates their behaviour in the surrounding environment. Hydrophilicity, surface charge, immunogenicity, in vivo circulation, bio-distribution and intracellular bioavailability are parameters that can be all modified by changing the arrangements of the chemical groups on the nanoparticles surface [131]. The ability to modify the NPs surface can be an effective way to control the interface between NPs and the biological systems they interact with. This can lead to the development of NPs able to maximise therapeutic efficacy while minimising unfavourable side effects. In this framework, Battaglia and co-workers showed that the modification of the external surface of polymersomes (obtained by changing the ratio of the two main polymers) significantly influences the cellular uptake through a super-selectivity process [92,132].

2.7 The body clearance of NPs

I have explored, in the previous sections, the many itineraries undertaken by circulating NPs. I described all the possible interactions occurring at molecular and supramolecular level, as well as we highlighted the features required to overcome innate biological barriers and bio-compartmentalisation. In the best-case scenario, 'perfectly designed' NPs will be able to: (*i*) repel plasma proteins, (*ii*) do not interact with undesired molecular targets, (*iii*) overcome membrane and tissue barriers, (*iv*) interact with the final target, and (*v*) eventually release its cargo. However, there is another big challenge that material scientists must interface with, namely the question of body clearance. Such topic is, honestly, not significantly evaluated among the nano-communities, where most of the investigations just try to characterise the biological effects of NPs, or to demonstrate the reliability of the systems in achieving the desired outcomes (e.g. tutor treatment, immune-modulatory effects, infections treatments). It is asked to the injected agent to be totally cleared in a reasonable amount of time, and this is rather unlikely for most of the NPs. The difficulty in releasing the NPs is one of the reasons why their clinical translation is still far to be seriously considered.

The first level of degradation is at cellular level, within the lysosomal compartments. The way this occurs, however, will strongly differ between hard and soft NPs. Soft NPs usually undergo disassembly of their polymeric structures, which may alternatively be integrated within the cellular membranes or be further degraded by cellular enzymes (in the case of biodegradable polymers) [133,134]. On the other side, hard NPs may undergo oxidation processes, with a consequent release of atoms from their surface that may, in turn, be the main cause of toxicity [116]. However, a complete degradation process is very unlikely. Hence, NPs may uncontrollably accumulate within the lysosomal compartments, even inducing alkalinisation and autophagosome accumulation, this latter being related to the blocking of autophagy flux, and not to the induction of autophagy [135]. In such conditions, the lysosomal storage disorders are then a concrete perspective, with the consequent occurrence and development of neurodegenerative manifestations [136,137].

NPs circulating in the body may be also cleared off again by the action of the immune system. In addition to the standard phagocytosis, already explained in the previous section, neutrophil granulocytes, monocytes and macrophages were demonstrated to produce an extracellular trap (consisting of DNA and protein) able to capture circulating NPs (also the PEO-modified) [138]. Together with phagocytosis, the immune cells-related extracellular trap significantly contributes to the clearance of NPs. Despite the cell-mediated detoxification, the NPs are however still present in the body, even lasting for more than 2 years without losing their optical activity [139], which is another reason why the regulatory approval of NPs in the clinics is very hard. In addition to this, this immune cells-controlled degradation often leads to accumulation in RES organs and the liver. Here NPs can be degraded and its quite surprizing how our liver can remove many chemicals. However, any liver degraded materials will be secreted via the biliary route, and this can take up to weeks to remove exogenous materials. A most favourable approach is to make sure that NPs either degrade or become smaller to be secreted via the renal route. Renal filtration is able to rapidly clear proteins with a hydrodynamic diameter of up to 10 nm, and represents indeed the only way to remove circulating NPs from the body via urinary excretion [140–142]. This is confirmed by recent evidences showing that NPs must have a maximum hydrodynamic diameter of 5.5 nm to be cleared, corresponding to the absolute value for the renal filtration threshold [143]. The size problem has been smartly overcome by exploiting luminescent porous silicon nanoparticles (LPSiNPs) that are able to shortly self-destroy in a small renally cleared components without any adverse effect [144].

3. Concluding remarks

The topics discussed in this chapter are probably the 'tip of the iceberg'. It is evident that NPs have the clear advantage (and yet the most challenging aspect) of an interdisciplinary area of research, which can simultaneously be dangerous: if not properly balanced it can be rather superficial, even overlooking critical details in favour to the final applications. Our goal is to translate the acquired knowledge to the clinic as soon as possible, without jumping from fundamental to applied science too quickly and without analytical control.

An additional aspect to be considered is that any new molecule will have to go through intensive clinical testing with considerable time and economic investment, typically between 5 and 20 years, and between few to several thousands of millions of pounds/dollars/euros [145]. Inevitably, together with the increase in the production of new medicines and devices, the large clinical data make future decisions even more stringent. This is quite evident in pharmaceutical industry, where the number of new drugs has been increasing steadily but the cost associated with new drugs has increased exponentially. In 1998, the average R&D cost for a new molecular entity was estimated around $26 billion (inflation corrected), while in 2008 it was already estimated to *c.a.* $50 billion [146].

NPs development for biomedical applications is still far from these numbers. Medicinal chemistry, nowadays, is not only a synthetic chemistry affair: drug design is continuously aided by bioinformatics, genomics, proteomics, cell-based screens and, moreover, by HTP approaches. Drugs are synthesised in libraries, and these are tested in outputs protocols that enable fast discovery and mapping out fundamental structure-to-function relations. Although there are few examples of HTP approaches providing new insights into biomaterial design, these do not still match with more mechanistic studies to create fundamental principles for future biomaterial design.

Clearly, when a specific material is selected for creating NPs for biomedical application, their final use, as well as the safety of the raw ingredients and the processing of production must be all a priori designed.

References

[1] M.A. Olayioye, B. Noll, A. Hausser, Spatiotemporal control of intracellular membrane trafficking by rho GTPases, Cells 8 (2019).

[2] M.J. Mitchell, et al., Engineering precision nanoparticles for drug delivery, Nature Reviews Drug Discovery 20 (2021) 101–124.

[3] J. Lee, H. Byun, S.K. Madhurakkat Perikamana, S. Lee, H. Shin, Current advances in immunomodulatory biomaterials for bone regeneration, Adv Healthc Mater 8 (2019) e1801106.

[4] M. Bordoni, et al., Biomaterials in neurodegenerative disorders: a promising therapeutic approach, International Journal of Molecular Sciences 21 (2020).

[5] M. Meyer, Processing of collagen based biomaterials and the resulting materials properties, BioMedical Engineering Online 18 (2019) 24.

[6] X. Li, et al., From precision synthesis of block copolymers to properties and applications of nanoparticles, Angewandte Chemie International Edition in English 57 (2018) 2046–2070.

[7] M.N. Aguilar, J.M. Perez-Aguilar, V.J. González-Coronel, J.G. Soriano Moro, B.L. Sanchez-Gaytan, Polymers as versatile players in the stabilization, capping, and design of inorganic nanostructures, ACS Omega 6 (2021) 35196–35203.

[8] X. Fu, et al., Top-down fabrication of shape-controlled, monodisperse nanoparticles for biomedical applications, Advanced Drug Delivery Reviews 132 (2018) 169–187.

[9] G. Liu, M. Hirtz, H. Fuchs, Z. Zheng, Development of dip-pen nanolithography (DPN) and its derivatives, Small 15 (2019) e1900564.

[10] M.A. Rose, J.J. Bowen, S.A. Morin, Emergent soft lithographic tools for the fabrication of functional polymeric microstructures, ChemPhysChem 20 (2019) 909–925.

[11] A. Fernández-Pacheco, et al., Writing 3D nanomagnets using focused electron beams, Materials 13 (2020).

[12] B.R. Karimadom, H. Kornweitz, Mechanism of producing metallic nanoparticles, with an emphasis on silver and gold nanoparticles, using bottom-up methods, Molecules 26 (2021).

[13] E.T. Sarcan, M. Silindir-Gunay, A.Y. Ozer, Theranostic polymeric nanoparticles for NIR imaging and photodynamic therapy, International Journal of Pharmaceutics 551 (2018) 329–338.

[14] X. Su, T. Wang, S. Guo, Applications of 3D printed bone tissue engineering scaffolds in the stem cell field, Regenerative Therapy 16 (2021) 63–72.

[15] A.A. Dayem, et al., The potential of nanoparticles in stem cell differentiation and further therapeutic applications, Biotechnology Journal 11 (2016) 1550–1560.

[16] I. Furxhi, F. Murphy, M. Mullins, A. Arvanitis, C.A. Poland, Nanotoxicology data for in silico tools: a literature review, Nanotoxicology 14 (2020) 612–637.

[17] M.R. Miller, C.A. Poland, Nanotoxicology: the need for a human touch? Small 16 (2020) e2001516.
[18] V.V. Chrishtop, A.Y. Prilepskii, V.G. Nikonorova, V.A. Mironov, Nanosafety vs. nanotoxicology: adequate animal models for testing in vivo toxicity of nanoparticles, Toxicology 462 (2021) 152952.
[19] A.L. Coolen, et al., Poly(lactic acid) nanoparticles and cell-penetrating peptide potentiate mRNA-based vaccine expression in dendritic cells triggering their activation, Biomaterials 195 (2019) 23–37.
[20] S. Senapati, A. Upadhyaya, S. Dhruw, D. Giri, P. Maiti, Controlled DNA delivery using poly(lactide) nanoparticles and understanding the binding interactions, Journal of Physical Chemistry B 125 (2021) 10009–10017.
[21] C. Grune, et al., Sustainable preparation of anti-inflammatory atorvastatin PLGA nanoparticles, International Journal of Pharmaceutics 599 (2021) 120404.
[22] S. Acharya, S.K. Sahoo, PLGA nanoparticles containing various anticancer agents and tumour delivery by EPR effect, Advanced Drug Delivery Reviews 63 (2011) 170–183.
[23] S. Liu, et al., Degradation behavior in vitro of carbon nanotubes (CNTs)/Poly(lactic acid) (PLA) composite suture, Polymers 11 (2019).
[24] I.C. Pereira, A.S. Duarte, A.S. Neto, J.M.F. Ferreira, Chitosan and polyethylene glycol based membranes with antibacterial properties for tissue regeneration, Materials Science & Engineering, C: Materials for Biological Applications 96 (2019) 606–615.
[25] X. Wan, et al., In vivo delivery of siRNAs targeting EGFR and BRD4 expression by peptide-modified redox responsive PEG-PEI nanoparticles for the treatment of triple-negative breast cancer, Molecular Pharmaceutics 18 (2021) 3990–3998.
[26] C. Andraos, I.J. Yu, M. Gulumian, Interference: a much-neglected aspect in high-throughput screening of nanoparticles, International Journal of Toxicology 39 (2020) 397–421.
[27] A. Choudhary, S. Singh, V. Ravichandiran, Toxicity, preparation methods and applications of silver nanoparticles: an update, Toxicology Mechanisms and Methods 1–12 (2022).
[28] A.K. Zhanataev, et al., Genotoxicity of cationic lipopeptide nanoparticles, Toxicology Letters 328 (2020) 1–6.
[29] S. Nallanthighal, R. Reliene, Evaluation of genotoxicity of nanoparticles in mouse models, Methods in Molecular Biology 1894 (2019) 301–312.
[30] G. Vales, E. Demir, B. Kaya, A. Creus, R. Marcos, Genotoxicity of cobalt nanoparticles and ions in Drosophila, Nanotoxicology 7 (2013) 462–468.
[31] M.S.J. Mangan, et al., Targeting the NLRP3 inflammasome in inflammatory diseases, Nature Reviews Drug Discovery 17 (2018) 588–606.
[32] A. Decout, J.D. Katz, S. Venkatraman, A. Ablasser, The cGAS-STING pathway as a therapeutic target in inflammatory diseases, Nature Reviews Immunology 21 (2021) 548–569.
[33] N. Leynen, et al., In vivo toxicity assessment of silver nanoparticles in homeostatic versus regenerating planarians, Nanotoxicology 13 (2019) 476–491.
[34] M.N. Croteau, S.K. Misra, S.N. Luoma, E. Valsami-Jones, Bioaccumulation and toxicity of CuO nanoparticles by a freshwater invertebrate after waterborne and dietborne exposures, Environmental Science & Technology 48 (2014) 10929–10937.

[35] C. Bai, M. Tang, Toxicological study of metal and metal oxide nanoparticles in zebrafish, Journal of Applied Toxicology 40 (2020) 37–63.
[36] J.S. Stine, B.J. Harper, C.G. Conner, O.D. Velev, S.L. Harper, In vivo toxicity assessment of chitosan-coated lignin nanoparticles in embryonic zebrafish (*Danio rerio*), Nanomaterials 11 (2021).
[37] S. Machado, et al., Toxicity in vitro and in zebrafish embryonic development of gold nanoparticles biosynthesized using cystoseira macroalgae extracts, International Journal of Nanomedicine 16 (2021) 5017–5036.
[38] A. Kocere, et al., Real-time imaging of polymersome nanoparticles in zebrafish embryos engrafted with melanoma cancer cells: localization, toxicity and treatment analysis, EBioMedicine 58 (2020) 102902.
[39] E. Cörek, et al., Shedding light on metal-based nanoparticles in zebrafish by computed tomography with micrometer resolution, Small 16 (2020) e2000746.
[40] S. Krimm, The hydrophobic effect: formation of micelles and biological membranes, Charles Tanford, Wiley-Interscience, New York, 1980, 233 pp. price: $18.50, Journal of Polymer Science: Polymer Letters Edition 18 (1980), 687-687.
[41] J.N. Israelachvili, G.E. Adams, Measurement of forces between two mica surfaces in aqueous electrolyte solutions in the range 0–100 nm, Journal of the Chemical Society, Faraday Transactions 1: Physical Chemistry in Condensed Phases 74 (1978) 975–1001.
[42] L. Vroman, Effect of adsorbed proteins on the wettability of hydrophilic and hydrophobic solids, Nature 196 (1962) 476–477.
[43] A.D. Bangham, B.A. Pethica, G.V. Seaman, The charged groups at the interface of some blood cells, Biochemical Journal 69 (1958) 12–19.
[44] I. Lynch, et al., The nanoparticle-protein complex as a biological entity; a complex fluids and surface science challenge for the 21st century, Advances in Colloid and Interface Science 134–135 (2007) 167–174.
[45] M. Hadjidemetriou, et al., In vivo biomolecule corona around blood-circulating, clinically used and antibody-targeted lipid bilayer nanoscale vesicles, ACS Nano 9 (2015) 8142–8156.
[46] M.P. Monopoli, C. Åberg, A. Salvati, K.A. Dawson, Biomolecular coronas provide the biological identity of nanosized materials, Nature Nanotechnology 7 (2012) 779–786.
[47] M.P. Monopoli, et al., Physical–Chemical aspects of protein corona: relevance to in vitro and in vivo biological impacts of nanoparticles, Journal of the American Chemical Society 133 (2011) 2525–2534.
[48] F. Chen, et al., Complement proteins bind to nanoparticle protein corona and undergo dynamic exchange in vivo, Nature Nanotechnology 12 (2017) 387–393.
[49] L. Gardner, K. Kostarelos, P. Mallick, C. Dive, M. Hadjidemetriou, Nano-omics: nanotechnology-based multidimensional harvesting of the blood-circulating cancerome, Nature Reviews Clinical Oncology (2022).
[50] G. Maiorano, et al., Effects of cell culture media on the dynamic formation of protein-nanoparticle complexes and influence on the cellular response, ACS Nano 4 (2010) 7481–7491.
[51] M. Hadjidemetriou, et al., The human in vivo biomolecule corona onto PEGylated liposomes: a proof-of-concept clinical study, Advances in Materials 31 (2019) e1803335.

[52] C. Reichert, G. Borchard, Noncovalent PEGylation, an innovative subchapter in the field of protein modification, Journal of Pharmaceutical Sciences 105 (2016) 386–390.
[53] J. Israelachvili, The different faces of poly(ethylene glycol), Proceedings of the National Academy of Sciences 94 (1997) 8378–8379.
[54] A.L. Lewis, Phosphorylcholine-based polymers and their use in the prevention of biofouling, Colloids and Surfaces B: Biointerfaces 18 (2000) 261–275.
[55] M. Aghajani, F. Esmaeili, Anti-biofouling assembly strategies for protein and cell repellent surfaces: a mini-review, Journal of Biomaterials Science, Polymer Edition 32 (2021) 1770–1789.
[56] S. Lowe, N.M. O'Brien-Simpson, L.A. Connal, Antibiofouling polymer interfaces: poly(ethylene glycol) and other promising candidates, Polymer Chemistry 6 (2015) 198–212.
[57] S. Schöttler, et al., Protein adsorption is required for stealth effect of poly(ethylene glycol)- and poly(phosphoester)-coated nanocarriers, Nature Nanotechnology 11 (2016) 372–377.
[58] M. Hadjidemetriou, K. Kostarelos, Evolution of the nanoparticle corona, Nature Nanotechnology 12 (2017) 288–290.
[59] S.T. Reddy, et al., Exploiting lymphatic transport and complement activation in nanoparticle vaccines, Nature Biotechnology 25 (2007) 1159–1164.
[60] A. Vonarbourg, C. Passirani, P. Saulnier, J.P. Benoit, Parameters influencing the stealthiness of colloidal drug delivery systems, Biomaterials 27 (2006) 4356–4373.
[61] A. Chanan-Khan, et al., Complement activation following first exposure to pegylated liposomal doxorubicin (Doxil®): possible role in hypersensitivity reactions, Annals of Oncology 14 (2003) 1430–1437.
[62] B.W. Neun, Y. Barenholz, J. Szebeni, M.A. Dobrovolskaia, Understanding the role of anti-PEG antibodies in the complement activation by Doxil in vitro, Molecules 23 (2018).
[63] S.J. Stachelek, et al., The effect of CD47 modified polymer surfaces on inflammatory cell attachment and activation, Biomaterials 32 (2011) 4317–4326.
[64] P.L. Rodriguez, et al., Minimal "self" peptides that inhibit phagocytic clearance and enhance delivery of nanoparticles, Science 339 (2013) 971–975.
[65] M. Merchant, et al., Monovalent antibody design and mechanism of action of onartuzumab, a MET antagonist with anti-tumor activity as a therapeutic agent, Proceedings of the National Academy of Sciences 110 (2013) E2987–E2996.
[66] E. Vigna, et al., Targeted therapy by gene transfer of a monovalent antibody fragment against the Met oncogenic receptor, Journal of Molecular Medicine 92 (2014) 65–76.
[67] C.B. Carlson, P. Mowery, R.M. Owen, E.C. Dykhuizen, L.L. Kiessling, Selective tumor cell targeting using low-affinity, multivalent interactions, ACS Chemical Biology 2 (2007) 119–127.
[68] M.J. Cloninger, et al., in: Supramolecular Chemistry, 2012.
[69] M. Delguste, et al., Multivalent binding of herpesvirus to living cells is tightly regulated during infection, Science Advances 4 (2018) eaat1273.
[70] A.M. Krachler, H. Ham, K. Orth, Turnabout is fair play, Virulence 3 (2012) 68–71.

[71] A.J. Ruthenburg, H. Li, D.J. Patel, C. David Allis, Multivalent engagement of chromatin modifications by linked binding modules, Nature Reviews Molecular Cell Biology 8 (2007) 983–994.
[72] A.M. Cuesta, N. Sainz-Pastor, J. Bonet, B. Oliva, L. Alvarez-Vallina, Multivalent antibodies: when design surpasses evolution, Trends in Biotechnology 28 (2010) 355–362.
[73] M. Mammen, S.-K. Choi, G.M. Whitesides, Polyvalent interactions in biological systems: implications for design and use of multivalent ligands and inhibitors, Angewandte Chemie International Edition 37 (1998) 2754–2794.
[74] F.J. Martinez-Veracoechea, D. Frenkel, Designing super selectivity in multivalent nano-particle binding, Proceedings of the National Academy of Sciences 108 (2011) 10963–10968.
[75] J. Tan, A. Thomas, Y. Liu, Influence of red blood cells on nanoparticle targeted delivery in microcirculation, Soft Matter 8 (2011) 1934–1946.
[76] Y. Cao, et al., The use of human umbilical vein endothelial cells (HUVECs) as an in vitro model to assess the toxicity of nanoparticles to endothelium: a review, Journal of Applied Toxicology 37 (2017) 1359–1369.
[77] M.S. Ehrenberg, A.E. Friedman, J.N. Finkelstein, G. Oberdörster, J.L. McGrath, The influence of protein adsorption on nanoparticle association with cultured endothelial cells, Biomaterials 30 (2009) 603–610.
[78] M.J. Ernsting, M. Murakami, A. Roy, S.D. Li, Factors controlling the pharmacokinetics, biodistribution and intratumoral penetration of nanoparticles, Journal of Controlled Release 172 (2013) 782–794.
[79] G. Song, J.S. Petschauer, A.J. Madden, W.C. Zamboni, Nanoparticles and the mononuclear phagocyte system: pharmacokinetics and applications for inflammatory diseases, Current Rheumatology Reviews 10 (2014) 22–34.
[80] Y. Yang, Z.K. Tu, X.K. Liu, P. Zhang, Mononuclear phagocyte system in hepatitis C virus infection, World Journal of Gastroenterology 24 (2018) 4962–4973.
[81] D.E. Owens 3rd, N.A. Peppas, Opsonization, biodistribution, and pharmacokinetics of polymeric nanoparticles, International Journal of Pharmaceutics 307 (2006) 93–102.
[82] J.A. Champion, S. Mitragotri, Role of target geometry in phagocytosis, Proceedings of the National Academy of Sciences of the U S A 103 (2006) 4930–4934.
[83] Y. Geng, et al., Shape effects of filaments versus spherical particles in flow and drug delivery, Nature Nanotechnology 2 (2007) 249–255.
[84] Ž. Krpetić, F. Porta, E. Caneva, V. Dal Santo, G. Scarì, Phagocytosis of biocompatible gold nanoparticles, Langmuir 26 (2010) 14799–14805.
[85] O. Lunov, et al., Differential uptake of functionalized polystyrene nanoparticles by human macrophages and a monocytic cell line, ACS Nano 5 (2011) 1657–1669.
[86] A. Akinc, G. Battaglia, Exploiting endocytosis for nanomedicines, Cold Spring Harbor Perspectives in Biology 5 (2013) a016980.
[87] I. Canton, G. Battaglia, Endocytosis at the nanoscale, Chemical Society Reviews 41 (2012) 2718–2739.
[88] Y.-R. Zhang, et al., Strategies to improve tumor penetration of nanomedicines through nanoparticle design, WIREs Nanomedicine and Nanobiotechnology 11 (2019) e1519.

[89] Z. Shen, H. Ye, X. Yi, Y. Li, Membrane wrapping efficiency of elastic nanoparticles during endocytosis: size and shape matter, ACS Nano 13 (2019) 215–228.
[90] M. Sousa de Almeida, et al., Understanding nanoparticle endocytosis to improve targeting strategies in nanomedicine, Chemical Society Reviews 50 (2021) 5397–5434.
[91] K. Shapero, et al., Time and space resolved uptake study of silica nanoparticles by human cells, Molecular BioSystems 7 (2011) 371–378.
[92] C. LoPresti, et al., Controlling polymersome surface topology at the nanoscale by membrane confined polymer/polymer phase separation, ACS Nano 5 (2011) 1775–1784.
[93] B.D. Chithrani, W.C. Chan, Elucidating the mechanism of cellular uptake and removal of protein-coated gold nanoparticles of different sizes and shapes, Nano Letters 7 (2007) 1542–1550.
[94] J.D. Robertson, et al., pH-sensitive tubular polymersomes: formation and applications in cellular delivery, ACS Nano 8 (2014) 4650–4661.
[95] H. Jin, D.A. Heller, R. Sharma, M.S. Strano, Size-dependent cellular uptake and expulsion of single-walled carbon nanotubes: single particle tracking and a generic uptake model for nanoparticles, ACS Nano 3 (2009) 149–158.
[96] A. Blanazs, J. Madsen, G. Battaglia, A.J. Ryan, S.P. Armes, Mechanistic insights for block copolymer morphologies: how do worms form vesicles? Journal of the American Chemical Society 133 (2011) 16581–16587.
[97] C. LoPresti, H. Lomas, M. Massignani, T. Smart, G. Battaglia, Polymersomes: nature inspired nanometer sized compartments, Journal of Materials Chemistry 19 (2009) 3576–3590.
[98] E. Ngandu Mpoyi, et al., Protein adsorption as a key mediator in the nanotopographical control of cell behavior, ACS Nano 10 (2016) 6638–6647.
[99] S. Guerrier, et al., The F-BAR domain of srGAP2 induces membrane protrusions required for neuronal migration and morphogenesis, Cell 138 (2009) 990–1004.
[100] F.C. Tsai, et al., Comparing physical mechanisms for membrane curvature-driven sorting of BAR-domain proteins, Soft Matter 17 (2021) 4254–4265.
[101] O. Daumke, A. Roux, V. Haucke, BAR domain scaffolds in dynamin-mediated membrane fission, Cell 156 (2014) 882–892.
[102] J.E. Hinshaw, Dynamin spirals, Current Opinion in Structural Biology 9 (1999) 260–267.
[103] K. He, et al., Dynamics of Auxilin 1 and GAK in clathrin-mediated traffic, The Journal of Cell Biology 219 (2020).
[104] S.L. Schmid, V.A. Frolov, Dynamin: functional design of a membrane fission catalyst, Annual Review of Cell and Developmental Biology 27 (2011) 79–105.
[105] M. Podinovskaia, A. Spang, The endosomal network: mediators and regulators of endosome maturation, Progress in Molecular & Subcellular Biology 57 (2018) 1–38.
[106] M. Vietri, M. Radulovic, H. Stenmark, The many functions of ESCRTs, Nature Reviews Molecular Cell Biology 21 (2020) 25–42.
[107] J.P. Luzio, Y. Hackmann, N.M.G. Dieckmann, G.M. Griffiths, The biogenesis of lysosomes and lysosome-related organelles, Cold Spring Harbor Perspectives in Biology 6 (2014).

[108] I. Milosevic, Revisiting the role of clathrin-mediated endoytosis in synaptic vesicle recycling, Frontiers in Cellular Neuroscience 12 (2018) 27.

[109] C. Mullins, J.S. Bonifacino, The molecular machinery for lysosome biogenesis, BioEssays 23 (2001) 333–343.

[110] S.R. Elkin, A.M. Lakoduk, S.L. Schmid, Endocytic pathways and endosomal trafficking: a primer, Wiener Medizinische Wochenschrift 166 (2016) 196–204.

[111] Y. Ju, H. Guo, M. Edman, S.F. Hamm-Alvarez, Application of advances in endocytosis and membrane trafficking to drug delivery, Advanced Drug Delivery Reviews 157 (2020) 118–141.

[112] V. Pietiäinen, et al., Echovirus 1 endocytosis into caveosomes requires lipid rafts, dynamin II, and signaling events, Molecular Biology of the Cell 15 (2004) 4911–4925.

[113] S. Sabharanjak, P. Sharma, R.G. Parton, S. Mayor, GPI-anchored proteins are delivered to recycling endosomes via a distinct cdc42-regulated, clathrin-independent pinocytic pathway, Developmental Cell 2 (2002) 411–423.

[114] C.C. Scott, J. Gruenberg, Ion flux and the function of endosomes and lysosomes: pH is just the start: the flux of ions across endosomal membranes influences endosome function not only through regulation of the luminal pH, BioEssays 33 (2011) 103–110.

[115] P. Saftig, J. Klumperman, Lysosome biogenesis and lysosomal membrane proteins: trafficking meets function, Nature Reviews Molecular Cell Biology 10 (2009) 623–635.

[116] S. Sabella, et al., A general mechanism for intracellular toxicity of metal-containing nanoparticles, Nanoscale 6 (2014) 7052–7061.

[117] V.M. Gouveia, et al., Targeting macrophages and synoviocytes intracellular milieu to augment anti-inflammatory drug potency (adv. Therap. 3/2022), Advanced Therapeutics 5 (2022) 2270005.

[118] F. Fenaroli, et al., Polymersomes eradicating intracellular bacteria, ACS Nano 14 (2020) 8287–8298.

[119] L. Su, et al., GRP75-driven, cell-cycle-dependent macropinocytosis of Tat/pDNA-Ca(2+) nanoparticles underlies distinct gene therapy effect in ovarian cancer, Journal of Nanobiotechnology 20 (2022) 340.

[120] X. Yang, et al., Probing the intracellular delivery of nanoparticles into hard-to-transfect cells, ACS Nano (2022).

[121] E.J. Kwon, J.M. Bergen, I.K. Park, S.H. Pun, Peptide-modified vectors for nucleic acid delivery to neurons, Journal of Controlled Release 132 (2008) 230–235.

[122] A.S. Verkman, Solute and macromolecule diffusion in cellular aqueous compartments, Trends in Biochemical Sciences 27 (2002) 27–33.

[123] G. Ruan, A. Agrawal, A.I. Marcus, S. Nie, Imaging and tracking of Tat peptide-conjugated quantum dots in living cells: new insights into nanoparticle uptake, intracellular transport, and vesicle shedding, Journal of the American Chemical Society 129 (2007) 14759–14766.

[124] S. Barua, S. Mitragotri, Challenges associated with penetration of nanoparticles across cell and tissue barriers: a review of current status and future prospects, Nano Today 9 (2014) 223–243.

[125] Y. Cheng, et al., Nanoparticulates reduce tumor cell migration through affinity interactions with extracellular migrasomes and retraction fibers, Nanoscale Horizons 7 (2022) 779–789.

[126] T. Stylianopoulos, et al., Diffusion of particles in the extracellular matrix: the effect of repulsive electrostatic interactions, Biophysical Journal 99 (2010) 1342–1349.
[127] A.B. Engin, et al., Mechanistic understanding of nanoparticles' interactions with extracellular matrix: the cell and immune system, Particle and Fibre Toxicology 14 (2017) 22.
[128] B.J. Lee, Y. Cheema, S. Bader, G.A. Duncan, Shaping nanoparticle diffusion through biological barriers to drug delivery, JCIS Open 4 (2021) 100025.
[129] T. Doane, C. Burda, Nanoparticle mediated non-covalent drug delivery, Advanced Drug Delivery Reviews 65 (2013) 607–621.
[130] A. Albanese, P.S. Tang, W.C. Chan, The effect of nanoparticle size, shape, and surface chemistry on biological systems, Annual Review of Biomedical Engineering 14 (2012) 1–16.
[131] M. Elsabahy, K.L. Wooley, Design of polymeric nanoparticles for biomedical delivery applications, Chemical Society Reviews 41 (2012) 2545–2561.
[132] S. Acosta-Gutiérrez, et al., A multiscale study of phosphorylcholine driven cellular phenotypic targeting, ACS Central Science 8 (2022) 891–904.
[133] J.K. Vasir, V. Labhasetwar, Biodegradable nanoparticles for cytosolic delivery of therapeutics, Advanced Drug Delivery Reviews 59 (2007) 718–728.
[134] H. Yamada, B. Loretz, C.-M. Lehr, Design of starch-graft-PEI polymers: an effective and biodegradable gene delivery platform, Biomacromolecules 15 (2014) 1753–1761.
[135] X. Ma, et al., Gold nanoparticles induce autophagosome accumulation through size-dependent nanoparticle uptake and lysosome impairment, ACS Nano 5 (2011) 8629–8639.
[136] F.M. Platt, Sphingolipid lysosomal storage disorders, Nature 510 (2014) 68–75.
[137] P. Tanpaiboon, Lysosomal storage disorders, Journal of Pediatric Biochemistry 4 (2014) 217–229.
[138] M. Bartneck, H.A. Keul, G. Zwadlo-Klarwasser, J. Groll, Phagocytosis independent extracellular nanoparticle clearance by human immune cells, Nano Letters 10 (2010) 59–63.
[139] B. Ballou, et al., Sentinel lymph node imaging using quantum dots in mouse tumor models, Bioconjugate Chemistry 18 (2007) 389–396.
[140] L.F. Prescott, J.A.N. McAuslane, S. Freestone, The concentration-dependent disposition and kinetics of inulin, European Journal of Clinical Pharmacology 40 (1991) 619–624.
[141] S.S. Olmsted, et al., Diffusion of macromolecules and virus-like particles in human cervical mucus, Biophysical Journal 81 (2001) 1930–1937.
[142] U. Lund, et al., Glomerular filtration rate dependence of sieving of albumin and some neutral proteins in rat kidneys 284 (2003) F1226–F1234.
[143] H. Soo Choi, et al., Renal clearance of quantum dots, Nature Biotechnology 25 (2007) 1165–1170.
[144] J.-H. Park, et al., Biodegradable luminescent porous silicon nanoparticles for in vivo applications, Nature Materials 8 (2009) 331–336.

[145] J.G. Lombardino, J.A. Lowe 3rd, The role of the medicinal chemist in drug discovery–then and now, Nature Reviews Drug Discovery 3 (2004) 853–862.
[146] J. Kling, Fresh from the biotech pipeline–2013, Nature Biotechnology 32 (2014) 121–124.

Molecular targets and pharmacodynamics for bactericidal and bacteriostatic activity

Pavani Cherukupally[1,2], Claudio Lourenco[3], Cher Farrugia[4,5], Diana Marcela Castillo[6] and Maja Sabalic-Schoener[7,8]

[1] *Schlumberger-Doll Research, One Hampshire St, Cambridge, MA, United States;* [2] *Department of Mechanical Engineering, Massachusetts Institute of Technology, Cambridge, MA, United States;* [3] *Department of Chemistry, University College London (UCL), London, United Kingdom;* [4] *Bristol Dental School, University of Bristol, Bristol, United Kingdom;* [5] *Bristol Dental Hospital, University Hospitals Bristol and Weston, Bristol, United Kingdom;* [6] *Unidad de Investigación Básica Oral-UIBO, Vicerrectoría de Investigaciones, Facultad de Odontología, Universidad El Bosque, Bogotá, Colombia;* [7] *The ADA Forsyth Institute, Cambridge, MA, United States;* [8] *Unit of Periodontology, UCL Eastman Dental Institute, London, United Kingdom*

1. Antimicrobial agents, mechanisms and modes of delivery

1.1 Clinical need for antimicrobial agents

Microorganisms are ubiquitous and have widespread effects on our daily lives. While some microorganisms are essential for our day-to-day functions, others significantly affect our well-being and healthcare systems. Nosocomial pathogens are a group of microorganisms that are notorious for their impact on both the developing and developed world. These pathogens are the cause of healthcare-associated infections (HAI) and are an ever-growing challenge compounded with increased antimicrobial resistance [1,2]. HAI are defined as infections acquired while patients are receiving healthcare [3]. HAI typically appear after 48 hours of hospitalisation or within 30 days of receiving health care [4]. A

Nanotechnology Tools for Infection Control **https://doi.org/10.1016/B978-0-12-823994-0.00009-8**

European study published in 2016 showed that HAI affect 1 in 20 patients admitted to hospital, or around 5% of patients [5]. Similarly, a study carried out in the United States reported HAI in 4% of patients admitted, highlighting the global burden of HAI [6].

An increasingly ageing population and increased availability of medical devices have also led to increased infections associated with medical devices, sometimes also referred to as foreign body-related/associated infections (FBRI) [7]. In the literature medical devices are sometimes also described as biomaterials and therefore their infections are at times also described as biomaterial-associated infections (BAI) [8]. Use of implantable devices continues to expand, particularly the use of catheters, prosthetic joints and breast implants. Despite only a small percentage of medical devices typically resulting in infection, FBRI pose increasing challenges to healthcare providers worldwide [7]. Between 40% and 75% of BAI have been associated with coagulase-negative staphylococci, *Staphylococcus epidermidis*. Staphylococci are not typically pathogenic but in the right conditions can pose a significant treat to medical device survival and can be a detriment to the affected patients' health due to the development of chronic infections [9]. These chronic infections result from attachment of the pathogenic microorganism to either the surface of the medical device or to the surrounding tissues. BAI form biofilms made up of several layers of communicating microorganisms, which are difficult to penetrate with antimicrobial agents. Research has also shown that pathogens can infiltrate macrophages, serving as an additional front for the advancing infection [8,9]. The mentioned features increase the complexity of medical device associated infections and as a result make them even more challenging to treat [7–9]. Challenges resulting from HAI and FBRI/BAI are compounded with ever-increasing antimicrobial resistance.

1.2 Modes of action of antimicrobial agents

The terms bacteriostatic and bactericidal are often used to describe the mode of action of different antibiotics and antimicrobial agents. These terms refer to the effect antimicrobial agents have on microbial cells. While bacteriostatic agents suppress microbial growth, bactericidal agents kill the target microorganism [10]. The mode of action is typically tested in vitro using several microbiological techniques including time-kill curves, the minimum bactericidal concentration (MBC) and serum bactericidal titres (SBT). Although these tests provide insights on how antimicrobial agents work against pathogenic organisms, the clinical interpretation and translation of such tests can at times be challenging. This is partly due to lack of standardisation of some of the methods used, which results in reproducibility challenges secondary to inter and intra-laboratory variability. Therefore, classification of activity (bacteriostatic or bactericidal) generally only applies to the pathogen and strain being tested, under the set conditions used for the test at that time. Since these tests are carried out in vitro, the role of the host response role is not investigated in these assessments, which further limits the clinical translation of such tests [11].

In the modern antibiotic era, since the use of antimicrobial agents has revolutionised clinical medicine, once lethal infections have become curable. Besides treatment of infections, antimicrobial agents have been used in the prevention of infections and complications, in cancer chemotherapy and surgery. Widespread use of antimicrobial agents in the treatment of humans, other animals and in agriculture [12–14] has also resulted in increased prevalence of antibiotic-resistant microorganisms. The identification of antimicrobial-resistant bacteria started soon after the discovery and isolation of penicillin [15]. Due to the high incidence of disease and deaths caused by antimicrobial resistance organism, in 2015, the World Health Organisation (WHO) published a global action plan on antimicrobial resistance and recommended each country to elaborate their own plan aligning with five strategic objectives and a framework for action [16] (see Table 7.1).

In 2019, in the European Union/European Economic Area (EU/EEA) were estimated more than 865,000 cases of antibiotic-resistant bacteria infections that lead to more than 38,000 deaths;

Table 7.1 WHO – global action plan on antimicrobial resistance.

WHO – global action plan on antimicrobial resistance Strategic objectives
Improve awareness and understanding of antimicrobial resistance through effective communication, education and training.
Strengthen the knowledge and evidence base through surveillance and research.
Reduce the incidence of infection through effective sanitation, hygiene and infection prevention measures.
Optimise the use of antimicrobial medicines in human and animal health.
Develop the economic case for sustainable investment that takes account of the needs of all countries, and increase investment in new medicines, diagnostic tools, vaccines and other interventions.

Table 7.2 2015 top 10 causes of death worldwide [19].

2015 top 10 causes of death
Ischaemic heart disease
Stroke
Lower respiratory infection
Chronic obstructive pulmonary disease
Trachea, bronchus lung cancers
Diabetes mellitus
Alzheimer disease and other dementias
Diarrhoeal diseases
Tuberculosis
Road injury

70.9% of the infections were attributed to healthcare acquired infections [17]. According to the World Health Organisation (WHO), among the top 10 causes of death three were antimicrobial resistance-related diseases, lower respiratory infection, diarrhoeal diseases and tuberculosis [18] (see Table 7.2).

To further address the burden on healthcare and problems created by bacterial infections and antimicrobial resistance among the general population, the WHO 'Development of New Antibiotics for Drug-Resistant Bacterial Infections, Including Tuberculosis' was published highlighting the need to develop and find coordinated strategies between its members to address and combat the antimicrobial resistance challenges and problems faced by healthcare worldwide [19].

Currently there are several classes or families of antibiotics used in healthcare, normally grouped by their chemical structure: β-lactams (sometimes referred as penicillin derivatives), fluoroquinolones, macrolides, tetracyclines, aminoglycosides, sulphonamides, glycopeptides, oxazolidinones, rifamycins, polymyxins, lipopeptides, nitrofurans, lincosamides, among others [22–26]. The modes of action of each family of antibiotics are quite specific and can be classified in damage to cell membrane, interference with cell wall synthesis, inhibition of metabolic pathways, interference with nucleic acid synthesis and inhibition/disruption of protein synthesis pathways [27]. A correlation between some antibiotics and their mode of action is shown in Table 7.3.

Table 7.3 Most used antibiotics and their mode of action [22–26].

Antibiotic	Mode of action
B-lactams	Inhibit cell wall synthesis
Fluoroquinolones	Disrupt DNA replication and repair
Macrolides	Inhibit protein synthesis by binding to the 23S unit of rRNA
Tetracyclines	Inhibit protein synthesis by interfering with the 30S ribosomal subunit preventing binding of aminoacyl-tRNA
Aminoglycosides	Inhibit protein synthesis by binding to the 30S ribosomal subunit causing error in the translation of mRNA
Sulphonamides	Disrupts DNA and RNA synthesis through inhibition of folic acid pathways
Glycopeptides	Inhibit effective cell wall synthesis by binding to peptidoglycan precursors
Oxazolidinones	Inhibit protein synthesis by interfering with the ribosomal 50S subunit
Rifamycins	Inhibit RNA polymerase
Polymyxins	Membrane disruption by interfering with phospholipids on gram negative cell membranes
Lipopeptides	Interfere with the cell membrane integrity acting like a detergent and creating pores
Nitrofurans	Multiple effects observed on inhibition of RNA and protein synthesis, DNA lesions
Lincosamides	Inhibit protein synthesis by binding to the peptidyl transferase centre on the 23S portion of the 50S subunit of bacterial ribosomes

Furthermore, some of the pathogenic bacteria have the capability to build up resistance against an antibiotic and subsequently pass relevant genes to other bacteria in their microenvironment, thus giving the resistance to a specific antibiotic to a wider population of microorganisms [29–31]. Such bacterial resistance arises from the need to survive and thrive by minimising or prevent the damage caused by the antibiotic. For example, β-lactams disrupt the cell wall synthesis by interacting with penicillin binding proteins. Bacteria can counter that by producing β-lactamases that can degrade penicillin and its derivates and/or modify its penicillin binding proteins to reduce antibiotic affinity [15,32]. Fluoroquinolones inhibit two enzymes [23], gyrase involved in chromosome elongation during replication and topoisomerase IV responsible for separating the daughter chromosomes in the final stages of DNA replication [33]. To counter such mechanisms, bacteria use efflux pumps systems to remove the antibiotic from their interior. Other mechanisms involve modification of the target site in the enzymes, thus reducing the antibiotic affinity [23]. Nitrofurans have a peculiar mode of action, only becoming active when reduced by bacterial enzymes. Their mode of action is not fully understood due to the complexity of the damage caused including DNA damage, inhibition of RNA and protein synthesis and oxidative stress [34]. The damage caused is a direct result of the generation of reactive oxygen species [35,36]. Despite being a very effective method, bacteria can also fight against the damage caused by reactive oxygen species, although it requires a quite complex approach by the microorganism because of the generation of multiple agents in the downstream of free radical generation. Indeed, the bacteria need to trigger specific antioxidant defences using specific proteins and enzymes [35,36]. The resistance against reactive oxygen damage in bacteria is generally accomplished through the expression of antioxidant enzymes such as dismutases, catalases, peroxidases and reductases that target reactive oxygen species and transfer or remove electrons; radical scavengers and or metal binding proteins that can scavenge free reactive oxygen species; and repair enzymes that mend the damage caused to proteins, enzymes and nucleic acids [35,37]. Microbial cells use these mechanisms to cope with the damage caused by reactive oxygen species under physiological conditions but if the mechanisms fail and reactive oxygen species concentration increases, the damage will be too extensive thus leading to oxidative stress and subsequent cell death [35–40]. Reactive oxygen species can be seen as an ideal antimicrobial due to its lack of specificity and broad range of targets, hindering the possibility of a microbe to develop resistance to it [35–37,41]. In summary, bacterial antimicrobial resistance mechanisms can be grouped in four modes of action: limiting uptake of a drug by modifications on its membrane structure or composition; modifying a drug target altering expression and translation patterns reducing antibiotic affinity; inactivating a drug with enzymes or proteins that bind to drugs; active drug efflux with over expression of pumps and channels [27,42,43]. Antimicrobial resistance mechanisms will be discussed in more detail in Section 1.4.1.

Another relevant fact to consider when treating a bacterial infection with antibiotics is the presence of persister cells [32]. Persister cells are a very small part of the bacterial population, roughly 1%, that appear to be in a deep dormant state and can evade antibiotic treatment [32,44]. It is implied the involvement of specific genes that regulate the expression of this type of cells among the microbial population, which appear to be related to quorum sensing and/or other external factors [45–48]. Inoculum age has an effect in the occurrence of persister cells [49]; in vitro experiments show that the length of stationary phase is directly correlated with an increase in the incidence of persister cells

[46,49], implying that well-established infections can also present a high incidence of persister cells.

The lack of effective global strategies for appropriate use of antibiotics lead to the development of a wide range of antimicrobial-resistant organisms and eventually lead the WHO to issue a list of critical pathogens that need urgent action and research [19,50] shown in Table 7.4.

1.3 Antimicrobial resistance mechanisms

1.3.1 Changes in permeability

In bacteria, all nutrients must enter through their envelope, which differs between Gram-positive and Gram-negative bacteria. The alteration in the permeability of bacterial envelopes is a well-described and important mechanism of antimicrobial resistance (AMR). In Gram-negative bacteria, a fundamental part of the external envelope are the porins, necessary for the entry of hydrophilic substances of less than 600 kDa. The structural modification of porins, decrease in number, narrowing in pore size and alteration in function are the main causes of AMR [53–55]. The OmpK35 and OmpK36 porins described in *Klebsiella pneumoniae* have been related to resistance to carbapenems due to their decreased size [56]. In the same sense, in *Escherichia coli* an increase in the transcription of the *ompC* gene and a reduction of *ompF* have been identified. This occurs due to the increased phosphorylation of OmpR that is part of a two-component system EnvZ-OmpR. The system regulates the expression of the OmpC and OmpF porins, and the increase in OmpR phosphorylation gives rise to smaller pores, making it easier for the bacteria to survive exposure to antibiotics such as carbapenems which favour OmpR mutations [54]. Another known example is in *Pseudomonas aeruginosa* involving the OprD porin, an altered porin that prevents the entry of antibiotics [53]. In Gram-positive bacteria, a decrease in the permeability of their envelope has also been reported, associated with alterations in the fluidity of the membrane reported in *Enterococcus faecalis* and *Enterococcus faecium*, due to alterations in the phospholipids and fatty acids of the bacterial membrane. These alterations give origin to daptomycin resistance [57].

1.3.2 Efflux pumps

Efflux pumps are transmembrane proteins naturally present in bacteria to transport different substances including antibiotics.

Table 7.4 2017 WHO global pathogens priority list (WHO publishes list of bacteria for which new antibiotics are urgently needed, 2017; [51]).

	Bacteria	Resistance	Major concerns
Priority 1: Critical	*Acinetobacter baumannii*	Carbapenem (β-lactam)	Spreads within hospitals and on surfaces. Leading cause of pneumonia, bloodstream and wound infections. Intrinsic and acquired resistance.
	Pseudomonas aeruginosa	Carbapenem (β-lactam)	Common cause of pneumonia, especially in immunocompromised patients.
	Enterobacteriaceae[a]	Carbapenem (β-lactam) Third-generation cephalosporins (β-lactam)	Worldwide increase of carbapenem resistance being reported.
Priority 2: High	*Enterococcus faecium*	Vancomycin (glycopeptide)	Persists in hospital environment. Common in hospital-acquired infections. High mortality. Very limited treatments.
	Staphylococcus aureus	Methicillin (β-lactam)	Methicillin-resistant *S. aureus* (MRSA) very common in hospital-acquired infections among immunocompromised patients.
		Vancomycin (Glycopeptide)	Vancomycin-resistant *S. aureus* incidence increasing partly to blame on its use in the treatment of MRSA infections [50a].
	Helicobacter pylori	Clarithromycin (macrolide)	Common cause of infection worldwide in adults and children. Limited treatment options available for children.
	Campylobacter spp.	Fluoroquinolones	Foodborne disease major cause of acute diarrhoea.
	Salmonella typhi	Fluoroquinolones	Most prevalent in regions with poor sanitation.
	Non-typhoidal Salmonella	Fluoroquinolones	Responsible for deaths from bacterial foodborne agents.
	Neisseria gonorrhoeae	Fluoroquinolone Third-generation cephalosporins (β-lactam)	Resistance to all recommended drugs for empirical monotherapy.
Priority 3: Medium	*Streptococcus pneumoniae*	Penicillin non-susceptible	Leading cause of pneumonia in children under 5 years. Major public health issue in low- and middle-income countries.
	Haemophilus influenzae	Ampicillin (β-lactam)	High morbidity in low-income countries.
	Shigella spp.	Fluoroquinolone	Major cause of morbidity and mortality worldwide with an estimation of one million deaths annually. High resistance to traditional first-line antibiotics.

[a]*Escherichia coli, Enterobacter* spp., *Klebsiella* ssp., *Citrobacter* spp., *Morganella* spp., *Providencia* spp., *Proteus* spp., *Serratia* spp.

These proteins are present in a wide variety of bacteria and have the ability to expel antibiotics and prevent their action on bacteria. They are considered important in intrinsic resistance to many antibiotics [54]. However, they have been implicated in resistance to different Gram-negative bacteria and in their virulence associated with the adaptive response that favours other resistance mechanisms. Efflux pumps are classified into superfamilies: ATP binding cassette (ABC) superfamily, the major facilitator superfamily (MFS), the resistance-nodulation-division (RND) superfamily and the multidrug and toxic compound extrusion (MATE) family [21]. It has been described that the RND efflux pumps are the most related to the multidrug resistance (MDR) phenotype in different Gram-negative bacteria [58]. Other important efflux pumps reported in anaerobic bacteria are the family of multidrug efflux transporter pumps (MATE), which have been associated with *Bacteroides fragilis* and resistance to β-lactam antibiotics, fluoroquinolones, tetracyclines, novobiocin and metronidazole [59].

1.3.3 Modification and protection of the target site

Antibiotics generally have specific affinity against bacterial structures favouring their action. Mutations in genes that code for structures that are considered the target site generate resistance to these antibiotics because they cannot bind to the bacteria. These mutations can be randomly generated in a timely manner and are expressed under antibiotic pressure. An example of this mechanism are mutations to PBPs (penicillin-binding proteins) such as those reported in *E. coli* that favour the insertion of amino acids, changing the affinity of these proteins and the antibacterial action of aztreonam/avibactam [60]. Additionally, by recombination of alleles present in the same cell or by transformation in competent bacteria, alterations of the target sites can be generated. Another example of this mechanism is associated with the mutation of the genes that code for DNA gyrase (*grlA* and *grlB*) and genes that code for topoisomerase IV (*parC*), target enzymes of fluoroquinolones, which results in resistance to these antibiotics. In this way, different mutations have been reported in genes associated with changes in the recognition sites with antibiotics, the genes of the erm family favouring the mutation of the 23S rRNA specifically by methylation of alanine 2058, which gives rise, for example, to the methylase-ErmC that could generate resistance to chloramphenicol, macrolides, lincosamides and streptogramins [55].

1.3.4 Inactivation or degradation of antibiotics

This mechanism of action is mediated by the action of different enzymes encoded in some cases in plasmids or in the bacterial chromosome. Different types of enzymes have been documented, and among the best known are β-lactamases. These enzymes are produced by different genera and bacterial species, especially Gram negatives, and can inactivate the action of these antibiotics by hydrolysis of the β-lactam ring of this group of antibiotics. Among these are serine-β-lactamases (SBLs) and metallo-β-lactamases (MBLs) [55]. These enzymes confer resistance to a wide range of extended spectrum antibiotics (ESBLs), such as carbapenems and cephamycins, but they can be inhibited by β-lactamase inhibitors such as clavulanic acid [61]. The presence of genes such as bla_{TEM}, bla_{SHV}, $bla_{CTX\text{-}M}$, among others, are related to this type of enzymes and the resistance associated with β-lactam antibiotics mainly in bacteria of the Enterobacteriaceae family [62]. However, some of these genes (bla_{TEM}) have also been detected in other Gram-negative bacteria such as those belonging to the genus Prevotella, a microorganism belonging to the normal microbiota of the oral cavity, although it is also associated with periodontitis [63]. AmpC β-lactamases are chromosomal or plasmid in type, confer resistance to penicillins, first to third generation cephalosporins, and aztreonam. They are not inhibited by clavulanic acid, sulbactam and tazobactam, but with new inhibitors such as avibactam, vaborbactam and relebactam, a good antimicrobial effect has been seen [64]. Additionally, carbapenemases are the β-lactamases that have the highest hydrolysis capacity over β-lactam antibiotics, since they include carbapenems and have been reported mainly in Enterobacterales such as *Klebsiella pneumoniae* and *E. coli*, among the most frequently related there are KPC, NDM, IMP, VIM and OXA-48-like, the presence of these β-lactamases are subject to epidemiological surveillance and are considered a global threat because they are associated with an increase in morbidity and mortality according to information from the WHO [65].

1.4 Novel modes of delivery of antimicrobial agents

One of the most promising strategies to overcome microbial drug resistance is use of nanoparticles [66]. Micro and nanoparticles are being commonly studied as a potential platform for the delivery of antibiotics in humans aiming to overcome limitations of conventional agents and modes of delivery. One of the main advantages of using nanoparticles is that they can help to improve the delivery of these agents to specific sites in the body. Nanoparticles can be designed to target specific cells, e.g. macrophages [67], tissues or organs, and they can be engineered to release antimicrobial cargo in a controlled manner. This can help to improve the effectiveness of the antimicrobial agents and reduce the risk of side effects. One example is development of polymersomes (nanosized block copolymer vesicles resulting from the self-assembly of amphiphilic poly[2-(methacryloyloxy) ethyl phosphorylcholine] (PMPC) and poly[2-(diisopropylamino) ethyl methacrylate] (PDPA) block copolymers) for dental applications. The nano and micro-sized vesicles demonstrated delivery of antibiotic to gingival keratinocytes and reduction of intracellular pathogens showing promising results for the application of polymersome-encapsulated antibiotics in dentistry [68]. Using fluorescent labelling, authors were able to visualise polymersome vesicles and both intracellular and extracellular bacteria. It was demonstrated that polymersome-encapsulated metronidazole can significantly reduce numbers of intracellular *P. gingivalis* in an organotypic oral mucosal model compared to free antibiotic or polymersome alone controls. Furthermore, it was shown in a zebrafish model that the pH-sensitive PMPC–PDPA polymersomes target macrophages and enhance antibiotic killing of intracellular pathogens in vivo without inducing toxicity.

Nanoparticles can be bactericidal and bacteriostatic depending on their properties such as particle size and concentration, and they have shown to be effective against both Gram-positive and Gram-negative bacteria. Mechanisms of antimicrobial nanoparticles vary according to their type. Some antimicrobial effect of nanoparticles are not fully understood, while others include prevention of biofilm formation, disruption or interaction with pathogen cell wall or membrane, production of reactive oxygen species and stimulation of intracellular effects such as DNA or protein damage and enzyme disruption [69,70].

2. Applications of antimicrobial nanoparticles, pharmacodynamics and safety

2.1 Nanoparticles

Nanoparticles are small, solid, stable particles with dimensions ranging from 1 to 100 nm. Their small size presents a significant advantage due to the significant increase in surface area to volume ratio and quantum effects that contribute to enhanced reactivity that differ from the material properties at a larger size. Nanoparticles can be composed of various materials, such as metals, semiconductors, ceramics, polymers or composites. They can be classified into organic, inorganic and carbon-based nanoparticles and can take on different shapes, including spheres, rods, tubes and more complex structures, depending on how they are synthesised and manipulated [52,71]. The use of nanoparticles has the potential to revolutionise the field of antimicrobials and present advantages against the well-established antimicrobials in use due to its broad-spectrum activity, capability to disrupt biofilms, potential inactivation of some bacterial spores, synergistic effects when used in combination with other antimicrobials and the diversity of their applications. Nanoparticles can be engineered into other materials that can be used in medical devices such as catheters and other invasive instruments, wound dressings plus in a wide range of coatings on everyday objects and surfaces [72–77]. Nanoparticles can interfere with functions of cell membranes like permeability and respiration; furthermore, once inside the cell, they can interfere with its the normal functioning [72,77,78].

2.1.1 Metal and metal oxide nanoparticles

Metal and metal oxide nanoparticles present an elegant efficacious alternative to combat antimicrobial-specific resistance towards antibiotics mainly due to the generation of reactive oxygen species and the broad range of targets for such reactive compounds [39,72,79,80]. This can also be directed towards a specific microorganism or treatment area by coating the nanoparticles with specific antibiotics and or antibodies [78,80–82]. Several studies have shown that the efficacy of some antibiotics can be enhanced when used in combination with nanoparticles targeting antibiotic-resistant bacteria [77,82]. The most widely studied nanoparticles and with many applications are silver, zinc, iron and gold nanoparticles. Several studies indicate direct correlation of nanoparticle size and antimicrobial activity with smaller sizes showing enhanced antimicrobial potential [75,80,82–86]. Silver antimicrobial potential is widely known, and this is also evident on its nanoparticles. Silver nanoparticles disrupt cell function, interact with nucleic acids, enzymes and cell membrane [80,81,85,87]. Zinc oxide nanoparticles generate reactive oxygen species and, like silver nanoparticles, can affect a wide range of cell structures [79,88,89]. Iron oxide nanoparticles damage cells through the generation of hydroxyl radical via a Fenton reaction mechanism [90]. Gold nanoparticles are known to interact with cell membranes by increasing its permeability, inhibiting enzyme activity and interacting with nucleic acids [91,92] with the added benefit of low toxicity towards animal cells. The mode of action of metallic nanoparticles can be directly connected to the oxidative stress caused by the generation of reactive oxygen species. Such compounds have low specificity, thus effectively targeting many different structures, in its vicinity, within the cell. The metal ions dissolved from the nanoparticles can also contribute to the antimicrobial activity by directly interacting with functional groups on enzymes, therefore impairing their normal function [77].

2.2 Pharmacodynamics and pharmacokinetics of antimicrobial nanoparticles

Pharmacodynamics is the study of the biochemical and physiological effects of drugs on the body or microorganism and its mechanism of action, while pharmacokinetics studies the effect that the organism has on the drug, such as absorption, distribution, metabolism and excretion. Route of administration, interpatient variability and the effect of physiologic or pathologic conditions such as pregnancy, ageing and disease are important considerations in pharmacokinetics. Most drugs are distributed to most body fluids and tissues except cerebrospinal fluid. Nanoparticles can overcome this limitation. However, the ability of silver nanoparticles to be transmitted across the blood–brain barrier and directly affecting the brain as well as crossing the placenta may be a safety concern [93,94]. Nanoparticles not only carry cargo, such as antimicrobials, but also exhibit drug-like effects with possible unanticipated effects on biological systems and their long-term implications [95]. One of the suggested benefits of downsizing to the nanoscale is increased bioavailability of poorly soluble drugs [96,97].

2.3 Emerging artificial intelligence applications

Antimicrobial treatment is effective when the drug is administered in an optimal dose that achieves a clinical response while minimising toxicity and drug resistance. However, there are various factors that can cause variability in pharmacokinetics, such as comorbidities and other medications, leading to different outcomes in treatment. While current approaches to antimicrobial dose optimisation address fixed variability, more precise methods are required to monitor and rapidly adjust antimicrobial dosing to further reduce the variability that occurs within and between individuals. We have reviewed the current challenges in implementing antimicrobial dose optimisation and upcoming computer-controlled closed-loop control systems that could provide potential solutions. These solutions promise to improve patient outcomes and are important for antimicrobial stewardship and the prevention of antimicrobial resistance.

2.3.1 Need for dose optimisation

The effectiveness of antimicrobial drugs depends on several factors, including patient, microbial and drug-related factors [98]. However, some factors that have an impact on the therapy are difficult to quantify and determine, such as the host immune response, size of the bacterial inoculum, biofilm formation, and hetero-resistance. Nevertheless, it is possible to optimise the exposure of the drug by adjusting and measuring its dose.

TDM (Therapeutic Drug Monitoring) can help improve clinical outcomes and reduce toxicity in cases where drugs like vancomycin, a glycopeptide antibiotic that causes nephrotoxicity, are used [99]. Furthermore, in vitro studies on levofloxacin, a fluoroquinolone used to treat *Pseudomonas aeruginosa* infections, have identified a pharmacokinetic-pharmacodynamic target that can prevent the emergence of resistant subpopulations upon antimicrobial exposure [100].

Achieving optimal doses that aim to meet pharmacokinetic–pharmacodynamic targets can help prevent the emergence of resistance, including the initial mechanisms like the upregulation of efflux pumps, and reduce the frequency of secondary mutational events [100]. Clinical studies have shown that achieving pharmacokinetic–pharmacodynamic targets for ciprofloxacin and *P. aeruginosa* can reduce the emergence of drug resistance [101,102]. This approach can also help reduce the development of decreased susceptibility and hetero-resistance in many other microorganisms [28]. For drugs with lower risks of toxicity, such as β-lactams, adjusting the dosing for critical care patients is crucial for better clinical outcomes and to reduce the development of drug resistance [103–105].

During the course of an infection, there are numerous factors that can cause intra-individual variation in antimicrobial pharmacokinetics. Some of these factors may not be immediately obvious. These factors include renal dysfunction, augmented renal clearance, fluid shifts due to inflammatory response, and the need for organ support, such as renal replacement therapy [106]. For instance, in critically ill patients receiving linezolid therapy for methicillin-resistant *Staphylococcus aureus*, there have been variations observed in the volume of distribution, clearance, and eventually, plasma and tissue pharmacokinetics [107]. Determining optimal dosing strategies for individual patients can be challenging due to these factors that drive variation [107].

2.3.2 Pharmacodynamic variables

To effectively combat invading microorganisms, it is important to ensure that drugs are administered in a manner that optimises their antimicrobial properties. The optimal exposure to drugs can be determined through various methods such as assessing the minimum inhibitory concentration (MIC) of the microorganism, measuring biomarkers like C-reactive protein (CRP) and galactomannan (in antifungal therapy), monitoring the rate of decline of bacterial colony-forming units per millilitre and observing host response indicators such as the white cell count or temperature [108–112].

The MIC is a laboratory test that determines the lowest concentration of an antibiotic needed to stop the visible growth of a microorganism [111]. However, different organisations use varying classifications of selected breakpoints, leading to varied interpretations of results [113,114]. In addition, using MIC to guide individualised dosing is challenging due to the accuracy of intra-laboratory variation in MIC determination and observed intra-sample variations. To determine pharmacokinetic–pharmacodynamic targets for individual patients, it is necessary to account for these factors [111]. Pharmacokinetic–pharmacodynamic indices aim to quantify the relationship between drug exposure and its effect on a microorganism. However, the MIC fails to provide information on in vivo microbial characteristics and host factors, such as immune response, and may not account for hetero resistance within a bacterial population [115–117]. MIC breakpoints also do not consider the site of infection, drug penetration, biofilm formation, inoculum load and local factors like pH [98,118].

The MIC of a drug is often unknown, especially when the invading pathogen is not identified, like in cases of sepsis that remain culture-negative throughout treatment [119,120]. To determine the effectiveness of antimicrobial pharmacodynamics, researchers measure a biomarker's response to a drug's exposure, such as CRP or galactomannan. For instance, in paediatric patients receiving teicoplanin, a glycopeptide antibiotic for gram-positive infections, the ratio of the area under the concentration–time curve (AUC) of teicoplanin to EC50 value (which indicates the drug concentration needed for a half-maximal response in CRP) was found to predict therapy response [110]. The AUC:EC50 ratio was compared with individual Bayesian posterior estimates obtained from the pharmacokinetic–pharmacodynamic model fitted to patient data [110]. The predictive ability of the AUC:EC50 for glycopeptide therapy response has also been studied in adult patients, and it demonstrates a good performance compared to the traditional AUC:MIC for vancomycin [112]. Additionally, voriconazole, a triazole antifungal widely used in treating invasive fungal infections, was linked to individual galactomannan–time profiles using AUC:EC50 to predict the treatment outcome in invasive aspergillosis patients [109].

2.3.3 Limitations of current methods

Optimising antimicrobial doses is crucial for effective treatment. One common method used for this purpose is a pharmacokinetic dosing nomogram, which is developed using pharmacokinetic models for the specific drug. These nomograms provide information on how a particular covariate (like weight) affects achieving the desired drug exposure target (such as concentration) [121,122]. For instance, a study developed a dosing nomogram for meropenem infusion in patients with varying renal function, which successfully achieved optimal pharmacokinetic–pharmacodynamic targets [123]. Dosing nomograms have been created for various antimicrobials and dosing regimens [121–124]. They are simple, can be combined with routine therapeutic drug monitoring and translate population pharmacokinetic modelling variables into clinical practice. However, nomograms use population-level estimates for dose optimisation based on single variables, which may not always be accurate in practice [125]. They also do not account for residual variability and thus do not provide a truly individualised approach to dose optimisation.

2.3.4 Closed-loop control systems

There are various clinical applications where closed-loop control systems are used, such as controlling blood glucose levels in patients with diabetes mellitus through automated insulin delivery [126], managing anaesthesia during surgery [127] and treating refractory epilepsy [128]. The use of continuous biosensing with closed-loop control systems has the potential to provide individualised antimicrobial therapy [112,129]. Automated drug delivery systems work on the principle of feedback, where a target signal such as target drug concentration or pharmacokinetic–pharmacodynamic target is compared to a real-time measurement determined through biosensing. The difference between the two readings is used to generate a corrective control action, which can be an increase or decrease in the rate of drug delivery from an infusion pump, to reduce the difference between the current measurement and the target value [129,130].

Automated drug delivery has successfully implemented three closed-loop control techniques that can also be used in automated continuous antimicrobial therapy. These techniques are proportional-integral-derivative (PID) control [131], model predictive control (MPC) [132] and reinforcement learning [133]. If intermittent dosing is required, such as a dose every 6 hours, other types of controllers such as iterative learning control, repetitive control and run-to-run control [132] can be used. The PID controller is a widely used controller in industrial applications due to its simplicity and effectiveness. In both simulated and real-world scenarios, PID control has demonstrated its capability to deliver antibiotics at precise concentrations, even within a narrow therapeutic window [131–134]. However, unlike PID control, MPC has a predictive ability that stems from its model-based nature. This attribute allows MPC to anticipate how changes in drug delivery will affect future target attainment and take appropriate action accordingly. MPC can handle multiple input and output variables, such as sensing multiple molecules and delivering multiple antibiotics, as well as constraints, such as drug infusion constraints. Additionally, MPC can handle nonlinear system dynamics better than traditional methods, such as PID control. MPC is currently a preferred choice for automatic insulin delivery in diabetes mellitus and is commercially available.

When using reinforcement learning, artificial intelligence interacts with its environment and is rewarded for performing well while being penalised for incorrect actions. This technique is especially useful in systems where rewards and penalties have a substantial delay and obtaining a reliable model of the system is difficult. Reinforcement learning has already been implemented in healthcare settings such as cancer therapy dosing and controlling blood glucose levels in diabetes [135,136].

Iterative learning control, repetitive control and run-to-run control play a crucial role in controlling repetitive processes such as automated batch production in the chemical and semiconductor industries. These techniques have also been successfully applied in medicine, specifically for insulin delivery in diabetes mellitus (ref.) Although their application to antimicrobial dosing is still in the proof-of-concept stage, they have great potential to support intermittent dosing, including the use of traditional TDM or continuous or intermittent biosensor-based sensing with oral antimicrobials. In the case of precision drug delivery, these techniques aim to improve pharmacokinetic–pharmacodynamic target attainment by adjusting the dose based on the deviation of observed drug exposure after past doses [137,138]. However, determining the optimal pharmacokinetic–pharmacodynamic index and target value still requires exploration and characterisation in many cases.

2.3.5 Decisions assisted by artificial intelligence systems

Decision support tools for optimising antimicrobial regimens have mainly focussed on Bayesian forecasting and mobile applications that contain traditional dose optimisation software [139–141]. These approaches have limited integration and connectivity with other aspects, such as diagnostics, electronic health records and surveillance systems [142], which are crucial for the wider adoption of optimised therapy. However, with the advances in artificial intelligence, connected data can be utilised to support real-time decision-making for individualised treatment [143–145].

Artificial intelligence has been successfully applied to optimise insulin delivery in diabetes [137], and closed-loop control techniques, such as reinforcement learning, have been demonstrated to support personalised therapy [146]. Thus, future work should explore connecting novel tools for the optimisation of antimicrobial dosing with wider decision support for antimicrobial therapy, which necessitates integration with electronic health records and other aspects of decision support for precision antimicrobial therapy [147]. This integration will increase adoption and provide individualised decision support at different points of antimicrobial management.

For instance, artificial intelligence systems supporting personalised antimicrobial selection have incorporated dose optimisation packages for individual drugs [145]. In conclusion, future decision-support approaches must focus on greater integration and connectivity with other aspects to promote the wider adoption of optimised therapy [142].

Antimicrobial dose optimisation is a crucial issue, and a significant question in this regard is whether the data generated by individual institutions and networks can be used for broader dosing recommendations for the population. However, there is a wide variation in practice and reporting, and hence, there is a need for improved curation and analysis of such data. Artificial intelligence can help in this aspect by analysing whether pooled population data can be applied to individualised dosing when TDM and biosensing technologies are not available in an area or when data is insufficient for the population in question. By pooling individual data into large artificially curated datasets, it may be possible to infer the optimal treatment strategies for the individual within this population in the future.

2.4 Clinical applications

Nanoparticle use in medicine has stretched a wide range of applications. This includes uses in antimicrobial coatings for implantable devices, integration in wound dressings, bone cement, maxillofacial devices and dental materials [148]. In this section, examples from the field of dentistry have been used to illustrate the potential of antimicrobial nanoparticles for clinical applications.

2.4.1 Preventative use and therapeutic application of antimicrobial nanoparticles in dentistry

Even though antimicrobial agents are not recommended for routine use in dentistry and oral care, there are a number of indications for their use in the treatment of oral infections and prevention and treatment of dental conditions caused by plaque biofilm in specific patient populations. Various types of nanoparticles have been investigated for prevention and treatment of oral infections, including nanometals (silver, copper, gold, titanium, zinc), nanoparticulate metal oxides, quaternary ammonium, chitosan, silica and silicon nanoparticles, hydroxyapatite and calcium phosphate-based systems and graphene-based nanomaterials [149,150].

Limitations for clinical application of antimicrobial particles include potential undesirable effects on the body and inconsistent antibacterial concentrations against biofilm [151]. The use of nanoparticles in dental products is a promising area of research, as they could be effective at preventing oral conditions and promoting oral health. However, more research is needed before their routine use to understand their pharmacokinetics and pharmacodynamics and to determine the optimal formulations and therapeutic regimens.

2.5 Safety of antimicrobial nanoparticles

Exposure to nanoparticles occurs via a number of cosmetic products, oral care products, topical medications and edible consumer products, and their effects on various human body systems and the microbiota are not well understood. It has been suggested that clinically and translationally relevant nanoparticles can exhibit effects on microbiome, coagulation, microvasculature, immune system as well as exhibit antitumour and protumourigenic effects. It is hypothesised that while many of the nanoparticle effects can be beneficial and employed in improving therapeutic outcomes, they may interact with human biology, tumours and microbiota in a harmful way [95].

Nanotoxicology research is increasingly being conducted using a range of in vitro and in vivo models, including microbes, plants, invertebrates and vertebrates, reporting on bioavailability and toxicity on nanoparticles [152]. Recently, a microfluidic chip model with *Caenorhabditis elegans* was developed and proposed as tool for toxicity analysis of silver nanoparticles [153]. In silico approaches are also increasingly used [154]. Studies have highlighted concerns regarding elimination from animals or humans after nanoparticle treatment. Some nanoparticles are coated with polymers, and this can result with them being in circulation for a wide period leading to accumulation in some organs. There is also the concern of heavy metal release that can be toxic to animal cells and the fact that reactive oxygen species can also damage animal cells [52,71,77]. Conflicting findings have been reported on the impact of one of the most widely used particles, silver nanoparticles on the host and microbiome. An animal study in rats investigated short-term (2 weeks), low-dose exposure to silver nanoparticles in the shape of cubes or spheres and reported behavioural changes (anxiety-like behaviour), a shift in gut microbiota and no apparent histopathological changes in the gastrointestinal system and brain compared to controls [93]. A study in mice reported long-term gut dysbiosis, body fat increase and neurobehavioral alterations in offspring following developmental exposure to silver nanoparticles 2 weeks prior to breeding and throughout gestation [94]. In a clinical study testing short-term in vivo exposure to commercially prepared solutions containing silver colloid nanoparticles for oral use, no important changes were observed in physical and laboratory findings or imaging (chest and abdomen magnetic resonance imaging) [155].

In summary, limited clinical testing of nanoparticles has been done to date. The toxicity of nanoparticles has been shown to be affected by many factors such as the type and shape of particles, dose, duration of application, distribution and interaction with other components [151]. Besides direct toxicity such as cell death and inflammatory response, nanoparticles may have effects on cell signalling, gene expression and cell behaviour such as differentiation or migration. This uncertainty about their long-term biological effects limits their clinical application [95].

3. Material antimicrobial testing

Shortcomings in standardisation and limited clinical relevance is an ongoing issue in antimicrobial testing, including in preclinical testing of novel antimicrobial agents and nanotechnology tools. Often tests do not mimic the complexity of the clinical scenario they are applied in which can result in false positives or negatives. A wide array of antimicrobial tests have been used throughout the literature and most of these have been adapted to test the efficacy of medical nanotechnology [148]. This section will highlight commonly used techniques in the scientific literature, highlighting their key features and use in nanotechnology assessment.

3.1 Colony forming unit assays

Static colony forming unit (CFU) assays have been traditionally considered to be a gold standard test in medical and dental material antimicrobial assessment [156]. In these tests the material is typically exposed to an organism or a mix of organisms with known concentration in broth form and later plated for counting to assess any changes in microorganism growth. Although this method provides essential information on how many live or viable organisms are left after exposure to the material or surface, one major limitation is that only organisms culturable in a laboratory environment can be tested. Variations of this assay have been used to assess the antimicrobial activity of nanoparticle applications including iron oxide and gold nanoparticles [157].

3.2 MIC: Minimum inhibitory concentration, MBC: Minimum bactericidal concentration and MBIC: Minimum biofilm inhibitory concentration

MIC is another fairly traditional way of assessing antimicrobial activity of antimicrobials. MIC is a method described by the Clinical and Laboratory Standards Institute of the United States of America [157a] and typically used to test concentrations of different antibiotics or antimicrobials. In this assay different concentrations of the tested agent are used against known concentrations of the relevant pathogen. The MIC determines the lowest concentration of the antimicrobial agent that can halt growth of an overnight incubation of the assessed pathogen [158]. A variation of this protocol is used to determine the MBC, which deduces the lowest concentration of antimicrobial agent required to kill the microorganism of interest [158]. MBIC on the other hand relates to assessment of biofilm inhibition, which is generally more clinically relevant than assessment of planktonic inhibition. MBIC is defined as the lowest concentration of antimicrobial agent required to halt increase in the mean number of biofilm viable cells [159]. The above-mentioned methods can also be found in literature assessing nanoparticles, such as silver nanoparticles assessment [160]. Nonetheless, these methods have their own limitations and are notorious for being subject to poor accuracy and significant intra and interlaboratory variations [161].

3.3 Viability staining kits

Viability staining kits offer a more rapid alternative to culture-based techniques. Kits such as the LIVE/DEAD BacLight Bacterial Viability Kit rely on fluorescent dyes that determine membrane integrity and potential, as a proxy for cell viability. These dyes are then adapted for use either in microscopy followed by fluorescent quantification comparisons or flow cytometry for quantification of differences in fluorescence following exposure to the antimicrobial agent of interest [162]. This method has been used to test several innovative nanotechnology advances including engineered nanoparticle combinations [163]. Even though this method boasts a simpler methodology, adequate optimisation is necessary for more accurate interpretation of the results since most dyes primarily reflect membrane damage [162].

3.4 Agar diffusion test and direct contact test

Both the agar diffusion and direct contact test are methods that test antimicrobial activity of materials on contact. The former also relies on the ability of the antimicrobial agent to diffuse and is tested by placing discs of either the material being tested or inoculated discs onto an agar plate inoculated with known concentrations of the microbe of interest [164]. In light of this, interpretation of results needs to consider whether solubility or diffusivity of the antimicrobial agent plays a role in the observed results [165], as well as the clinical implications of agent diffusion if the antimicrobial nanoparticle is toxic [164]. The direct contact test on the other hand tests material antimicrobial activity by contact with a liquid bacterial inoculum after allowing the inoculum a set amount of time of contact with the material. This quantitative test provides information about the initial interaction of the material with the studied microorganism [166]. The direct contact test is frequently used in the assessment of antimicrobial activity of dental endodontic sealers including sealers with incorporated nanosilver as an antimicrobial agent [167].

3.5 Molecular techniques

Molecular techniques have also been used to assess antimicrobial properties of novel nanotechnology [163]. Techniques such as polymerase chain reaction (PCR), DNA microarray, whole-genome sequencing and metagenomics, and matrix-assisted laser desorption ionisation—time of flight mass spectrometry are methods where the genetic mechanism is characterised. These techniques have been traditionally used to study antimicrobial resistance [167a] and later been adapted to quantify antimicrobial activity [163]. Although one of the main advantages of molecular techniques is that unculturable microorganisms can be assessed, Bankier et al. in 2018 highlighted that these techniques are amongst the ones with the lowest quantification potential (amongst the one they tested in their work) due to the difficulty in distinguishing between live and dead cells [163].

As highlighted in this section each method has its limitations and it is therefore important to interpret pre-clinical antimicrobial assays in light of the method's limitations. While fixed standards have been in use for biocompatibility testing of medical materials and devices through the use of ISO 10993, development of medical and dental device antimicrobial and/or infection risk assessment has to date been less established [156,168,169]. As result, inter-laboratory or facility comparisons as well as assessments of pre-clinical testing of newly developed materials have been quite challenging. This has transpired in several initiatives by groups worldwide to highlight the need for increased standardisation, including the development of a new standard for assessing the antibacterial activity of dental restorative materials, ISO 3990 [156]. Development of clinically relevant standards will aid reproducibility and more predictable antimicrobial assessment of medical materials including those incorporating novel nanotechnology developments.

3.6 Emerging analytical techniques for antimicrobial susceptibility testing

The primary goal of antimicrobial susceptibility testing (AST) is to quickly and accurately predict the effectiveness of antibiotics in treating infections. Currently, this is achieved through manual methods or automated systems like the Becton, Dickinson Phoenix, the Siemens Micoscan WalkAway or the bioMérieux Vitek 2, all of which use broth microdilution (BMD) testing. However, these methods have several limitations, including the need for large amounts of viable organisms, complex preanalytical processing, limited organism range, variation in results, lengthy turnaround times and high costs. Table 7.5 provides a brief overview of upcoming analytical techniques, along with their respective advantages and current state, designed to overcome the traditional, laborious and time-consuming AST methods.

Time-of-flight mass spectrometry (TOF-SIMS) is a powerful tool to quickly detect cells that are essential for medical applications and can become a valuable AST method [12,20]. Several approaches on the TOF-SIMS to detect the live/dead cells have been explored, including (i) identifying the antibiotic-inactivating enzymes (e.g. β-lactamases), verifying the PCR products that indicate antimicrobial resistance (e.g. *vanA*, *mecA*, or NDM-1), and monitoring the variation in protein spectrum of cells with and without the use of the antimicrobial agent that correlate with live/dead cells. Another major advantage of the TOF-SIMS is that it can visualise the biofilm growth and live/dead cells on complex 3D structures, such as implants, foams and nanoneedles, that are essential to test the emerging nanotechnologies for practical medical applications [170].

We can weigh microbial cells by using vibrating cantilevers. These cantilevers have small canals that help the bacteria to pass through. By making them vibrate continuously, the weight of the bacteria (in the femtogram range) can be measured, which

Table 7.5 Automated bacterial viability tests [20].

Test name	Test principal	[a]Test time (h)	Commercial or laboratory test
Calorimetry	Heat produced or consumed by the bacteria over time	Rapid: 2–12 Slow: 24–72	Laboratory
Cantilever	High sensitivity of the cantilever vibration to bacterial mass changes or stress changes	Rapid: 1–2 Slow: 12–24	Laboratory
Fluorescence	Staining bacteria with fluorescent dyes that distinguish live and dead cells due to variation in size and intensity of fluorescence	Rapid: 3–6 Slow: 6–12	Both
Magnetic	Monitoring changes in bead spin within a magnetic field in relation to the quantity of adhered bacteria	Rapid: 4–8 Slow: 8–24	Laboratory
Droplet	Tracking growth and substrate conversion in nanoliter droplets	Rapid: 4–8 Slow: 8–24	Laboratory
Calorimetric respirometry	Active respiration of the cells is identified from substrate or indicator colour changes	Rapid: 2–12 Slow: 24–72	Laboratory
Acoustics-based method	Studying the vibrational frequency changes between living and dead bacteria	Rapid: 6–12 Slow: 12–24	Laboratory
Impedance spectroscopy	Variation in the electrical properties of live and dead bacteria in suspensions	Rapid: 6–12 Slow: 12–24	Laboratory
Infrared spectroscopy	Absorption characteristics of bacteria upon exposure to infrared radiation	Rapid: 8–12 Slow: 12–24	Laboratory
Raman spectroscopy	The absorption properties of bacteria under laser exposure	Rapid: 6–12 Slow: 12–24	Laboratory
Secondary mass spectroscopy	Identifies antibiotic degradation in products with precision	Rapid: 8–12 Slow: 24–48	Laboratory
Nuclear magnetic resonance spectrometry	Analysing the molecular composition of intricate heterogeneous mixtures allows obtaining metabolic profiles	Rapid: 8–12 Slow: 24–48	Laboratory

[a]Test time included sample preparation, actual testing time, and data analysis.

causes a change in the frequency of cantilever movement [171]. The density of less-dense and more-dense cells causes a different change. When antimicrobial agents are used to treat the cells, their buoyant mass density changes, which can be measured [172]. This principle has been tested and proven using ampicillin-resistant and -susceptible variants of *Citrobacter rodentium*. It has also been demonstrated that after osmotic shock, the resuscitation of both phenotypes in the presence or absence of ampicillin allows for rapid differentiation in a reduced time span. Cantilevers can be multiplexed using nanotechnology, multiple antibiotics in various concentrations can be tested for a single growing culture simultaneously.

A biosensor that facilitates the rapid detection of bacterial growth has been developed using vibrating cantilevers [173]. These cantilevers contain a certain number of fixed but still viable bacteria. The detection scheme is based on the change in resonance frequency as the mass on the cantilever increases. The mass sensitivity of the cantilever sensor is approximately 50 pg/Hz according to its mechanical properties. This mass corresponds to about 100 *E. coli* cells. The sensor can detect the active growth of *E. coli* cells within 1 hour. On average, 1000 *E. coli* cells are initially attached to the cantilever. Moreover, the cantilever technology has been used to measure the binding of vancomycin to cell wall precursors and to evaluate the effects of colistin on *P. aeruginosa* [174,175]. The growth of resistant cells can also be detected within 2 hours after the addition of antibiotics [176].

4. Conclusions

Overall, the use of nanoparticles for the delivery of antimicrobials as well as direct antimicrobial action in humans is a promising area of research, and there is evidence to suggest that these particles can be effective at improving antimicrobial activity. Besides, development of antimicrobial nanoparticles is a promising strategy for combating antimicrobial resistance. However, more research is needed to fully understand the mechanisms of action of these nanoparticles and to determine the appropriate administration route, optimal concentrations, dose and formulations for their use. It is also important to consider the potential harmful effects of nanoparticles with short- and long-term exposure, as their application may cause adverse effects in humans.

References

[1] World Health Organization, Prevention of Hospital-Acquired Infections: A Practical Guide, second ed., 2002. Available at: https://apps.who.int/iris/bitstream/handle/10665/67350/WHO_CDS_CSR_EPH_2002.12.pdf.

[2] N.C.T. Dadi, et al., Impact of healthcare-associated infections connected to medical devices—an update, Microorganisms 9 (11) (2021) 2332, https://doi.org/10.3390/microorganisms9112332.

[3] A.S. Collins, Preventing health care–associated infections, in: Patient Safety and Quality: An Evidence-Based Handbook for Nurses, 2009.

[4] M. Haque, et al., Health care-associated infections - an overview, Infection and Drug Resistance 11 (2018) 2321–2333, https://doi.org/10.2147/IDR.S177247.
[5] A. Cassini, et al., Burden of six healthcare-associated infections on European population health: estimating incidence-based disability-adjusted life years through a population prevalence-based modelling study, in: S. Harbarth (Ed.), PLoS Medicine 13 (10) (2016) e1002150, https://doi.org/10.1371/journal.pmed.1002150.
[6] S.S. Magill, et al., Multistate point-prevalence survey of health care–associated infections for the emerging infections program healthcare-associated infections and antimicrobial use prevalence survey team, New England Journal of Medicine 37013370 (27) (2014) 1198–1208.
[7] P.S. Stewart, T. Bjarnsholt, Risk factors for chronic biofilm-related infection associated with implanted medical devices, Clinical Microbiology and Infection 26 (8) (2020) 1034–1038, https://doi.org/10.1016/j.cmi.2020.02.027.
[8] M. Riool, et al., Staphylococcus epidermidis originating from titanium implants infects surrounding tissue and immune cells, Acta Biomaterialia 10 (12) (2014) 5202–5212, https://doi.org/10.1016/j.actbio.2014.08.012.
[9] J.J. Boelens, et al., Biomaterial-associated persistence of Staphylococcus epidermidis in pericatheter macrophages, The Journal of Infectious Diseases 181 (4) (2000) 1337–1349, https://doi.org/10.1086/315369.
[10] S. Bernatová, et al., Following the mechanisms of bacteriostatic versus bactericidal action using Raman spectroscopy, Molecules 18 (11) (2013) 13188–13199, https://doi.org/10.3390/molecules181113188.
[11] G.A. Pankey, L.D. Sabath, Clinical relevance of bacteriostatic versus bactericidal mechanisms of action in the treatment of gram-positive bacterial infections, Clinical Infectious Diseases 38 (6) (2004) 864–870, https://doi.org/10.1086/381972.
[12] K. Kumar, et al., Antibiotic use in agriculture and its impact on the terrestrial environment, in: Advances in Agronomy, 2005, pp. 1–54, https://doi.org/10.1016/S0065-2113(05)87001-4.
[13] G.D. Wright, Q& a: antibiotic resistance: where does it come from and what can we do about it? BMC Biology 8 (1) (2010) 123, https://doi.org/10.1186/1741-7007-8-123.
[14] C. Manyi-Loh, et al., Antibiotic use in agriculture and its consequential resistance in environmental sources: potential public health implications, Molecules 23 (4) (2018) 795, https://doi.org/10.3390/molecules23040795.
[15] E.P. Abraham, E. Chain, An enzyme from bacteria able to destroy penicillin, Nature 146 (3713) (1940), https://doi.org/10.1038/146837a0, 837–837.
[16] World Health Organization, WHO Library Cataloguing-In-Publication Data Global Action Plan on Antimicrobial Resistance, 2015.
[17] European Centre for Disease Prevention and Control (ECDC), Assessing the Health Burden of Infections with Antibiotic-Resistant Bacteria in the EU/EEA, 2022, pp. 2016–2020.
[18] Prioritization of Pathogens to Guide Discovery, Research and Development of New Antibiotics for Drug-resistant Bacterial Infections, Including Tuberculosis, World Health Organization, Geneva, 2017. WHO/EMP/IAU/2017.12).

[19] World Health Organization, Global Action Plan on Antimicrobial Resistance, World Health Organization, 2017, pp. 1–28.
[20] A. Van Belkum, W.M. Dunne, Next-generation antimicrobial susceptibility testing, Journal of Clinical Microbiology (2013), https://doi.org/10.1128/JCM.00313-13.
[21] I. Alav, et al., Structure, assembly, and function of tripartite efflux and type 1 secretion systems in gram-negative bacteria, Chemical Reviews (2021), https://doi.org/10.1021/acs.chemrev.1c00055.
[22] R. Leclercq, Mechanisms of resistance to macrolides and lincosamides: nature of the resistance elements and their clinical implications, Clinical Infectious Diseases 34 (4) (2002) 482–492, https://doi.org/10.1086/324626.
[23] W.M. Scheld, Maintaining fluoroquinolone class efficacy: review of influencing factors, Emerging Infectious Diseases 9 (1) (2003) 1–9, https://doi.org/10.3201/eid0901.020277.
[24] J. Spížek, T. Řezanka, Lincosamides: chemical structure, biosynthesis, mechanism of action, resistance, and applications, Biochemical Pharmacology 133 (2017) 20–28, https://doi.org/10.1016/j.bcp.2016.12.001.
[25] K.E. Greber, et al., Characterization of antimicrobial and hemolytic properties of short synthetic cationic lipopeptides based on QSAR/QSTR approach, Amino Acids 50 (3–4) (2018) 479–485, https://doi.org/10.1007/s00726-017-2530-2.
[26] S. Kırmusaoğlu, N. Gareayaghi, B. S. Kocazeybek, Introductory chapter: the action mechanisms of antibiotics and antibiotic resistance, in: Antimicrobials, Antibiotic Resistance, Antibiofilm Strategies and Activity Methods, IntechOpen, 2019, https://doi.org/10.5772/intechopen.85211.
[27] W. C Reygaert, An overview of the antimicrobial resistance mechanisms of bacteria, AIMS Microbiology 4 (3) (2018) 482–501, https://doi.org/10.3934/microbiol.2018.3.482.
[28] R. Álvarez, et al., Optimizing the clinical use of vancomycin, Antimicrobial Agents and Chemotherapy 60 (5) (2016), https://doi.org/10.1128/AAC.03147-14.
[29] M. Griffith, M. Postelnick, M. Scheetz, Antimicrobial stewardship programs: methods of operation and suggested outcomes, Expert Review of Anti-Infective Therapy 10 (1) (2012) 63–73, https://doi.org/10.1586/eri.11.153.
[30] N. Matsunaga, K. Hayakawa, Estimating the impact of antimicrobial resistance, Lancet Global Health 6 (9) (2018) e934–e935, https://doi.org/10.1016/S2214-109X(18)30325-5.
[31] WHO Europe and European Centre for Disease Prevention and Control, Surveillance of Antimicrobial Resistance in Europe, 2020 Data, 2021.
[32] G.L. Hobby, K. Meyer, E. Chaffee, Observations on the mechanism of action of penicillin, Experimental Biology and Medicine 50 (2) (1942) 281–285, https://doi.org/10.3181/00379727-50-13773.
[33] C. Levine, H. Hiasa, K.J. Marians, DNA gyrase and topoisomerase IV: biochemical activities, physiological roles during chromosome replication, and drug sensitivities, Biochimica et Biophysica Acta (BBA) - Gene Structure and Expression 1400 (1–3) (1998) 29–43, https://doi.org/10.1016/S0167-4781(98)00126-2.
[34] V.V.H. Le, J. Rakonjac, Nitrofurans: revival of an “old” drug class in the fight against antibiotic resistance, in: J.M. Leong (Ed.), PLoS Pathogens 17 (7) (2021) e1009663, https://doi.org/10.1371/journal.ppat.1009663.

[35] S.Y. Kim, et al., Antibacterial strategies inspired by the oxidative stress and response networks, Journal of Microbiology 57 (3) (2019) 203–212, https://doi.org/10.1007/s12275-019-8711-9.
[36] A. Vaishampayan, E. Grohmann, Antimicrobials functioning through ros-mediated mechanisms: current insights, Microorganisms 10 (1) (2022), https://doi.org/10.3390/microorganisms10010061.
[37] A.F. Seixas, et al., Bacterial response to oxidative stress and RNA oxidation, Frontiers in Genetics 12 (January) (2022) 1–12, https://doi.org/10.3389/fgene.2021.821535.
[38] F.C. Fang, Antimicrobial reactive oxygen and nitrogen species: concepts and controversies, Nature Reviews Microbiology 2 (10) (2004) 820–832, https://doi.org/10.1038/nrmicro1004.
[39] Y. Li, et al., Mechanism of photogenerated reactive oxygen species and correlation with the antibacterial properties of engineered metal-oxide nanoparticles, ACS Nano 6 (6) (2012) 5164–5173, https://doi.org/10.1021/nn300934k.
[40] L. Sun, et al., Honokiol induces reactive oxygen species-mediated apoptosis in Candida albicans through mitochondrial dysfunction, in: G. López Lluch (Ed.), PLoS One 12 (2) (2017) e0172228, https://doi.org/10.1371/journal.pone.0172228.
[41] F.C. Fang, Antimicrobial actions of reactive oxygen species, mBio 2 (5) (2011), https://doi.org/10.1128/mBio.00141-11.
[42] G. Kapoor, S. Saigal, A. Elongavan, Action and resistance mechanisms of antibiotics: a guide for clinicians, Journal of Anaesthesiology Clinical Pharmacology 33 (3) (2017) 300, https://doi.org/10.4103/joacp.JOACP_349_15.
[43] C.J.L. Murray, et al., Global burden of bacterial antimicrobial resistance in 2019: a systematic analysis, The Lancet 399 (10325) (2022) 629–655, https://doi.org/10.1016/S0140-6736(21)02724-0.
[44] J.W. Bigger, Treatment of staphylococcal infections with penicillin by intermittent sterilisation, The Lancet 244 (6320) (1944), https://doi.org/10.1016/S0140-6736(00)74210-3.
[45] T. Nyström, MicroReview Conditional senescence in bacteria : death of, Molecular Microbiology 48 (2003) 17–23.
[46] I. Keren, et al., Persister cells and tolerance to antimicrobials, FEMS Microbiology Letters 230 (1) (2004) 13–18, https://doi.org/10.1016/S0378-1097(03)00856-5.
[47] Y. Li, Y. Zhang, PhoU is a persistence switch involved in persister formation and tolerance to multiple antibiotics and stresses in *Escherichia coli*, Antimicrobial Agents and Chemotherapy 51 (6) (2007) 2092–2099, https://doi.org/10.1128/AAC.00052-07.
[48] T.K. Wood, S.J. Knabel, B.W. Kwan, Bacterial persister cell formation and dormancy, Applied and Environmental Microbiology 79 (23) (2013) 7116–7121, https://doi.org/10.1128/AEM.02636-13.
[49] H. Luidalepp, et al., Age of inoculum strongly influences persister frequency and can mask effects of mutations implicated in altered persistence, Journal of Bacteriology 193 (14) (2011) 3598–3605, https://doi.org/10.1128/JB.00085-11.
[50] I. Singh, P.C. Jain, Current status of dental plaque, International Journal of Pharma and Bio Sciences 3 (3) (2012).
[50a] Y. Cong, S. Yang, X. Rao, Vancomycin resistant *Staphylococcus aureus* infections: A review of case updating and clinical features, Journal of

Advanced Research 21 (2019) 169–176, https://doi.org/10.1016/j.jare.2019.10.005. PMID: 32071785; PMCID: PMC7015472.
[51] G. Asokan, et al., WHO global priority pathogens list: a bibliometric analysis of medline-PubMed for knowledge mobilization to infection prevention and control practices in Bahrain, Oman Medical Journal 34 (3) (2019) 184–193, https://doi.org/10.5001/omj.2019.37.
[52] Z. Alhalili, Metal oxides nanoparticles: general structural description, chemical, physical, and biological synthesis methods, role in pesticides and heavy metal removal through wastewater treatment, Molecules (2023), https://doi.org/10.3390/molecules28073086.
[53] J.M. Munita, C.A. Arias, Mechanisms of antibiotic resistance, in: Virulence Mechanisms of Bacterial Pathogens, 2016, https://doi.org/10.1128/9781555819286.ch17.
[54] E.M. Darby, et al., Molecular mechanisms of antibiotic resistance revisited, Nature Reviews Microbiology 21 (5) (2023) 280–295, https://doi.org/10.1038/s41579-022-00820-y.
[55] T. Li, et al., Bacterial resistance to antibacterial agents: mechanisms, control strategies, and implications for global health, Science of The Total Environment 860 (2023) 160461, https://doi.org/10.1016/j.scitotenv.2022.160461.
[56] J.L.C. Wong, et al., OmpK36-mediated Carbapenem resistance attenuates ST258 *Klebsiella pneumoniae* in vivo, Nature Communications 10 (1) (2019) 3957, https://doi.org/10.1038/s41467-019-11756-y.
[57] N.N. Mishra, et al., Daptomycin resistance in enterococci is associated with distinct alterations of cell membrane phospholipid content, in: T. Msadek (Ed.), PLoS One 7 (8) (2012) e43958, https://doi.org/10.1371/journal.pone.0043958.
[58] D. Du, et al., Multidrug efflux pumps: structure, function and regulation, Nature Reviews Microbiology 16 (9) (2018) 523–539, https://doi.org/10.1038/s41579-018-0048-6.
[59] R. Ghotaslou, M. Yekani, M.Y. Memar, The role of efflux pumps in Bacteroides fragilis resistance to antibiotics, Microbiological Research 210 (2018) 1–5, https://doi.org/10.1016/j.micres.2018.02.007.
[60] H. Periasamy, et al., High prevalence of *Escherichia coli* clinical isolates in India harbouring four amino acid inserts in PBP3 adversely impacting activity of aztreonam/avibactam, Journal of Antimicrobial Chemotherapy 75 (6) (2020) 1650–1651, https://doi.org/10.1093/jac/dkaa021.
[61] C.-H. Tseng, C.-W. Liu, P.-Y. Liu, Extended-spectrum β-lactamases (ESBL) producing bacteria in animals, Antibiotics 12 (4) (2023) 661, https://doi.org/10.3390/antibiotics12040661.
[62] M. Castanheira, P.J. Simner, P.A. Bradford, Extended-spectrum β -lactamases: an update on their characteristics, epidemiology and detection, JAC-Antimicrobial Resistance 3 (3) (2021), https://doi.org/10.1093/jacamr/dlab092.
[63] Y. Castillo, et al., Antibiotic susceptibility and resistance genes in oral clinical isolates of Prevotella intermedia, Prevotella nigrescens, and Prevotella melaninogenica, Antibiotics 11 (7) (2022) 888, https://doi.org/10.3390/antibiotics11070888.
[64] S. Meini, et al., AmpC β-lactamase-producing Enterobacterales: what a clinician should know, Infection (2019), https://doi.org/10.1007/s15010-019-01291-9.

[65] R. Han, et al., Dissemination of carbapenemases (KPC, NDM, OXA-48, IMP, and VIM) among carbapenem-resistant Enterobacteriaceae isolated from adult and children patients in China, Frontiers in Cellular and Infection Microbiology 10 (2020), https://doi.org/10.3389/fcimb.2020.00314.
[66] R.Y. Pelgrift, A.J. Friedman, Nanotechnology as a therapeutic tool to combat microbial resistance, Advanced Drug Delivery Reviews 65 (13–14) (2013) 1803–1815, https://doi.org/10.1016/j.addr.2013.07.011.
[67] F. Fenaroli, et al., Polymersomes eradicating intracellular bacteria, ACS Nano 14 (7) (2020) 8287–8298, https://doi.org/10.1021/acsnano.0c01870.
[68] K. Wayakanon, et al., Polymersome-mediated intracellular delivery of antibiotics to treat Porphyromonas gingivalis -infected oral epithelial cells, The FASEB Journal 27 (11) (2013) 4455–4465, https://doi.org/10.1096/fj.12-225219.
[69] S. Sharmin, et al., Nanoparticles as antimicrobial and antiviral agents: a literature-based perspective study, Heliyon (2021), https://doi.org/10.1016/j.heliyon.2021.e06456.
[70] M. Ozdal, S. Gurkok, Recent advances in nanoparticles as antibacterial agent, ADMET and DMPK 10 (2) (2022), https://doi.org/10.5599/admet.1172.
[71] A.M. Ealias, M.P. Saravanakumar, A review on the classification, characterisation, synthesis of nanoparticles and their application, IOP Conference Series: Materials Science and Engineering 263 (3) (2017), https://doi.org/10.1088/1757-899X/263/3/032019.
[72] E. Taylor, T.J. Webster, Reducing infections through nanotechnology and nanoparticles, International Journal of Nanomedicine 6 (12) (2011) 1463–1473, https://doi.org/10.2147/IJN.S22021.
[73] T.J. Macdonald, et al., Thiol-capped gold nanoparticles swell-encapsulated into polyurethane as powerful antibacterial surfaces under dark and light conditions, Scientific Reports 6 (1) (2016) 39272, https://doi.org/10.1038/srep39272.
[74] S. Sehmi, Antibacterial Surfaces with Nanoparticle Incorporation for Prevention of Hospital-Acquired Infections', *Doctoral Thesis*, UCL (University College London), 2016.
[75] S.K. Sehmi, et al., Enhancing the antibacterial activity of light-activated surfaces containing crystal violet and ZnO nanoparticles: investigation of nanoparticle size, capping ligand, and dopants, ACS Omega 1 (3) (2016) 334–343, https://doi.org/10.1021/acsomega.6b00017.
[76] S.K. Sehmi, et al., Antibacterial surfaces with activity against antimicrobial resistant bacterial pathogens and endospores, ACS Infectious Diseases 6 (5) (2020) 939–946, https://doi.org/10.1021/acsinfecdis.9b00279.
[77] S. Shaikh, et al., Mechanistic insights into the antimicrobial actions of metallic nanoparticles and their implications for multidrug resistance, International Journal of Molecular Sciences 20 (10) (2019) 2468, https://doi.org/10.3390/ijms20102468.
[78] A.M. Allahverdiyev, et al., Coping with antibiotic resistance: combining nanoparticles with antibiotics and other antimicrobial agents, Expert Review of Anti-infective Therapy 9 (11) (2011) 1035–1052, https://doi.org/10.1586/eri.11.121.
[79] A.A. Tayel, et al., Antibacterial action of zinc oxide nanoparticles against foodborne pathogens, Journal of Food Safety 31 (2) (2011), https://doi.org/10.1111/j.1745-4565.2010.00287.x.

[80] E.O. Mikhailova, Silver nanoparticles: mechanism of action and probable bio-application, Journal of Functional Biomaterials 11 (4) (2020) 84, https://doi.org/10.3390/jfb11040084.
[81] D.P. Gnanadhas, et al., Interaction of silver nanoparticles with serum proteins affects their antimicrobial activity in vivo, Antimicrobial Agents and Chemotherapy 57 (10) (2013) 4945–4955, https://doi.org/10.1128/AAC.00152-13.
[82] N.-Y. Lee, W.-C. Ko, P.-R. Hsueh, Nanoparticles in the treatment of infections caused by multidrug-resistant organisms, Frontiers in Pharmacology 10 (October) (2019) 1–10, https://doi.org/10.3389/fphar.2019.01153.
[83] S. Perni, et al., Antibacterial activity of light-activated silicone containing methylene blue and gold nanoparticles of different sizes, Journal of Cluster Science 21 (3) (2010) 427–438, https://doi.org/10.1007/s10876-010-0319-5.
[84] K.R. Raghupathi, R.T. Koodali, A.C. Manna, Size-dependent bacterial growth inhibition and mechanism of antibacterial activity of zinc oxide nanoparticles, Langmuir 27 (7) (2011) 4020–4028, https://doi.org/10.1021/la104825u.
[85] Y. Jeong, D.W. Lim, J. Choi, Assessment of size-dependent antimicrobial and cytotoxic properties of silver nanoparticles, Advances in Materials Science and Engineering 2014 (2014) 1–6, https://doi.org/10.1155/2014/763807.
[86] S. Noimark, et al., Functionalised gold and titania nanoparticles and surfaces for use as antimicrobial coatings, Faraday Discussions 175 (2014) 273–287, https://doi.org/10.1039/C4FD00113C.
[87] S. Pal, Y.K. Tak, J.M. Song, Does the antibacterial activity of silver nanoparticles depend on the shape of the nanoparticle? A study of the gram-negative bacterium *Escherichia coli*, Applied and Environmental Microbiology 73 (6) (2007), https://doi.org/10.1128/AEM.02218-06.
[88] Y. Xie, et al., Antibacterial activity and mechanism of action of zinc oxide nanoparticles against Campylobacter jejuni, Applied and Environmental Microbiology 77 (7) (2011), https://doi.org/10.1128/AEM.02149-10.
[89] E. Ozkan, et al., The use of zinc oxide nanoparticles to enhance the antibacterial properties of light-activated polydimethylsiloxane containing crystal violet, RSC Advances 5 (12) (2015) 8806–8813, https://doi.org/10.1039/C4RA13649G.
[90] R.J. Wydra, et al., Accelerated generation of free radicals by iron oxide nanoparticles in the presence of an alternating magnetic field, RSC Advances 5 (24) (2015), https://doi.org/10.1039/c4ra13564d.
[91] S. Shamaila, et al., Gold nanoparticles: an efficient antimicrobial agent against enteric bacterial human pathogen, Nanomaterials 6 (4) (2016) 71, https://doi.org/10.3390/nano6040071.
[92] E.-K. Tian, et al., Gold nanoparticle: recent progress on its antibacterial applications and mechanisms, in: L. Balan (Ed.), Journal of Nanomaterials (2021) 1–18, https://doi.org/10.1155/2021/2501345.
[93] A.B. Javurek, et al., Gut dysbiosis and neurobehavioral alterations in rats exposed to silver nanoparticles, Scientific Reports 7 (1) (2017), https://doi.org/10.1038/s41598-017-02880-0.
[94] Z. Lyu, et al., Developmental exposure to silver nanoparticles leads to long term gut dysbiosis and neurobehavioral alterations, Scientific Reports 11 (1) (2021), https://doi.org/10.1038/s41598-021-85919-7.

[95] E.P. Stater, et al., The ancillary effects of nanoparticles and their implications for nanomedicine, Nature Nanotechnology (2021), https://doi.org/10.1038/s41565-021-01017-9.
[96] L. Jia, Nanoparticle formulation increases oral bioavailability of poorly soluble drugs: approaches, experimental evidences and theory, Current Nanoscience 1 (3) (2005), https://doi.org/10.2174/157341305774642939.
[97] T. Gunasekaran, et al., Nanotechnology: an effective tool for enhancing bioavailability and bioactivity of phytomedicine, Asian Pacific Journal of Tropical Biomedicine (2014), https://doi.org/10.12980/APJTB.4.2014C980.
[98] N.J. Onufrak, A. Forrest, D. Gonzalez, Pharmacokinetic and pharmacodynamic principles of anti-infective dosing, Clinical Therapeutics (2016), https://doi.org/10.1016/j.clinthera.2016.06.015.
[99] M.N. Neely, et al., Are vancomycin trough concentrations adequate for optimal dosing? Antimicrobial Agents and Chemotherapy 58 (1) (2014) https://doi.org/10.1128/AAC.01653-13.
[100] G.L. Drusano, et al., Suppression of emergence of resistance in pathogenic bacteria: keeping our powder dry, part 1, Antimicrobial Agents and Chemotherapy 60 (3) (2016), https://doi.org/10.1128/AAC.02177-15.
[101] J.K. Thomas, et al., Pharmacodynamic evaluation of factors associated with the development of bacterial resistance in acutely ill patients during therapy, Antimicrobial Agents and Chemotherapy 42 (3) (1998), https://doi.org/10.1128/aac.42.3.521.
[102] J.M. Hyatt, J.J. Schentag, Pharmacodynamic modeling of risk factors for ciprofloxacin resistance in *Pseudomonas aeruginosa*, Infection Control & Hospital Epidemiology 21 (S1) (2000), https://doi.org/10.1086/503167.
[103] J.A. Roberts, et al., Therapeutic drug monitoring of β-lactams in critically ill patients: proof of concept, International Journal of Antimicrobial Agents 36 (4) (2010), https://doi.org/10.1016/j.ijantimicag.2010.06.008.
[104] J.A. Roberts, S.K. Paul, et al., DALI: defining antibiotic levels in intensive care unit patients: are current ß-lactam antibiotic doses sufficient for critically ill patients? Clinical Infectious Diseases 58 (8) (2014) 1072–1083, https://doi.org/10.1093/cid/ciu027.
[105] A.H. Holmes, et al., Understanding the mechanisms and drivers of antimicrobial resistance, The Lancet (2016), https://doi.org/10.1016/S0140-6736(15)00473-0.
[106] A.A. Udy, J.A. Roberts, J. Lipman, Antibiotic Pharmacokinetic/pharmacodynamic Considerations in the Critically Ill, Antibiotic Pharmacokinetic/Pharmacodynamic Considerations in the Critically Ill, 2017, https://doi.org/10.1007/978-981-10-5336-8.
[107] C. Buerger, et al., Pharmacokinetics of unbound linezolid in plasma and tissue interstitium of critically ill patients after multiple dosing using microdialysis, Antimicrobial Agents and Chemotherapy 50 (7) (2006), https://doi.org/10.1128/AAC.01468-05.
[108] P. Liu, M. Müller, H. Derendorf, Rational dosing of antibiotics: the use of plasma concentrations versus tissue concentrations, in: International Journal of Antimicrobial Agents, 2002, https://doi.org/10.1016/S0924-8579(02)00024-9.
[109] L.J. Huurneman, et al., Pharmacodynamics of voriconazole in children: further steps along the path to true individualized therapy, Antimicrobial Agents and Chemotherapy 60 (4) (2016), https://doi.org/10.1128/AAC.03023-15.

[110] V. Ramos-Martín, et al., Population pharmacokinetics and pharmacodynamics of teicoplanin in neonates: making better use of C-reactive protein to deliver individualized therapy, Journal of Antimicrobial Chemotherapy 71 (11) (2016), https://doi.org/10.1093/jac/dkw295.
[111] J.W. Mouton, et al., MIC-based dose adjustment: facts and fables, Journal of Antimicrobial Chemotherapy 73 (3) (2018), https://doi.org/10.1093/jac/dkx427.
[112] T.M. Rawson, E. Charani, et al., Exploring the use of C-reactive protein to estimate the pharmacodynamics of vancomycin, Therapeutic Drug Monitoring 40 (3) (2018) 315–321, https://doi.org/10.1097/FTD.0000000000000507.
[113] The Clinical & Laboratory Standards Institute (CLSI). CLSI Breakpoints, CLSI', 2020. Available at: https://clsi.org/standards/products/free-resources/access-our-free-resources.
[114] European Committee on Antimicrobial Susceptibility Testing. Clinical Breakpoints - Breakpoints and Guidance, EUCAST', 2020. Available at: https://eucast.org/clinical_ breakpoints/.
[115] D.I. Andersson, D. Hughes, Antibiotic resistance and its cost: is it possible to reverse resistance? Nature Reviews Microbiology (2010) https://doi.org/10.1038/nrmicro2319.
[116] D.I. Andersson, D. Hughes, Evolution of antibiotic resistance at non-lethal drug concentrations, Drug Resistance Updates 15 (3) (2012), https://doi.org/10.1016/j.drup.2012.03.005.
[117] T.M. Rawson, D. O'Hare, et al., Delivering precision antimicrobial therapy through closed-loop control systems, Journal of Antimicrobial Chemotherapy 73 (4) (2018) 835–843, https://doi.org/10.1093/jac/dkx458.
[118] P.G. Ambrose, et al., Pharmacokinetics-pharmacodynamics of antimicrobial therapy: it's not just for mice anymore, Clinical Infectious Diseases (2007), https://doi.org/10.1086/510079.
[119] P. Zarb, H. Goossens, European surveillance of antimicrobial consumption (ESAC): value of a point-prevalence survey of antimicrobial use across Europe, Drugs 71 (6) (2011), https://doi.org/10.2165/11591180-000000000-00000.
[120] J. Phua, et al., Characteristics and outcomes of culture-negative versus culture-positive severe sepsis, Critical Care 17 (5) (2013), https://doi.org/10.1186/cc12896.
[121] C. Bartal, et al., Pharmacokinetic dosing of aminoglycosides: a controlled trial, The American Journal of Medicine 114 (3) (2003), https://doi.org/10.1016/S0002-9343(02)01476-6.
[122] P. Williams, et al., Antimicrobial dosing in critical care: a pragmatic adult dosing nomogram, International Journal of Antimicrobial Agents 55 (2) (2020), https://doi.org/10.1016/j.ijantimicag.2019.10.018.
[123] I.K. Minichmayr, et al., Development of a dosing nomogram for continuous-infusion meropenem in critically ill patients based on a validated population pharmacokinetic model, Journal of Antimicrobial Chemotherapy 73 (5) (2018), https://doi.org/10.1093/jac/dkx526.
[124] F. Pea, et al., TDM coupled with Bayesian forecasting should be considered an invaluable tool for optimizing vancomycin daily exposure in unstable critically ill patients, International Journal of Antimicrobial Agents 20 (5) (2002), https://doi.org/10.1016/S0924-8579(02)00188-7.

[125] E. Charani, et al., Lack of weight recording in patients being administered narrow therapeutic index antibiotics: a prospective cross-sectional study, BMJ Open 5 (4) (2015), https://doi.org/10.1136/bmjopen-2014-006092.
[126] S.A. Brown, et al., Six-month randomized, multicenter trial of closed-loop control in type 1 diabetes, New England Journal of Medicine 381 (18) (2019), https://doi.org/10.1056/nejmoa1907863.
[127] J. Sethu Madhavan, G.D. Puri, P.J. Mathew, Closed-loop isoflurane administration with bispectral index in open heart surgery: randomized controlled trial with manual control, Acta Anaesthesiologica Taiwanica 49 (4) (2011), https://doi.org/10.1016/j.aat.2011.11.007.
[128] M.T. Salam, et al., An implantable closedloop asynchronous drug delivery system for the treatment of refractory epilepsy, IEEE Transactions on Neural Systems and Rehabilitation Engineering 20 (4) (2012), https://doi.org/10.1109/TNSRE.2012.2189020.
[129] J. Li, et al., Clinical opportunities for continuous biosensing and closed-loop therapies, Trends in Chemistry (2020), https://doi.org/10.1016/j.trechm.2020.02.009.
[130] K. Scholten, E. Meng, A review of implantable biosensors for closed-loop glucose control and other drug delivery applications, International Journal of Pharmaceutics 544 (2) (2018), https://doi.org/10.1016/j.ijpharm.2018.02.022.
[131] P. Herrero, et al., Closed-loop control for precision antimicrobial delivery: an in silico proof-of-concept, IEEE Transactions on Biomedical Engineering 65 (10) (2018), https://doi.org/10.1109/TBME.2017.2787423
[132] M.A. Johnson, et al., PID control: new identification and design methods, PID Control: New Identification and Design Methods (2005), https://doi.org/10.1007/1-84628-148-2.
[133] R.S. Sutton, A.G. Barto, Reinforcement learning: an introduction, IEEE Transactions on Neural Networks 9 (5) (1998), https://doi.org/10.1109/tnn.1998.712192.
[134] N. Arroyo-Currás, et al., High-precision control of plasma drug levels using feedback-controlled dosing, ACS Pharmacology & Translational Science 1 (2) (2018), https://doi.org/10.1021/acsptsci.8b00033.
[135] R. Padmanabhan, N. Meskin, W.M. Haddad, Reinforcement learning-based control of drug dosing for cancer chemotherapy treatment, Mathematical Biosciences 293 (2017), https://doi.org/10.1016/j.mbs.2017.08.004.
[136] M. Tejedor, A.Z. Woldaregay, F. Godtliebsen, Reinforcement learning application in diabetes blood glucose control: a systematic review, Artificial Intelligence in Medicine (2020), https://doi.org/10.1016/j.artmed.2020.101836.
[137] M. Reddy, et al., Clinical safety and feasibility of the advanced bolus calculator for type 1 diabetes based on case-based reasoning: a 6-week nonrandomized single-arm pilot study, Diabetes Technology & Therapeutics 18 (8) (2016), https://doi.org/10.1089/dia.2015.0413.
[138] M. Cescon, et al., Using iterative learning for insulin dosage optimization in multiple-daily-injections therapy for people with type 1 diabetes, IEEE Transactions on Biomedical Engineering 68 (2) (2021), https://doi.org/10.1109/TBME.2020.3005622.
[139] J.A. Roberts, M.H. Abdul-Aziz, et al., Individualised antibiotic dosing for patients who are critically ill: challenges and potential solutions, The

Lancet Infectious Diseases (2014), https://doi.org/10.1016/S1473-3099(14)70036-2.
[140] C.C. Bulik, et al., PK–PD Compass: bringing infectious diseases pharmacometrics to the patient's bedside, Journal of Pharmacokinetics and Pharmacodynamics 44 (2) (2017), https://doi.org/10.1007/s10928-017-9518-0.
[141] M.L. Avent, B.A. Rogers, Optimising antimicrobial therapy through the use of Bayesian dosing programs, International Journal of Clinical Pharmacy (2019), https://doi.org/10.1007/s11096-019-00886-4.
[142] D. Ming, et al., Connectivity of rapid-testing diagnostics and surveillance of infectious diseases, Bulletin of the World Health Organization (2019), https://doi.org/10.2471/BLT.18.219691.
[143] M. Komorowski, et al., The Artificial Intelligence Clinician learns optimal treatment strategies for sepsis in intensive care, Nature Medicine 24 (11) (2018), https://doi.org/10.1038/s41591-018-0213-5.
[144] T.M. Rawson, et al., Supervised machine learning for the prediction of infection on admission to hospital: a prospective observational cohort study, Journal of Antimicrobial Chemotherapy 74 (4) (2019), https://doi.org/10.1093/jac/dky514.
[145] T.M. Rawson, et al., A real-world evaluation of a case-based reasoning algorithm to support antimicrobial prescribing decisions in acute care, Clinical Infectious Diseases 72 (12) (2021), https://doi.org/10.1093/cid/ciaa383.
[146] B. Ribba, et al., Model-informed artificial intelligence: reinforcement learning for precision dosing, Clinical Pharmacology and Therapeutics (2020), https://doi.org/10.1002/cpt.1777.
[147] T.M. Rawson, et al., Mapping the decision pathways of acute infection management in secondary care among UK medical physicians: a qualitative study, BMC Medicine 14 (1) (2016), https://doi.org/10.1186/s12916-016-0751-y.
[148] L. Wang, C. Hu, L. Shao, The antimicrobial activity of nanoparticles: present situation and prospects for the future, International Journal of Nanomedicine (2017), https://doi.org/10.2147/IJN.S121956.
[149] R.P. Allaker, The use of antimicrobial nanoparticles to control oral infections, in: Nano-Antimicrobials: Progress and Prospects, 2012, https://doi.org/10.1007/978-3-642-24428-5_14.
[150] R.P. Allaker, K. Memarzadeh, Nanoparticles and the control of oral infections, International Journal of Antimicrobial Agents (2014), https://doi.org/10.1016/j.ijantimicag.2013.11.002.
[151] W. Song, S. Ge, Application of antimicrobial nanoparticles in dentistry, Molecules 24 (6) (2019) 1033, https://doi.org/10.3390/molecules24061033.
[152] J. Choi, et al., A micro-sized model for the in vivo study of nanoparticle toxicity: what has *Caenorhabditis elegans* taught us? Environmental Chemistry (2014) 227–246, https://doi.org/10.1071/EN13187.
[153] J.H. Kim, et al., C. elegans-on-a-chip for in situ and in vivo Ag nanoparticles' uptake and toxicity assay, Scientific Reports 7 (1) (2017) 40225, https://doi.org/10.1038/srep40225.
[154] J.C. Madden, et al., A review of in silico tools as alternatives to animal testing: principles, resources and applications, ATLA, Alternatives to Laboratory Animals (2020), https://doi.org/10.1177/0261192920965977.
[155] M.A. Munger, et al., In vivo human time-exposure study of orally dosed commercial silver nanoparticles, Nanomedicine: Nanotechnology,

Biology and Medicine 10 (1) (2014), https://doi.org/10.1016/j.nano.2013.06.010.
[156] F. Cieplik, et al., Development of standard protocols for biofilm-biomaterial interface testing, JADA Foundational Science 1 (2022), https://doi.org/10.1016/j.jfscie.2022.100008.
[157] S. Chatterjee, A. Bandyopadhyay, K. Sarkar, Effect of iron oxide and gold nanoparticles on bacterial growth leading towards biological application, Journal of Nanobiotechnology 9 (2011), https://doi.org/10.1186/1477-3155-9-34.
[157a] CLSI, The Clinical & Laboratory Standards Institute (CLSI). CLSI Breakpoints, CLSI, 2020, Available at: https://clsi.org/standards/products/free-resources/access-our-free-resources, 2020.
[158] I.A. Hassounah, et al., Designing and testing single tablet for tuberculosis treatment through electrospinning, in: Fabrication and Self-Assembly of Nanobiomaterials: Applications of Nanobiomaterials, 2016, https://doi.org/10.1016/B978-0-323-41533-0.00011-8.
[159] L. Thieme, et al., MBEC versus MBIC: the lack of differentiation between biofilm reducing and inhibitory effects as a current problem in biofilm methodology, Biological Procedures Online (2019), https://doi.org/10.1186/s12575-019-0106-0.
[160] P. Parvekar, et al., The minimum inhibitory concentration (MIC) and minimum bactericidal concentration (MBC) of silver nanoparticles against *Staphylococcus aureus*, Biomaterial Investigations in Dentistry 7 (1) (2020), https://doi.org/10.1080/26415275.2020.1796674.
[161] C.B. Landersdorfer, R.L. Nation, Limitations of antibiotic MIC-based PK-PD metrics: looking back to move forward, Frontiers in Pharmacology (2021), https://doi.org/10.3389/fphar.2021.770518.
[162] J. Robertson, et al., Optimisation of the protocol for the liVE/DEAD®BacLightTM bacterial viability kit for rapid determination of bacterial load, Frontiers in Microbiology 10 (APR) (2019), https://doi.org/10.3389/fmicb.2019.00801.
[163] C. Bankier, et al., A comparison of methods to assess the antimicrobial activity of nanoparticle combinations on bacterial cells, PLoS One 13 (2) (2018), https://doi.org/10.1371/journal.pone.0192093.
[164] A. Kourmouli, et al., Can disc diffusion susceptibility tests assess the antimicrobial activity of engineered nanoparticles? Journal of Nanoparticle Research 20 (3) (2018) 62, https://doi.org/10.1007/s11051-018-4152-3.
[165] C. Farrugia, et al., Clinical relevance of antimicrobial testing results for dental restorative materials, Journal of Applied Biomaterials & Functional Materials 15 (2) (2017), https://doi.org/10.5301/jabfm.5000337.
[166] M.T. Arias-Moliz, J. Camilleri, The effect of the final irrigant on the antimicrobial activity of root canal sealers, Journal of Dentistry 52 (2016), https://doi.org/10.1016/j.jdent.2016.06.008.
[167] Y. Huang, et al., The in vitro antimicrobial activities of four endodontic sealers, BMC Oral Health 19 (1) (2019), https://doi.org/10.1186/s12903-019-0817-2.
[167a] M.F. Anjum, E. Zankari, H. Hasman, Molecular methods for detection of antimicrobial resistance, Microbiology Spectrum 5 (6) (2017), https://doi.org/10.1128/microbiolspec.ARBA-0011-2017. PMID: 29219107.
[168] M. Ramstedt, et al., Evaluating efficacy of antimicrobial and antifouling materials for urinary tract medical devices: challenges and

recommendations, Macromolecular Bioscience (2019), https://doi.org/10.1002/mabi.201800384.
[169] J. Camilleri, et al., Standardization of antimicrobial testing of dental devices, Dental Materials 36 (3) (2020) e59–e73, https://doi.org/10.1016/j.dental.2019.12.006.
[170] S.K. Davies, et al., Visualizing antimicrobials in bacterial biofilms: three-dimensional biochemical imaging using TOF-SIMS, mSphere 2 (4) (2017), https://doi.org/10.1128/msphere.00211-17.
[171] M. Godin, et al., Using buoyant mass to measure the growth of single cells, Nature Methods 7 (5) (2010), https://doi.org/10.1038/nmeth.1452.
[172] S.M. Knudsen, et al., Determination of bacterial antibiotic resistance based on osmotic shock response, Analytical Chemistry 81 (16) (2009), https://doi.org/10.1021/ac900968r.
[173] K.Y. Gfeller, N. Nugaeva, M. Hegner, Rapid biosensor for detection of antibiotic-selective growth of *Escherichia coli*, Applied and Environmental Microbiology 71 (5) (2005b), https://doi.org/10.1128/AEM.71.5.2626-2631.2005.
[174] J.W. Ndieyira, et al., Nanomechanical detection of antibiotic-mucopeptide binding in a model for superbug drug resistance, Nature Nanotechnology 3 (11) (2008), https://doi.org/10.1038/nnano.2008.275.
[175] N.P. Mortensen, et al., Effects of colistin on surface ultrastructure and nanomechanics of pseudomonas aeruginosa cells, Langmuir 25 (6) (2009), https://doi.org/10.1021/la803898g.
[176] K.Y. Gfeller, N. Nugaeva, M. Hegner, Micromechanical oscillators as rapid biosensor for the detection of active growth of *Escherichia coli*, Biosensors and Bioelectronics 21 (3) (2005a), https://doi.org/10.1016/j.bios.2004.11.018.

How to fight bacteria without inducing drug resistance?

Alessandra M. Martorana, Paola Sperandeo and Alessandra Polissi
Department of Pharmacological and Biomolecular Sciences, University of Milano, Milano, Italy

1. Introduction

The discovery of antibiotics and their therapeutic use can be considered as one of the greatest medical breakthroughs of the 20th century. Antibiotics not only have saved countless lives but have also made possible many modern medical procedures including surgery, organ transplants and cancer treatments. However, a non-appropriate usage of antibiotics together with the extraordinary ability of bacteria to develop resistance mechanisms and to spread them by horizontal gene transfer have led to the so-called 'antibiotic crisis' with the emergence of bacterial pathogens resistant to all antimicrobial drugs in clinical use [1]. Antimicrobial Resistance (AMR) is therefore a global health threat which, if not tackled appropriately, can lead to negative clinical, economic and societal consequences in the near future [2]. The recent COVID-19 pandemic has further aggravated this scenario due to the high risk of secondary infections, often associated to multidrug-resistant bacteria, in hospitalised patients [3]. Indeed, the massive use of antibiotics worldwide as COVID19 co-treatment is likely to have a negative impact on AMR.

2. The antimicrobial resistance crisis: Why are we there?

The serendipitous discovery of penicillin as a metabolite of *Penicillium notatum* by Alexander Fleming [4] made scientists to realise that microorganisms (bacteria and fungi) can produce molecules capable to kill or arrest growth of other

Nanotechnology Tools for Infection Control. https://doi.org/10.1016/B978-0-12-823994-0.00001-3

microorganisms. This led to the setting up in the 1940s of the Waksman platform (named after microbiologist Selman Waksman who discovered streptomycin) as the first platform for antibiotic discovery based on the ability of soil microbes to produce their own antibiotics, which they use to out-compete each other. This method, widely adopted by pharmaceutical companies, led to the discovery of the main classes of antibiotics in over the next 20 years, the so-called 'golden era of antibiotic discovery' [5,6] (Fig. 8.1). In the 1960s, the Waksman platform was progressively abandoned due to the persistent rediscovery of known compounds in the screening campaigns. In the 1970s and 1980s, antibiotic discovery shifted from the identification of active molecules produced by environmental isolates to the chemical modification of known drugs to improve their properties (i.e. spectrum) and overcome resistance mechanisms that inevitably developed due to drug clinical use. In the same period, there was some success in identifying synthetic compounds with antimicrobial properties such as the broad-spectrum class of fluoroquinolones [5]. Synthetic compounds as isoniazid, pyrazinamide and ethambutol were also discovered as potent drugs against *Mycobacterium tuberculosis* transforming tuberculosis from a predictably fatal disease to a curable disease [7]. While these discoveries allowed

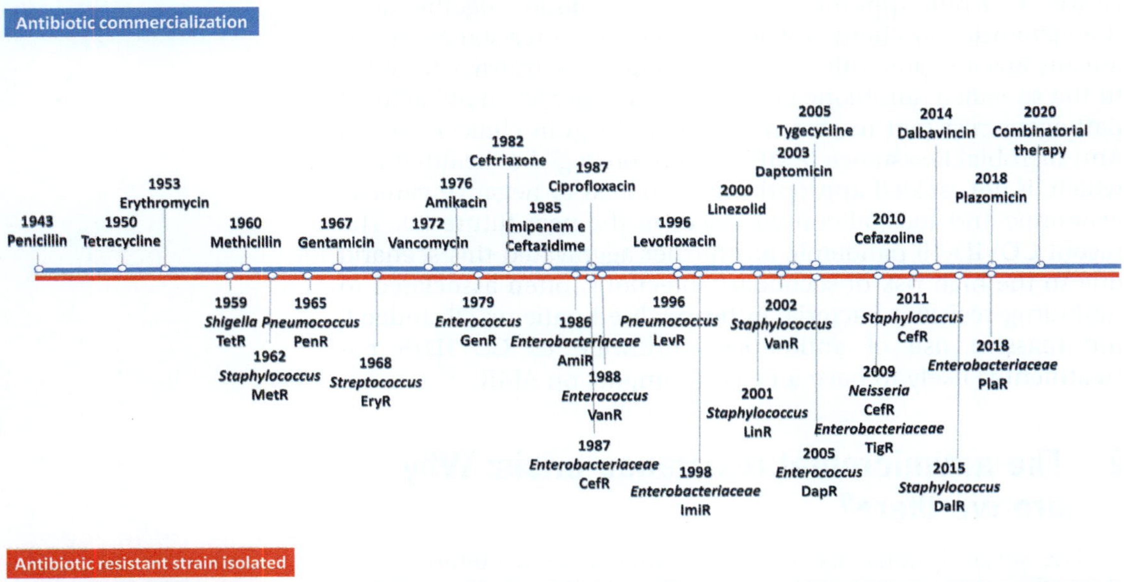

Figure 8.1 Timeline of commercialisation of main classes of antibiotics and antibiotic resistance identification. The upper line shows when a given antibiotic/antibiotic class was introduced in clinical use, whereas the lower line indicates when antibiotic resistance was identified. Modified from https://amr.biomerieux.com/en/challenges/a-lack-of-antibiotics/.

introduction of several useful drugs in clinics, no systematic antibiotic discovery platforms were developed to feed the antibiotic discovery pipeline (Fig. 8.1).

In the mid of 1990s, the sequencing of the first complete genome of a microorganism, *Hemophilus influenzae* [8], changed completely the approach for antibiotic discovery. The possibility to explore hundreds of new genes as potential targets combined with the ability of creating large libraries of synthetic compounds by combinatorial chemistry, renewed the interest of pharmaceutical companies in the antibacterial field. Novel high-tech discovery platforms based on genomics-derived target-based approaches were therefore set up to screen for new classes of drugs with novel modes of action. However, the results were far below the expectations, one of the major issues being to identify molecules with a reasonable spectrum of activity able to penetrate through the bacteria envelope to reach their targets [6,9,10]. Overall, failure of these antibacterial programmes made pharmaceutical companies to divest again from antibacterial research.

The current lack of new antibacterials with novel mechanisms of action is further aggravated by the rapid increase and spread of antimicrobial resistance (Fig. 8.1). Antibiotics typically target essential cellular processes (i.e. cell wall biogenesis, protein synthesis, nucleic acids synthesis), thus inhibiting bacterial growth under all conditions and posing a high selective pressure [11]. Moreover, bacteria can also be intrinsically resistant to certain antibiotics. As an example, Gram-negative bacteria, because of the highly impermeable outer membrane (OM) [12], are insensitive to vancomycin, an antibiotic that targets peptidoglycan synthesis and that is very efficacious against Gram-positive bacteria [13]. Another example of intrinsic resistance in an individual species results from the absence of a susceptible target of a specific antibiotic. The antibacterial compound triclosan targets the enoyl-acyl carrier protein (ACP) reductase that catalyses the last step of the fatty acid elongation cycle. Some bacteria are naturally resistant to triclosan due to the presence of triclosan-resistant ACP reductase isoforms [14,15]. Bacteria can also develop resistance to antibiotics or acquire it via horizontal gene transfer, by three major mechanisms [16]:

i) by enzymatic inactivation of the antibiotic, due to hydrolysis or chemical modification of a key structural element of the antibiotic (for example, β-lactam ring opening by β-lactamases);

ii) by reduction of drug influx or increase of its efflux through the deletion of porin genes or the induction of efflux pump expression, respectively;

iii) through mechanisms or mutations resulting in the modification of the drug target (such as the resistance to vancomycin, that implies the synthesis of a different stem peptide in the peptidoglycan that is no longer recognised by the antibiotic) [17]. The efficacy and efficiency of these mechanisms together with a global poor antibiotic stewardship have led to a rapid global increase of infections caused by multidrug-resistant bacteria with the spectre of untreatable infections becoming a reality [18,19].

It is therefore becoming urgent not only to identify innovative antibacterial strategies, based on unexplored targets and new mechanisms of actions and active against multidrug-resistant pathogens, but also to develop novel therapeutic options that minimise the evolution of resistance and increase the clinical lifespan of newly identified drugs.

In the past few years, several cell-based screening systems have been developed in an effort to isolate new classes of bacterial growth inhibitors from large libraries of molecules, and a few promising lead compounds have been identified (for some examples on Gram-negative bacteria see Refs. [20–23]). While these molecules have the potential to overcome existing antibiotic resistance mechanisms, we expect resistance to evolve against these traditional growth inhibitors once released for clinical use.

3. How to develop antibiotic therapies with low selective pressure

In the past years, great effort has been set on approaches that overcome or minimise the emergence of resistance to existing antibiotics, trying to extend their lifespan in the market. Such approaches are based on the combination of the established antibiotics with molecules that either repress the known mechanism of resistance or augment the potency of the antibiotics themselves. These booster molecules are collectively defined as 'antibiotic adjuvants' and the co-formulation of drugs is defined 'combination therapy'.

Combination therapy offers a general strategy to counteract the resistance mechanisms and has multiple applications. The most common application is to directly target the resistance mechanism, making drug-resistant pathogens sensitive to the antibiotics again (Fig. 8.2A and B). But the combination therapy is also exploited to widen the spectrum of activity of an antibiotic (e.g. to make the treatment of Gram-negative infections possible using antibiotics otherwise efficacious only against Gram-

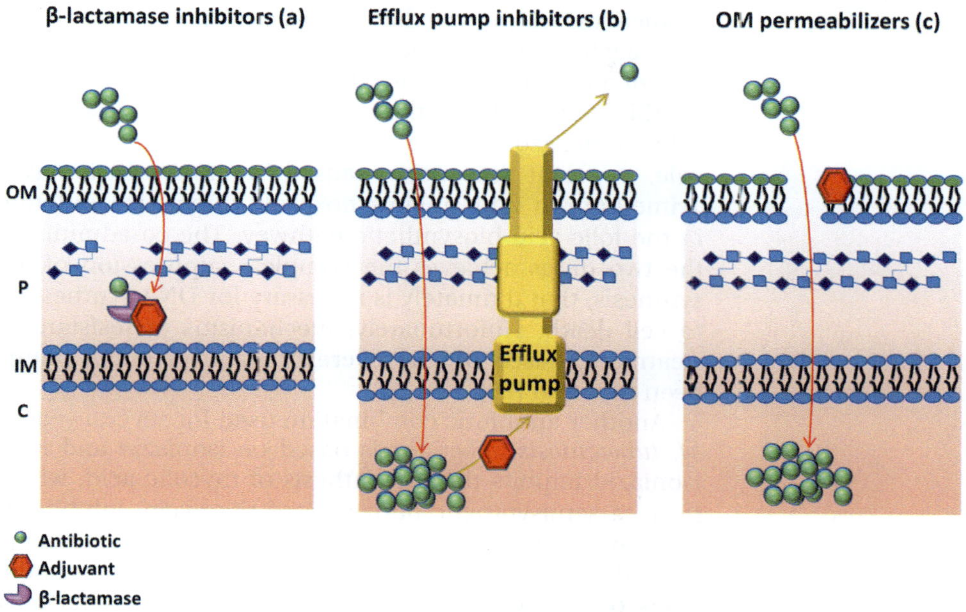

Figure 8.2 Schematic representation of modes of action of antibiotic adjuvants. Class IA adjuvants directly prevent antibiotic resistance by inhibiting the hydrolytic activity of β-lactamase enzymes on antibiotics (A) or enhancing the intracellular accumulation of antibiotics by inhibiting their extrusion by efflux pumps (B). Class IB increases antibiotic activity by facilitating their permeation across the outer membrane (C). The double-membrane cell envelope of gram-negative bacteria is depicted with the peptidoglycan layer embedded in the periplasm. *C,* cytoplasm; *IM,* inner membrane; *OM,* outer membrane; *P,* periplasm.

positive bacteria) or to lower the effective dose of a drug that shows toxicity against human cells, mitigating the potential side effects (such as the case of colistin) [24]. Most importantly, when the adjuvant molecule is devoid of bactericidal effect, the combination therapy has the potential to reduce the evolutive pressure to select for resistance, thus preserving the efficacy of the antibiotic itself [25].

3.1 Antibiotic combination therapy

Antibiotic combination therapy has long been used in the clinic [26]. In this therapeutic approach, two or more antibiotics with different modes of action are empirically combined to achieve a broad-spectrum activity and cover all possible resistance profiles, especially when the causative agent of an infection is unknown. This approach has the potential to achieve synergism between the drug partners (each drug results effective at lower doses than when used in monotherapy) and ensure the complete eradication of intermediate resistance phenotypes that might arise against each antibiotic, eventually resulting in the suppression of antibiotic resistance development. A well-known example of this approach is the combination of trimethoprim and sulfamethoxazole, in use since 1969 with the name of cotrimoxazole, to treat infections caused by *Enterobacteriaceae* [27]. Trimethoprim and sulfamethoxazole target two different steps in the folic acid biosynthetic pathway. The co-administration of the two drugs achieves the complete suppression of folic acid synthesis, that ultimately is necessary for DNA synthesis, leading to cell death. Unfortunately, mechanisms of resistance to this treatment, based on the overexpression of efflux pumps have been reported [28].

Another antibiotic combination used for several years to treat *M. tuberculosis* infections is based on isoniazid and rifampicin. Isoniazid inhibits the biosynthesis of mycolic acid, while rifampicin, a semisynthetic derivative of rifamycin, inhibits the RNA polymerase. Unfortunately, the extensive use of rifampicin in monotherapy has led to the emergence of resistance and the first cases of multidrug-resistant *M. tuberculosis* strains have been described in 2005, highlighting the importance to explore other antibiotic combinations to treat such infections [29].

Another notable example of this approach is the drug combination employed for the treatment of vancomycin-resistant and methicillin resistant (MRSA) *Staphylococcus aureus* strains. This therapy involves vancomycin and oxacillin and has proven useful to overcome resistance to both antibiotics. The mechanism of synergy between vancomycin and oxacillin is intriguing. Resistance to the β-lactam methicillin (oxacillin) involves the production of an alternative penicillin-binding protein, PBP2a (encoded by the *mecA* gene), insensitive to β-lactams, whereas resistance to the glycopeptide vancomycin implicates the reprogramming of peptidoglycan synthesis (encoded by *vanHAX* operon) leading to the production of an alternative peptidoglycan precursor ending in D-alanine-D-lactate, instead of the canonical D-alanine-D-alanine. The mechanism of synergy relies on the low affinity of PBP2a towards the peptidoglycan produced by vancomycin-resistant strains and the inability of PBP2a to use peptidoglycan precursor D-alanine-D-lactate as the substrate for the transpeptidation reaction, thus failing to complete peptidoglycan synthesis. As PBP2a and the alternative peptidoglycan precursor D-alanine-D-lactate are produced only in the presence of oxacillin and vancomycin, respectively, the bacterial cell will not be able to survive expression of *mecA* and *vanHAX* simultaneously. The combination of vancomycin and oxacillin represents a good example of how synergy between antibiotics can overcome the development of resistance against each drug separately [30].

The above examples highlight the power of antibiotic combination therapy that, however, is still mostly empirical. In an effort to identify general principles of antibacterial drug combinations and understand their potential, Typas and co-workers profiled almost 3000 combinations of antibiotics, food additives and human-targeted drugs in six selected Gram-negative bacterial pathogens [31]. The generated database of pairwise drug combinations can be a powerful resource to explore drug combinations on more rational bases and to identify effective synergies against multidrug-resistant clinical isolates.

Besides the combination of established antibiotics, several bioactive molecules devoid of antibacterial activity can also be exploited as adjuvants of antibiotics in combination therapies.

According to the classification of Wright, antibiotic adjuvants can be divided into two groups based on target profile. Class I adjuvants comprises molecules that synergise with the antibiotic directly on the bacterial cell, whereas Class II comprises molecules that act on the host defence system boosting the action of the antibiotic [25].

Within the Class I adjuvants, it is possible to discriminate two main sub-classes: Class IA comprises agents that directly inhibit antibiotic resistance (such as the β-lactamase inhibitors, the only adjuvant family in clinical use, or efflux pump inhibitors) (Fig. 8.2A and B). Whereas Class IB comprises agents that enhance the activity of the antibiotic, for example, by facilitating the permeation of the antibiotic into the cell (OM permeabilizers) (Fig. 8.2C). Besides these classes of adjuvants, an innovative strategy that is emerging to enhance the potency of antimicrobial drugs and falls in between of them, targets the ability of the pathogens to establish infection in vivo [32,33]. This option implies the attenuation of bacterial virulence and has the effect of making the pathogens more susceptible to the clearance action of the host immune response or to antibiotics. This strategy will be discussed in detail in Section 3.2.

The following paragraphs will cover the basic concepts and the best-studied examples of antibiotic adjuvants belonging to Class I that collectively show a proof of concept for their efficacy in combination therapy to fight antibiotic resistance.

3.1.1 Class IA adjuvants: β-lactamase inhibitors

The most significant and clinically successful adjuvants used in combination therapy are the inhibitors of β-lactamases, enzymes responsible of antibiotic resistance associated with the hydrolytic inactivation of the β-lactams antibiotics (penicillin, cephalosporins and carbapenems drugs).

β-lactamases are widespread in bacterial strains due to their transmission among pathogens through horizontal gene transfer. Based on protein sequence similarity, β-lactamases have been grouped into four classes named A, B, C and D. These four classes can also be distinguished by fundamental differences in the hydrolytic mechanism that leads to β-lactams inactivation. Class A, C and D are Ser β-lactamases that use a serine residue in their active site to covalently bind the antibiotic and release it in the inactive form. Class B are a heterogeneous group of zinc metallo-β-lactamases, that coordinate Zn^{2+} atoms in their catalytic site and activate a water molecule to induce the hydrolysis of the β-lactam ring [34,35]. Class A includes the classical β-lactamases (comprising the extended-spectrum β-lactamases, ESBL, and several carbapenemases); class C β-lactamases are widespread on the chromosomes of many Gram-negative species and usually do not possess carbapemenase activity; class D β-lactamases are the most diverse, encompassing enzymes active against penicillins, cephalosporins and carbapenems. Finally, the zinc-dependent class B β-lactamases are able to hydrolyse all classes of β-lactams with the exception of monobactams [34,35].

Adjuvants belonging to the group of β-lactamase inhibitors are classified as reversible or irreversible based on the type of inhibition.

Irreversible. The first β-lactam-based β-lactamase inhibitors identified and introduced into the clinic in 1970 were clavulanic acid [36] and sulbactam [37], the last was tazobactam, approved in 1993 to be co-administered with piperacillin [38]. These three inhibitors are commercialised according to the following combinations: amoxicillin and clavulanate (Augmentin), ticarcillin and clavulanate (Timentine), ampicillin and sulbactam (Unasyn) and piperacillin and tazobactam (Zosyn). The general mechanism of these inhibitors, whose antibacterial activity per se is poor, involves the covalent interaction of their β-lactam structures with the active site of the β-lactamases. As an example, clavulanic acid prevents the hydrolysis of amoxicillin by several types of β-lactamases belonging to the family of ESBL [39].

It is noteworthy that no β-lactamase inhibitors in clinical use are active against classes A and D β-lactamases and, among them, carbapenem-hydrolysing class D β-lactamases, also referred to as oxacillinases (OXAs), are rapidly spreading among most clinically challenging species, generating great concern [40]. In 2019, a novel diazabicyclooctanones, ETX2514 has shown promise in combination with sulbactam for the treatment of *Acinetobacter* infections [41]. Another diazabicyclooctanone that is worth mentioning is relebactam, that displays inhibitory activity against β-lactamases from different families and potentiates the activity of imipenem when co-administered (MK-7655) [42].

Reversible. This group of adjuvants do not covalently bind to the active site of the β-lactamases and the activity of the enzymes can be restored by diluting the inhibitor, lowering the pressure for the emergence of resistance. Adjuvants belonging to this group of molecules are avibactam, the first diazabicyclooctanone to be approved by the Food and Drug Administration agency (FDA) in 2014 in combination with ceftazidime [43], and vaborbactam, belonging to the group of boronic acid-containing inhibitors, recently approved in the United States in combination with meropenem (Carbavance) [44].

No inhibitors of zinc metallo-β-lactamases are currently in clinical use. However, recently, a metabolite produced by the fungus *Aspergillus versicolour*, the Aspergillomarasmine A, has been shown to resuscitate the activity of meropenem by inhibiting NDM-1 and VIM metallo-β-lactamases produced by carbapenem-resistant *Klebsiella pneumoniae* in a mouse model of infection [45]. The inhibitor irreversibly inactivates the β-lactamase possibly by sequestration of the zinc ions from its active site [46].

Finally, three combinations of penicillin antibiotics with inhibitors that do not belong to the group of β-lactam-based inhibitors are currently in the final stage of clinical development. One of these combinations involves the stigmasterol steroid as adjuvant of ampicillin. However, the mechanism of potentiation of the antibiotic activity against resistant pathogens by this molecule is still unknown [47].

Resistance to β-lactamase inhibitors has been observed. For example, it has been reported a decreased sensitivity of *E. coli*-resistant strains to β-lactamase inhibitors when used in combination with cephalosporins [48]. This observation should encourage researchers to identify more potent adjuvant molecules to counteract bacterial evolution.

3.1.2 Class IA adjuvants: Efflux pump inhibitors

In addition to the direct resistance mechanism associated to the inactivation of β-lactamase enzymes, pathogens have also evolved a general system to expel antibiotics from the cell at the expense of metabolic energy (Fig. 8.2B). The existence of such a mechanism was first shown in 1980, when it was demonstrated that energy-mediated export is the general feature of bacterial resistance to tetracycline [49]. This resistance mechanism is based on a variety of membrane carrier proteins, called efflux pumps [50,51]. The most common efflux systems found in pathogens belong to the superfamilies of the tripartite Resistance-Nodulation-Division (RND) or Major Facilitator (MFS). The overexpression of these efflux pumps by bacterial strains allows them to acquire resistance to antibiotics belonging to several and different classes [50]. Each single pump can be selective for a specific substrate or can be non-selective and handling a wide range of structurally diverse substrates, leading to the emergence of multidrug-resistant strains. In the contest of combination therapy, the inhibition of efflux pumps is therefore expected to improve the entry of antibiotics into the cells, counteracting their expulsion and restoring drug sensitivity (Fig. 8.2B). Importantly, the inhibition of the efflux system is a direct way to lower the dosage of the antibiotic and limit the emergence of new resistant strains. However, the lack of substrate specificity of several of these pumps hampers the development of suitable inhibitors. Efflux pump inhibitors (EPIs) are small molecules that block the activity of the multidrug efflux pump exploiting four different mechanisms: (i) By inhibiting the expression of the efflux pump genes; (ii) by inhibiting the assembly of the pump in the membrane; (iii) by obstructing the channel; (iv) by depleting the metabolic energy necessary for drug expulsion [52].

Although no inhibitor for efflux pumps has been approved for clinical use till now due to toxicity issues, some promising examples of this strategy have been reported. Phenilalanine-Arginine β-Naphtylamide (PAβN) is one of the first and the most studied inhibitors of RND efflux pumps active in several bacteria, among which *Pseudomonas aeruginosa* [53]. For the high number of redundant efflux systems in this pathogen, PAβN is a promising broad-spectrum adjuvant for suppressing the emergence of resistance.

EPIs have been also exploited for the design of strategies to treat Mycobacterial infections. In this case, several natural products have also been investigated for their ability to counteract the action of efflux pumps, among which bonducellin, a metabolite purified from *Caesalpinia digyna* roots that has been shown to synergise with the fluorescent dye ethidium bromide for the entry in resistant *M. smegmatis* cells [54]. In the case of EPIs, the use of new sources has been shown to be a good strategy to widen the pool of bioactive molecules to screen. Another plant-derived molecule proven to have efflux pump inhibitory activity is the polyphenolic compound epigallocatechin-3-gallate (EGCG) extracted from tea plants, that has been shown not only to increase the susceptibility of multidrug-resistant *P. aeruginosa* and MRSA strains to several antibiotics but also to synergise with PAβN [55].

The increasing attention in this class of adjuvants to restore antibiotic sensitivity in clinically relevant multidrug-resistant pathogens is demonstrated by the current administration of the efflux pump inhibitor MP-601 as an aerosol in combination with antibiotic therapy for the treatment of infections in cystic fibrosis patients [56].

3.1.3 Class IB adjuvants: Outer membrane permeabilizers

The effect of efflux pump overexpression is greatly augmented in Gram-negative bacteria by the presence of an additional external membrane, the OM, that further limits the activity of many classes of antibiotics [57]. In the pathogens belonging to this group, permeation of hydrophobic antibiotics, that gain access to the cytoplasm by passive diffusion through the lipid bilayer (such as macrolides or rifampicin), is blocked by an external asymmetric membrane whose outer layer is constituted by the polyanionic amphipathic molecule lipopolysaccharide (LPS) [58]. The LPS layer is stabilised by the bridging action of divalent cations that contribute to preventing the flux of hydrophobic drugs [12]. The passage of antibiotics across the OM is possible only through channel-forming proteins (porins), whose diameter is small and limit the overall rate of the uptake, increasing the effectiveness of other resistance mechanisms, such as multidrug efflux pumps and antibiotic-modifying enzymes [59]. All these features contribute to the intrinsic resistance of Gram-negative pathogens to many classes of antibiotics, that make this group of bacteria particularly difficult to treat with antibiotics that display potent activity against Gram-positive pathogens. However, molecules that displace divalent cations have the dual ability to locally destabilise the membrane, gaining access across it (exploiting the so-called 'self-promoted uptake mechanism'), and also to make the membrane more permeable to other compounds enhancing their passage [60] (Fig. 8.2C). Drugs that exploit the self-promoted uptake mechanism are polycationic molecules containing polyamine functional groups like polymyxins, antimicrobial peptides, aminoglycosides and dibasic macrolides like azithromycin [61]. Among these, polymyxin B and E (colistin) act as permeabilizers, because of their synergy with hydrophobic drugs, but cannot be considered as adjuvants because of their high bactericidal activity. On the contrary, the polymyxin B deacylated derivative PMBN (polymyxin B nonapeptide), devoid of much of its antibacterial activity, is one of the best-known antibiotic adjuvant [62]. PMBN has been shown to sensitise efflux pumps-expressing *P. aeruginosa* strains to nalidixic acid, ciprofloxacin and carbenicillin [63]. Another polymyxin derivative lacking the fatty acid tail that shows promise as antibiotic adjuvant is SPR741, a tricationic molecule developed by Evotec AG and Spero Therapeutic that has been reported to sensitise Enterobacteriaceae and *Acinetobacter baumannii* to several antibiotics such as clarithromycin, rifampicin and fusidic acid [64,65]. Interestingly, the EPI PAβN has been shown to behave like PMBN in *E. coli* and to sensitise the class C β-lactamase AmpC-producing *P. aeruginosa* strains towards β-lactam antibiotics, disclosing an additional permeabilising function for this EPI drug [66].

Several non-polymyxin derived permeabilising adjuvants have also been reported, such as cationic peptides and their derivatives, cationic steroids, small molecules approved for non-antibiotic applications and several plant-derived compounds [67]. Recently, the importance to target OM permeability has been further highlighted by the design of new hybrid systems wherein the OM permeabilizer aminoglycoside tobramycin is linked to other antibiotics achieving a double effect by increasing the antibacterial potency of the hybrid molecules against *P. aeruginosa* and simultaneously synergising with other antibiotics [67].

Despite their great potential in increasing antibiotic activity, a major obstacle in the development of antibiotic adjuvants is the understanding of their mode of action. A recent work dissected the mechanism of action of AI-1 (aryl 2-aminoimidazole), a compound which sensitises *A. baumannii* to vancomycin and clarithromycin. By looking at mutations that make cells 'adjuvant blind' it was shown that the AI-1 targets determinants for maintaining OM structural integrity, such as genes involved in LPS biogenesis and in phospholipid trafficking [68]. This approach offers a rationale for the characterisation and development of OM permeabilizers able to rescue antibiotics from resistance.

3.2 Anti-virulence strategies

Another strategy to minimise the evolution of resistance implies targeting virulence pathways rather than growth [32]. These pathways include not only virulence factors that cause damage to host cells and tissues (i.e. bacterial toxins) but also structures and strategies that facilitate pathogen colonisation, invasion and immune evasion [33]. Since anti-virulence agents do not target bacterial growth, it is hypothesised that they might apply a milder evolutionary pressure for the development of resistance [69]. Moreover, they should not affect the composition of the natural host microbiota whose disruption is increasingly recognised to have a role in the aetiology of various diseases [70]. Anti-virulence compounds are expected to decrease bacterial virulence thus potentially enhancing susceptibility to antibiotics and helping the host immune system in eliminating the infection. In the following paragraphs we will discuss the development of anti-virulence strategies against (i) adhesion process; (ii) functions required for bacterial survival and/or persistence during the infection, like biofilm and its maintenance; (iii) microbial communication; (iv) toxins and secretion systems and (v) microbial signal transduction and regulation. The most promising molecules and/or those in clinical development will be considered.

3.2.1 Targeting bacterial invasion

Bacterial adhesion is a crucial step for bacterial pathogenesis which requires surface structures of both the bacteria and the host cells [71]. In many Gram-negative and Gram-positive pathogens, the adhesion process is mediated by pili, multi-subunit proteinaceous hair-like structures, anchored to the cell envelope and assembled via sophisticated nanomachineries. The adhesin subunit responsible for the recognition/attachment to a specific host cell receptor is located at the tip of the pilus fibre. Anti-adhesion strategies would prevent the association between the pathogen and the host cell, causing the clearance of pathogen by the host immune system [72]. Bacterial adherence can be targeted at two different levels: (i) by disrupting the pilus assembly pathway; and (ii) by blocking the binding between the bacterial adhesin and host receptor (Fig. 8.3A).

In most Gram-positives, pilus assembly is mediated by membrane-anchored sortase enzyme.

Gram-positive sortases are a family of cysteine transpeptidases that catalyse the attachment of pili to the cell wall and drive the secretion of them on bacterial surface [73]. Inhibition of sortase activity impairs virulence in several pathogens such *S. aureus*, *Listeria monocytogenes*, *Streptococcus pneumoniae*, *Streptococcus suis* and *Streptococcus mutans* [74,75], strongly suggesting that sortase activity inhibitors could act as anti-virulence molecules that interfere with pathogen adhesion/invasion process without affecting cell growth. Among the sortase inhibitor peptidomimetic molecules, the small-molecule inhibitors diarylacrylonitriles

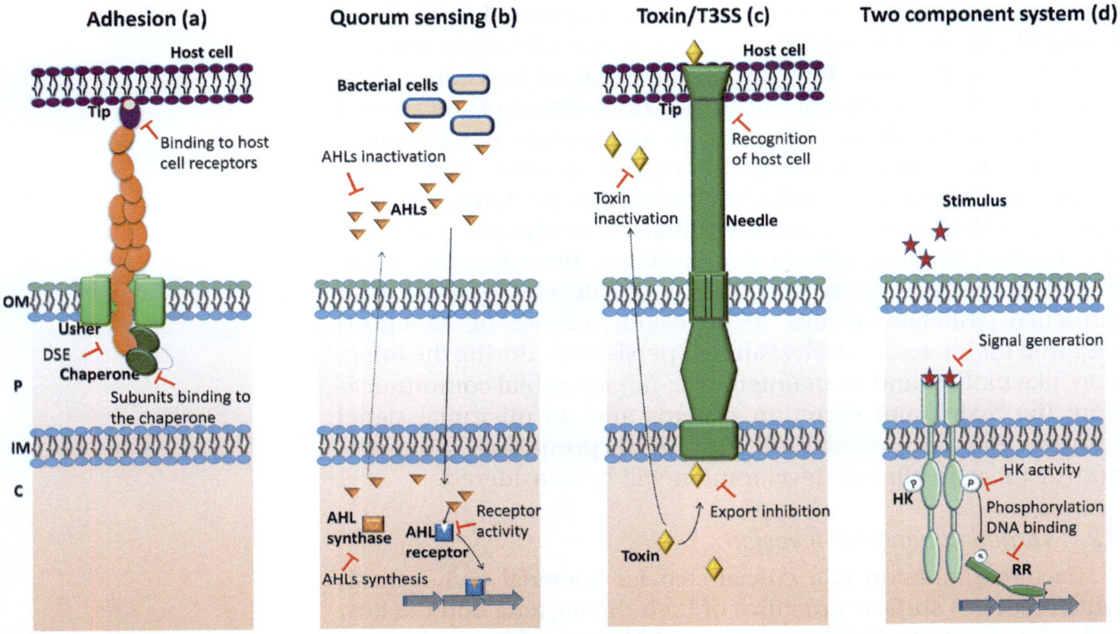

Figure 8.3 Overview of current anti-virulence strategies to combat bacterial infections. (A) Anti-adhesive agents reduce bacterial host-surface attachment and colonisation. Inhibitors can target adhesin biogenesis or host receptor–adhesin interaction. The assembly of type 1 pilus is schematically shown. The pili subunits (grey ovals) polymerise to form the pilus. Inhibitors of biogenesis are mimics of the pilin subunits that can prevent elongation by competing with the chaperones (bright grey ovals) or usher translocon (light grey rectangles) or the DSE step during the assembly of the pilus. Binding to the host receptor can be inhibited by host-surface receptor analogues, that bind to the tip (dark grey oval) of the pilus. (B) Quorum sensing (QS) inhibitors can degrade autoinducers (AHLs; bright grey triangles) or interfere with synthesis by blocking AHL synthases or by competitively binding to AHLs receptors. All these mechanisms prevent QS signalling, thus decreasing virulence gene expression (grey block arrows). Dashed and solid grey lines show release (from producer cell) and uptake (by target cell), respectively, of autoinducer molecules. (C) Secreted toxins (light grey diamonds) can be targeted directly in the extracellular milieu or by inhibiting the secretion system (T3SS, grey needle-like structure) that delivers them in the cytosol of the host cell. T3SS can be targeted by blocking export function or by inhibiting recognition of host cell surface receptor by needle tip protein. (D) Two-component systems (TCS) inhibitors target the HK sensory domain or its interaction with RR, which prevents phosphotransfer, and the downstream activation of virulence gene expression (grey block arrows). The double-membrane cell envelope of Gram-negative bacteria is depicted. The peptidoglycan layer is omitted for neatness. *AHLs,* N-acylhomoserine lactones; *C,* cytoplasm; *DSE,* donor-strand exchange; *HK,* histidine kinase; *IM,* inner membrane; *OM,* outer membrane; *P,* periplasm; *RR,* response regulator.

flavonols and the compound (2-(2,3-dihydro-1H-perimidin-2-yl)-phenoxy)-acetic acid, were found to effectively inhibit the sortase A of *S. aureus,* protecting mice from bacteraemia [76–78]. Very recently, it has been identified an *S. aureus* sortase A inhibitor,

2-(2-amino-3-chloro-benzoylamino)-benzoic acid, that displays antibacterial and antibiofilm activity by reducing planktonic cells and biofilm thickness [79].

In Gram-negatives, pili are assembled via the Chaperone-usher (CU) pathway [80]. The major elements of the CU pathway are pilin subunits, periplasmic chaperones and an OM usher protein [71]. Pilin subunits are transported across the inner membrane (IM) and reach the periplasm where their folding is assisted by periplasmic chaperones before they are polymerised via Donor Strand Exchange (DSE) mechanism and translocated across the OM via the usher channel.

FimH in type 1 pilus or PapG in P pilus are the adhesins assembled on the tip of the pilus structure and are responsible for binding their specific receptors on the host cell surface. FimH binds mannosylated receptors, whereas PagG binds galabiosylated receptors [80].

Several small molecules that target the pilus assembly by the CU pathway and prevent pilus fibres assembly on the bacterial surface have been identified (Fig. 8.3A). One such class of small-molecule CU pilus inhibitors, known as pilicides, consists of molecules with a 2-pyridine scaffold [81]. Pilicides compete for the binding of pilus subunits to the periplasmic chaperone and have been demonstrated not only to impair the biogenesis of either type 1 or type P pili in uropathogenic *E. coli* (UPEC) but also to inhibit haemagglutination mediated by type 1 or type P pili, adherence to bladder cells, and biofilm formation in laboratory and clinical isolates [82]. The data suggest that the mechanism of action and effect of pilicides could be broader than initially envisioned. Indeed, it has been demonstrated that these compounds also affect flagellar motility [83]. Treatment of UPEC with one such pilicide reduced biofilm formation and attenuated bacterial colonisation in the mouse model, confirming the ability of pilicides to interfere in vivo with the infection process [84].

Additional pilicides-derived molecules have been developed that inhibit pilus assembly by interfering with the DSE mechanism of pilin subunit polymerisation. Notably, this small pilicide-derived molecule, named AL1, is active against type 1 pilus biogenesis in UPEC, reducing bacterial adhesion to human bladder epithelial cells [85].

The second approach to block pathogen adhesion/invasion is the development of molecules that competitively inhibit adhesins–host receptors interaction (Fig. 8.3A). Soluble receptor analogues, the so-called mannosides, are promising molecules to inhibit the FimH adhesin of type 1 pili [86,87]. Mannosides bind to the FimH receptor-binding site and behave as antiadhesives by preventing bacterial colonisation. Accordingly, these molecules prevent bacterial invasion of the bladder following urinary tract infection in a mouse model [88]. Moreover, mannosides can be administered orally and have been shown to act in synergy with traditional antibiotic treatments in their capacity to reduce urinary tract UPEC infection in mice [89]. To inhibit bacterial adhesion mediated by P pili, galabiose-based inhibitors are as well being developed [90].

3.2.2 Targeting cell–cell communication: Quorum Sensing

Quorum Sensing (QS), a form of bacterial communication, is crucial for the establishment of a successful infection process and consequently is an attractive, largely explored target for developing anti-virulence therapeutic strategies [91]. The QS communication systems are commonly based on a sequence of common events: (i) the production of a signalling molecule, the so-called autoinducer; (ii) the secretion and accumulation of the autoinducer molecule in the external medium until a threshold of concentration that can be detected by bacteria; (iii) the expression of a subset of genes as a consequence of the detection of the signalling molecules [92–95]. This message transmission system among cells of the same species (self-communication) or among different species regulates the expression of genes responsible for biofilm formation, antibiotic resistance and of many virulence factors [96]. Thus, QS is an ideal target for anti-virulence drug development (Fig. 8.3B). QS has been identified in both Gram-negative and Gram-positive bacteria. In Gram-positive bacteria, the signal molecules are secreted oligopeptides, while Gram-negative bacteria produce N-acylhomoserine lactones (AHLs) or quinolones (PQS) or 2-heptyl-4-hydroxyquinoline (HHQ) as autoinducers.

Anti-QS strategies aim at blocking autoinducer biosynthesis, inactivating the signal molecules and disrupting signal detection [97] (Fig. 8.3B). Selected examples are discussed below.

Blocking autoinducers synthases with the use of autoinducer structural analogues has been found a successful option to disable bacterial QS [92]. The biosynthesis of AHLs occurs via the enzyme AHL synthase and requires a suitable acyl chain (from fatty acid biosynthesis) and S-adenosyl methionine (SAM). Newly synthesised AHLs are exported outside of the cell by specific efflux pumps [98]. Analogues of SAM (for example, S-adenosyl-homocysteine) can act as inhibitors of AHL synthases [99]. Moreover, the inhibition of certain autoinducer-producing enzymes could affect multiple QSs, such it is the case of 5′-methylthioad-enosine/Sadenosylhomocysteine nucleosidase (MTAN nucleosidase) that is involved in the production several type of autoinducers [100]. *P. aeruginosa* QS signal-producing enzymes have been extensively explored to identify QS inhibitors. *P. aeruginosa* uses *Pseudomonas* quinolone signal (PQS) and 2-heptyl-4-hydroxyquinoline (HHQ) as signalling molecules [92,95]. The biosynthesis of PQS depends on anthranilate as an intermediate, and its production can be inhibited by the anthranilate analogue, methyl-anthranilate. A screen for inhibitors of *P. aeruginosa* LasI and RhlI autoinducer-producing enzymes, identified salicylic acid, tannic acid and *trans*-cinnamaldehyde [95].

Another largely explored strategy to disable QS relies on inactivation of QS signals molecules (Fig. 8.3B) [92]. This strategy exploits the ability of several bacterial species to produce enzymes capable of degrading AHL molecules [101]. For instance, *Bacillus subtilis* produces an acyl-homoserine lactonase, which hydrolyzes the lactone ring of AHL molecules, making the hydrolysed product inactive. This is one of the most characterised QS inhibiting enzyme together with acyl-HSL acylases, and acyl-HSL oxidoreductases [101]. Interestingly, the heterologous expression of acyl-homoserine lactonase in numerous pathogenic bacteria, including *P. aeruginosa*, reduced AHL accumulation altering QS signalling and markedly decreasing expression and production of several virulence factors [102]. The potential for using inactivation of QS signalling molecules in clinical infection treatment is supported by several studies [103]. For example, the intranasal administration of purified PvdQ acylase, a *P. aeruginosa* AHL-hydrolysing enzyme, and engineered lactonase *Sso*Pox-W263I in animal models of pulmonary *P. aeruginosa* infection, hamper *P. aeruginosa* virulence [104,105]. This strategy is more advantageous than the inhibition of autoinducer production because these enzymes do not need to penetrate the bacteria and it is less likely to select resistant bacteria.

QS signalling can also be inhibited by preventing autoinducer binding to the cognate-receptor at the cell surface (Fig. 8.3B). QS signal inhibitors can be either structural analogues that compete with the signal molecule by binding the receptor [106] or not related molecules that act in a non-competitive fashion (e.g. halogenate furanones and flavonoids) [107–109]. The binding of inhibitors to the receptors could affect the signalling cascade at different levels: by blocking signal molecule binding, by destabilising the receptor, by inhibiting the binding of transcriptional factors to the DNA or by impairing interaction with RNA polymerase [103]. Several compounds, both natural and synthetic, have been studied. One of such natural compounds is (5Z)-4-bromo-5-

(bromomethylene)-3-butyl-2(5H)-furanone, isolated from marine algae that has been shown to have a dramatic effect on QS of several bacteria, by inhibiting biofilm formation and swarming thus causing cells to aggregate and die [110]. Synthetic AHL receptor antagonists have also been investigated, through modification of the acyl chain or the lactone moiety. Structural analogues of AHL, like N-decanoyl-L-homoserine benzyl ester, are able to reduce the production of virulence factors, such as elastase and rhamnolipids, by blocking the AHL receptors in *P. aeruginosa* [111,112]. Another receptor antagonist, meta-bromo-thiolactone (mBLT), is able to prevent *P. aeruginosa* infection by decreasing the pyocyanin production and inhibiting the biofilm formation via binding to LasR receptor. The treatment of *P. aeruginosa* with mBLT reduces bacterial virulence in *Caenorhabditis elegans* and human lung carcinoma cell line [113]. Although the use of molecules that interfere with signal molecule–receptor binding is supported by several in vivo studies, this QS inhibition approach has several drawbacks. Some of AHL receptor antagonists are structurally unstable and degradable under alkaline conditions [114,115]. Moreover, these inhibitors could be potentially degraded by enzymes and/or targeted by efflux pumps [116,117].

3.2.2.1 Targeting biofilm formation and maintenance

Another possible strategy to inhibit virulence is targeting biofilm formation. In biofilm bacteria live on surfaces in a three-dimensional community that is enclosed within an extracellular polymeric matrix produced by bacteria themselves, composed of hydrated polysaccharides, proteins and DNA [118]. The biophysical characteristics of biofilms render bacterial cells resistant not only to antibiotics but also to stress such us UV, acidity, toxic metal exposure and host immune clearance and phagocytosis [119,120]. Moreover, the successful establishment of pathogenic biofilm on human surfaces is the cause of chronic infections by limiting the success of antibiotic therapy [121]. In addition to preventing biofilm formation by interfering with QS systems (as describe above), biofilms can be disrupted by physical–mechanical approaches [122], by preventing extracellular matrix production [123] or by controlling bacterial adhesion on surfaces [124,125].

Existing biofilms can be disrupted by enzymatically destroying the extracellular matrix, such DNA, proteins and carbohydrates [122]. It has been demonstrated that human DNAse I is able to degrade extracellular DNA stimulating biofilm removal [126,127], and bacteria released from biofilm are more susceptible to conventional antibiotics [126,128].

Natural molecules, such us coumarin, prevent bacterial biofilm formation without affecting bacterial growth [129]. In particular, it has been demonstrated that coumarin represses expression of genes involved in fimbriae production, swarming motility, and biofilm formation [129]. Conversely a chemical compound, the TCS (3, 3′, 4′, 5-tetrachlorosalicylanilide) has been identified as able to inhibit biofilm formation by reducing extracellular matrix production [130].

3.2.3 Toxins and secretion systems

Toxin production by pathogens results in severe tissue damage, cellular malfunction or destruction [131]. Anti-virulence strategies targeting toxin function do not exert direct selective pressure on individual bacteria; but instead interfere with host–pathogen interactions, thus possibly reducing the chance of developing resistance (Fig. 8.3C). Therefore, toxin neutralisation compromises bacterial proliferation and survival in the host [132].

A major anti-virulence strategy to neutralise toxins makes use of antibodies. Currently, there are a couple of antitoxin drugs approved by FDA, which are primarily Monoclonal Antibody (MAb)-based or compound-based inhibitors [133]. These drugs not only help the eradication of the infections but also control the inflammatory response triggered by the toxins released by the pathogen. The BabyBIG, BAT, Raxibacumab, Bezlotoxumab and Obiltoxaximab are all FDA-approved antitoxins that reduce the damages imposed by the pathogen on the host tissues [134].

Screening assays have also been designed to identify small-molecule compounds that inhibit the action of the specific toxins (Fig. 8.3C). A notable example is Ebselen (2-phenyl-1,2-benzoselenazol-3-one), a lipid-soluble membrane-penetrating organoselenium compound. Ebselen has been independently identified as an inhibitor of *Clostridium difficile* TcdB toxin in two different high-throughput screening. Ebselen protects fibroblats and mice against TcdA/TcdB toxins-mediated killing [135], reduces recurrence rate and decreases the severity of colitis in animal models [136]. Although Ebselen is an active antitoxin molecule, it has generic antioxidant properties [137] and for this function it has already advanced to Phase III clinical trials in diseases unrelated to *C. difficile* infection (NCT00762671) [134]. It remains to establish if Ebselen works on *C. difficile* infection because of its generic anti-inflammatory properties and/or its anti-TcdB functions, but to date it should be considered a very promising anti-virulence molecule.

Alongside anti-toxin antibodies and small molecules in anti-virulence therapies, studies have also underscored the potentiality of engineered nanoparticles mimicking cell membranes for sequestering cytotoxic bacterial toxins. For example, artificial liposomes made of natural lipids have been demonstrated to be able to sequester bacterial toxins in vitro, preserving the integrity of mammalian cells. Moreover, administration of artificial liposomes in mice demonstrated the recovering from septicaemia caused by *S. aureus* and *S. pneumoniae*, as well as mice protection from pneumonia. In the same work, the combination of artificial liposomes with conventional antibiotics, like vancomycin and penicillin, improved mice survival compared to mono-therapies [138], suggesting a potential combinatorial therapy option.

Toxins are synthesised in the pathogenic organisms and then released by specialised secretion systems which are ideal targets for anti-virulence therapies. Many pathogens developed sophisticated secretory systems named type III, IV and VI, that are used to inject toxic proteins directly into the cytoplasm of the host cell [139].

The type III secretion system (T3SS) is one of the most validated anti-virulence targets, with many inhibitory compounds in development (Fig. 8.3C) [140]. T3SS consists of a multiprotein machine that forms a needle-type structure allowing bacteria to inject toxic effectors directly from the bacterial cytoplasm into the cytosol of the host cell. T3SS is employed by many Gram-negative pathogens to cause and maintain an infection [141,142] and in pathogens with a non-functional T3SS virulence, but not viability, is compromised. As T3SS is found mainly in bacterial pathogens, its targeting should not affect commensal bacteria [143].

A lot of molecules have been shown to interfere with T3SS activity, increasing survival of animals infected with otherwise lethal doses of pathogen cells [144]. Among them a linear polyketide compound, Aurodox, has been shown to impair T3SS-mediated haemolysis of enteropathogenic *Escherichia coli* (EPEC). Aurodox is a promising molecule, as in an in vivo mouse model, the administration of Aurodox allowed the mice to survive a lethal dose of *Citrobactor rodentium*, a model bacterium for human pathogens such as EPEC [145].

The most promising therapeutics targeting T3SS are monoclonal antibodies-based drugs that target the PrcV needle tip protein and whose clinical development is in progress. One of these, the KB001-A, is a human PEGylated IgG monoclonal anti-PcrV Fab that blocks T3SS secretion in *P. aeruginosa*. KB001-A has undergone phase I and II clinical trials for both ventilator-associated *P. aeruginosa* and treatment of chronic pneumonia in cystic fibrosis patients but unfortunately it was not progressed to phase

III trials due to lack of efficacy [140]. Another anti-PcrV mAb MEDI3902 has found to be effective in a rabbit model of pneumonia and when administered in combination with sub-MIC doses of meropenem it significantly protects *P. aeruginosa*-infected animals from death. MEDI3902 is currently under clinical evaluation for the prevention of pneumonia in ventilated patients [146].

3.2.4 Targeting microbial signal transduction

Two-component systems (TCSs) enable cells to sense environmental changes and to modulate gene expression to adapt to environmental signals. TCSs are ubiquitous in bacteria (but absent in eukaryotes) and typically consist of a homo-dimeric membrane-bound histidine kinase (HK) and a cognate cytoplasmic response regulator (RR). Under appropriate stimuli, the sensor HK protein auto-phosphorylates at the conserved histidine residue, then the phosphoryl group is moved to a conserved aspartate residue of the RR, tuning on its affinity for specific DNA sequences [147]. TCSs regulate many bacterial functions, such as envelope biogenesis and cell division, drug resistance and virulence [148]. While essential TCSs modulate cell envelope-associated functions in response to external signals [149,150], non-essential TCSs often control the expression of factors involved in virulence, antibiotic-resistance mechanisms, expression of efflux pumps, antibiotic-degrading enzyme induction [151]. Therefore, TCSs represent additional targets to develop therapies that contrast bacterial infections, without killing the bacteria (Fig. 8.3D) [152]. As TCSs are absent in host cells, molecules targeting TCSs are predicted to have low toxicity in humans [153]. The proof of concept that TCSs are good candidates for blocking bacterial infections comes from evidence that strains deleted of certain TCSs are attenuated in virulence and can be used in a vaccination strategy. For example, *Salmonella typhi* mutants deleted for *phoP/phoQ* TCS are attenuated in virulence and have been used in animal model for immunogenic live-attenuated vaccine against typhoid fever [154].

Independently on the signal sensing mechanism and the downstream regulated functions, HK's ATP-binding domain (CA) and dimerisation and histidine phosphorylation (DHp) domains are conserved [153], and these common features of TCSs are the basis for the design of broad-spectrum antimicrobial/anti-virulence agents.

TCSs functioning can be targeted by inhibiting (i) sensor HK activity, (ii) response regulator activity, (iii) signal generation (Fig. 8.3D). Few examples of some promising inhibitors are described below. For a comprehensive summary of TCSs inhibitors, the reader is directed to recent reviews on the topic [155–157].

Inhibition of sensor HK activity. Many molecules found to inhibit HK activity act as ATP competitors and exhibit poor selectivity and 'non-specific' inhibition mechanisms. A selective sensor HK inhibitor is radicicol, a diarylpyrazole-derived compound, shown to inhibit the auto-phosphorylation activity of PhoQ [158]. Although radicicol inhibitory effect was moderate, it can be used as scaffold to design more potent sensor HK inhibitors [156]. PhoQ is on the top of a regulatory cascade that activates also the response regulator PmrA, which contributes to the resistance to cationic antimicrobial peptides, such as polymyxin B [159]. Polymixins are last resort antibiotics employed in the treatment of infections caused by Gram-negative bacteria that are resistant to standard of care antibiotics [160]. Therefore, resorcin is a promising prototype molecule that could be used in combinatorial therapy with polymyxin B [156].

A benzenesulfonamide compound, named LED209, identified by screening a library of small organic molecules was found to be a specific inhibitor of QseC [161], a sensor HK present in several Gram-negative bacterial pathogens including enterohaemorrhagic *E. coli* (EHEC), uropathogenic *E. coli* (UPEC) and *Salmonella enterica*. LED209 treatment lowers the QseC-induced expression of virulence factors without affecting bacterial growth. Finally, LED209 decreases mortality in mice infected with *S. enterica* [162].

Inhibition of response regulator activity. There are two events that can be targeted at the level of RR: the phosphorylation of its conserved aspartate residue and the binding to the target DNA (Fig. 8.3D). For example, Lactoferricin B, originally characterised as a cationic antimicrobial peptide, and able to cross the bacterial membrane, impairs *E. coli* BasR and CreB RR phosphorylation but does not affect their binding to the target DNA [163]. Recently, seven natural flavonoids were found to interact with the amino acids involved in forming the helix-turn-helix DNA-binding motif of phosphorylated *Helicobacter pylori* HsrA inhibiting the in vitro DNA-binding activity of HsrA. Four of them showed bactericidal activity against *H. pylori* [164].

Inhibition of signal generation. Analogues of competence-stimulating peptide (CSP) of *S. pneumoniae*, the so-called 'COM-blockers', were tested for their ability to compete for binding to the sensor ComD (HK) without triggering the expression of factors for competence and virulence. CSP is a small molecule secreted by the *S. pneumoniae* used by the bacterium as a QS signal. When CSP concentration reaches a threshold, ComD/ComE TCS triggers the expression of competence and virulence factors [165]. Some CSP analogues reduce the expression of ComD/ComE-regulated genes as well as mouse mortality in an *S. pneumoniae* model of lung infection [166]. Savirin, a small molecule inhibitor, reduces the expression of AgrCA TCS regulated genes in *S. aureus*, leading to a reduction of virulence without affecting the skin commensal *Staphylococcus epidermidis* [167].

3.3 Search for conventional antibiotics with low susceptibility to resistance: The example of teixobactin

As outlined in the above paragraphs, development of resistance to antimicrobial compounds targeting bacterial essential pathways seems inevitable. The recently discovered teixobactin antimicrobial compound challenged this assumption. Teixobactin is a natural product synthesised by the previously uncultured Gram-negative soil bacterium *Eleftheria terrae* that displays excellent activity against Gram-positive pathogens including drug resistant strains. Teixobactin inhibits cell wall synthesis by binding to lipid I and lipid II, the precursors of peptidoglycan. The molecule is a promising therapeutic as it is efficacious in different mouse models of infections [168]. Surprisingly, resistance is not developed even after serial passages of the Gram-positive *S. aureus* in the presence of sub-MIC levels of the compound. It has been proposed that lack of detectable resistance to teixobactin is the consequence of its binding to multiple non-protein targets [168]. It is well known that resistance may also arise from horizontal gene transfer of immunity/resistance mechanisms from the antibiotic producer. However, for teixobactin, this is unlikely as the producer strain is a Gram-negative bacterium which is protected from the compound by the impermeable OM [168]. Resistance to vancomycin, an antibiotic that, as teixobactin, binds lipid II and inhibits peptidoglycan synthesis, took almost 30 years to appear (Fig. 8.1). Notably, the genes responsible for reprogramming lipid II synthesis (*vanHAX*) resulting in vancomycin resistance, likely originated in the antibiotic producer strain [169,170]. These findings suggest that it would likely take even longer for teixobactin resistance to appear, making this molecule very appealing for development into a clinically useful drug. While the dissection of the mode of action of teixobactin at the molecular level led us to understand the rationale of the low susceptibility to resistance of this compound, it will be challenging to translate this knowledge into a discovery platform to identify other natural products with similar properties.

4. Conclusions

There is no doubt that antimicrobial resistance is and will be a major health threat of the 21st century. The number of antibiotics efficacious against multi-resistant pathogens is being dramatically reducing and there are no new molecules under development to fill the antibiotic discovery pipeline. In this scenario alternative therapeutic options are urgently required with the objective not only to find and develop novel antimicrobials but also to minimise the evolution of resistance thus increasing the lifespan of the newly developed drugs.

An alternative approach to overcome the inherent difficulty in finding new antimicrobials and minimise resistance development is to search for antibiotic adjuvants, namely molecules that can either restore the susceptibility of resistant strains or extend the spectrum of Gram-positive antibiotics to Gram-negative bacteria. Indeed, several β-lactamase inhibitors discussed in this chapter are currently in clinical use. In addition, new classes of antibiotic adjuvants that act as membrane permeabilizers are currently under study and look promising. It is possible that these molecules, when used in combinatorial therapies, also increase the susceptibility of bacteria to host defences thus overall exerting lower evolutionally pressure.

Anti-virulence drugs represent an additional alternative strategy to face antimicrobial resistance. By definition, these compounds are narrow spectrum. The idea of narrow-spectrum antibiotics is becoming much more attractive. It is believed that resistance to narrow-spectrum drugs may emerge more slowly, as the normal flora will not provide a reservoir for resistance determinants. Further, narrow-spectrum antibiotics are not expected to damage the microbiota, therefore their use should not induce the dysbiosis that is associated with broad-spectrum antibiotics. However, the number of anti-virulence agents that are under clinical development is very limited and restricted to monoclonal antibodies that bind to bacterial cell surface antigens (i.e. T3SS of *P. aeruginosa*).

Overall, drug combination and anti-virulence therapies seem promising strategies to face the tremendous clinical need for new antibiotics and to counteract bacterial resistance.

Acknowledgements

PS was supported by PRIN 2020 (grant protocol 20208LLXEJ) from the Italian Ministry of University and Research (MUR, Italy).

References

[1] C.L. Ventola, The antibiotic resistance crisis: part 1: causes and threats, P and T 40 (2015) 277–283.
[2] M. Bassetti, D.R. Giacobbe, A look at the clinical, economic, and societal impact of antimicrobial resistance in 2020, Expert Opinion on Pharmacotherapy 21 (2020) 2067–2071.
[3] S.A. Omoush, J.A.M. Alzyoud, The prevalence and impact of coinfection and superinfection on the severity and outcome of COVID-19 infection: an updated literature review, Pathogens 11 (2022).
[4] A. Fleming, On the antibacterial action of cultures of a penicillium, with special reference to their use in the isolation of B. influenzae, British Journal of Experimental Pathology 10 (1929) 226–236.
[5] K. Lewis, Antibiotics: recover the lost art of drug discovery, Nature 485 (2012) 439–440.
[6] K. Lewis, Platforms for antibiotic discovery, Nature Reviews Drug Discovery 12 (2013) 371–387.
[7] S. Chakraborty, K.Y. Rhee, Tuberculosis drug development: history and evolution of the mechanism-based paradigm, Cold Spring Harbor Perspectives in Medicine 5 (2015) a021147.
[8] R.D. Fleischmann, et al., Whole-genome random sequencing and assembly of Haemophilus influenzae Rd, Science 269 (1995) 496–512.
[9] D.J. Payne, M.N. Gwynn, D.J. Holmes, D.L. Pompliano, Drugs for bad bugs: confronting the challenges of antibacterial discovery, Nature Reviews Drug Discovery 6 (2007) 29–40.
[10] R. Tommasi, D.G. Brown, G.K. Walkup, J.I. Manchester, A.A. Miller, ESKAPEing the labyrinth of antibacterial discovery, Nature Reviews Drug Discovery 14 (2015) 529–542.
[11] M. Baym, L.K. Stone, R. Kishony, Multidrug evolutionary strategies to reverse antibiotic resistance, Science 351 (2016) aad3292.
[12] H. Nikaido, Molecular basis of bacterial outer membrane permeability revisited, Microbiology and Molecular Biology Reviews 67 (2003) 593–656.
[13] T. Tsuchido, M. Takano, Sensitization by heat treatment of *Escherichia coli* K-12 cells to hydrophobic antibacterial compounds, Antimicrobial Agents and Chemotherapy 32 (1988) 1680–1683.
[14] R.P. Massengo-Tiassé, J.E. Cronan, *Vibrio cholerae* FabV defines a new class of enoyl-acyl carrier protein reductase, Journal of Biological Chemistry 283 (2008) 1308–1316.
[15] L. Zhu, J. Lin, J. Ma, J.E. Cronan, H. Wang, Triclosan resistance of *Pseudomonas aeruginosa* PAO1 is due to FabV, a triclosan-resistant enoyl-acyl carrier protein reductase, Antimicrobial Agents and Chemotherapy 54 (2010) 689–698.
[16] J.M. Blair, M.A. Webber, A.J. Baylay, D.O. Ogbolu, L.J. Piddock, Molecular mechanisms of antibiotic resistance, Nature Reviews Microbiology 13 (2015) 42–51.
[17] T.D. Bugg, et al., Molecular basis for vancomycin resistance in *Enterococcus faecium* BM4147: biosynthesis of a depsipeptide

peptidoglycan precursor by vancomycin resistance proteins VanH and VanA, Biochemistry 30 (1991) 10408–10415.
[18] R.J. Fair, Y. Tor, Antibiotics and bacterial resistance in the 21st century, Perspectives in Medicinal Chemistry 6 (2014) 25–64.
[19] Global burden of bacterial antimicrobial resistance in 2019: a systematic analysis, Lancet 399 (2022) 629–655.
[20] N.N. Nickerson, et al., A novel inhibitor of the LolCDE ABC transporter essential for lipoprotein trafficking in gram-negative bacteria, Antimicrobial Agents and Chemotherapy 62 (2018).
[21] X. Zhang, et al., Identification of an anti-Gram-negative bacteria agent disrupting the interaction between lipopolysaccharide transporters LptA and LptC, International Journal of Antimicrobial Agents 53 (2019) 442–448.
[22] M. Steenhuis, et al., Combining cell envelope stress reporter assays in a screening approach to identify BAM complex inhibitors, ACS Infectious Diseases 7 (2021) 2250–2263.
[23] M.K. Alexander, et al., Disrupting gram-negative bacterial outer membrane biosynthesis through inhibition of the lipopolysaccharide transporter MsbA, Antimicrobial Agents and Chemotherapy 62 (2018).
[24] R.J. Melander, C. Melander, The challenge of overcoming antibiotic resistance: an adjuvant approach? ACS Infectious Diseases 3 (2017) 559–563.
[25] G.D. Wright, Antibiotic adjuvants: rescuing antibiotics from resistance: (Trends in Microbiology 24, 862–871; October 17, 2016), Trends in Microbiology 24 (2016) 928.
[26] M. Hilf, et al., Antibiotic therapy for *Pseudomonas aeruginosa* bacteremia: outcome correlations in a prospective study of 200 patients, Americas Journal of Medicine 87 (1989) 540–546.
[27] D.S. Reeves, Sulphamethoxazole-trimethoprim: the first two years, Journal of Clinical Pathology 24 (1971) 430–437.
[28] P. Huovinen, Resistance to trimethoprim-sulfamethoxazole, Clinical Infectious Diseases 32 (2001) 1608–1614.
[29] J.P. Cegielski, Extensively drug-resistant tuberculosis: "there must be some kind of way out of here", Clinical Infectious Diseases 50 (Suppl. 3) (2010) S195–S200.
[30] L. Kalan, G.D. Wright, Antibiotic adjuvants: multicomponent anti-infective strategies, Expert Reviews in Molecular Medicine 13 (2011) e5.
[31] A.R. Brochado, et al., Species-specific activity of antibacterial drug combinations, Nature 559 (2018) 259–263.
[32] A.E. Clatworthy, E. Pierson, D.T. Hung, Targeting virulence: a new paradigm for antimicrobial therapy, Nature Chemical Biology 3 (2007) 541–548.
[33] D.A. Rasko, V. Sperandio, Anti-virulence strategies to combat bacteria-mediated disease, Nature Reviews Drug Discovery 9 (2010) 117–128.
[34] C.L. Tooke, et al., beta-Lactamases and beta-Lactamase Inhibitors in the 21st Century, Journal of Molecular Biology 431 (2019) 3472–3500.
[35] K. Tehrani, N.I. Martin, beta-lactam/beta-lactamase inhibitor combinations: an update, MedChemComm 9 (2018) 1439–1456.
[36] C. Reading, M. Cole, Clavulanic acid: a beta-lactamase-inhiting beta-lactam from Streptomyces clavuligerus, Antimicrobial Agents and Chemotherapy 11 (1977) 852–857.

[37] J.D. Williams, beta-Lactamase inhibition and in vitro activity of sulbactam and sulbactam/cefoperazone, Clinical Infectious Diseases 24 (1997) 494–497.
[38] K. Bush, Beta-lactamase inhibitors from laboratory to clinic, Clinical Microbiology Reviews 1 (1988) 109–123.
[39] D.L. Paterson, R.A. Bonomo, Extended-spectrum beta-lactamases: a clinical update, Clinical Microbiology Reviews 18 (2005) 657–686.
[40] D.A. Leonard, R.A. Bonomo, R.A. Powers, Class D beta-lactamases: a reappraisal after five decades, Accounts of Chemical Research 46 (2013) 2407–2415.
[41] T.F. Durand-Reville, et al., ETX2514 is a broad-spectrum beta-lactamase inhibitor for the treatment of drug-resistant Gram-negative bacteria including *Acinetobacter baumannii*, Nature Microbiology 2 (2017) 17104.
[42] T.A. Blizzard, et al., Discovery of MK-7655, a beta-lactamase inhibitor for combination with Primaxin(R), Bioorganic & Medicinal Chemistry Letters 24 (2014) 780–785.
[43] P. Lagace-Wiens, A. Walkty, J.A. Karlowsky, Ceftazidime-avibactam: an evidence-based review of its pharmacology and potential use in the treatment of Gram-negative bacterial infections, Core Evidence 9 (2014) 13–25.
[44] S.J. Hecker, et al., Discovery of a cyclic boronic acid beta-lactamase inhibitor (RPX7009) with utility vs class A serine carbapenemases, Journal of Medicinal Chemistry 58 (2015) 3682–3692.
[45] A.M. King, et al., Aspergillomarasmine A overcomes metallo-beta-lactamase antibiotic resistance, Nature 510 (2014) 503–506.
[46] F. von Nussbaum, G. Schiffer, Aspergillomarasmine A, an inhibitor of bacterial metallo-beta-lactamases conferring blaNDM and blaVIM resistance, Angewandte Chemie International Edition in English 53 (2014) 11696–11698.
[47] T.W. Yenn, et al., Stigmasterol: an adjuvant for beta lactam antibiotics against beta-lactamase positive clinical isolates, Steroids 128 (2017) 68–71.
[48] A. Ripoll, et al., Detection of resistance to beta-lactamase inhibitors in strains with CTX-M beta-lactamases: a multicenter external proficiency study using a well-defined collection of *Escherichia coli* strains, Journal of Clinical Microbiology 52 (2014) 122–129.
[49] L.J. Piddock, Multidrug-resistance efflux pumps - not just for resistance, Nature Reviews Microbiology 4 (2006) 629–636.
[50] F. Van Bambeke, Y. Glupczynski, P. Plesiat, J.C. Pechere, P.M. Tulkens, Antibiotic efflux pumps in prokaryotic cells: occurrence, impact on resistance and strategies for the future of antimicrobial therapy, Journal of Antimicrobial Chemotherapy 51 (2003) 1055–1065.
[51] G.P. Tegos, et al., Microbial efflux pump inhibition: tactics and strategies, Current Pharmaceutical Design 17 (2011) 1291–1302.
[52] J.M. Bolla, et al., Strategies for bypassing the membrane barrier in multidrug resistant Gram-negative bacteria, FEBS Letters 585 (2011) 1682–1690.
[53] O. Lomovskaya, et al., Identification and characterization of inhibitors of multidrug resistance efflux pumps in *Pseudomonas aeruginosa*: novel agents for combination therapy, Antimicrobial Agents and Chemotherapy 45 (2001) 105–116.

[54] S.K. Roy, et al., 7-Hydroxy-(E)-3-phenylmethylene-chroman-4-one analogues as efflux pump inhibitors against *Mycobacterium smegmatis* mc(2) 155, European Journal of Medicinal Chemistry 66 (2013) 499–507.
[55] R. Kanagaratnam, R. Sheikh, F. Alharbi, D.H. Kwon, An efflux pump (MexAB-OprM) of *Pseudomonas aeruginosa* is associated with antibacterial activity of Epigallocatechin-3-gallate (EGCG), Phytomedicine 36 (2017) 194–200.
[56] H. Douafer, V. Andrieu, O.t. Phanstiel, J.M. Brunel, Antibiotic adjuvants: make antibiotics great again!, Journal of Medicinal Chemistry 62 (2019) 8665–8681.
[57] H.I. Zgurskaya, C.A. Lopez, S. Gnanakaran, Permeability barrier of gram-negative cell envelopes and approaches to bypass it, ACS Infectious Diseases 1 (2015) 512–522.
[58] T.J. Silhavy, D. Kahne, S. Walker, The bacterial cell envelope, Cold Spring Harbor Perspectives in Biology 2 (2010) a000414.
[59] S.P. Denyer, J.Y. Maillard, Cellular impermeability and uptake of biocides and antibiotics in Gram-negative bacteria, Journal of Applied Microbiology 92 (Suppl. l) (2002) 35S–45S.
[60] E.B. Breidenstein, C. de la Fuente-Nunez, R.E. Hancock, *Pseudomonas aeruginosa*: all roads lead to resistance, Trends in Microbiology 19 (2011) 419–426.
[61] C. Li, et al., Incremental conversion of outer-membrane permeabilizers into potent antibiotics for gram-negative bacteria, Journal of the American Chemical Society 121 (1999) 931–940.
[62] M. Vaara, T. Vaara, Polycations sensitize enteric bacteria to antibiotics, Antimicrobial Agents and Chemotherapy 24 (1983) 107–113.
[63] R.E. Hancock, P.G. Wong, Compounds which increase the permeability of the *Pseudomonas aeruginosa* outer membrane, Antimicrobial Agents and Chemotherapy 26 (1984) 48–52.
[64] T.P. Zabawa, M.J. Pucci, T.R. Parr Jr., T. Lister, Treatment of Gram-negative bacterial infections by potentiation of antibiotics, Current Opinion in Microbiology 33 (2016) 7–12.
[65] D. Corbett, et al., Potentiation of antibiotic activity by a novel cationic peptide: potency and spectrum of activity of SPR741, Antimicrobial Agents and Chemotherapy 61 (2017).
[66] R.P. Lamers, J.F. Cavallari, L.L. Burrows, The efflux inhibitor phenylalanine-arginine beta-naphthylamide (PAbetaN) permeabilizes the outer membrane of gram-negative bacteria, PLoS One 8 (2013) e60666.
[67] C.M.J. Wesseling, N.I. Martin, Synergy by perturbing the gram-negative outer membrane: opening the door for gram-positive specific antibiotics, ACS Infectious Diseases 8 (2022) 1731–1757.
[68] J. Bailey, et al., Genetic dissection of antibiotic adjuvant activity, mBio (2022) e0308421.
[69] S. Mühlen, P. Dersch, Anti-virulence strategies to target bacterial infections, Current Topics in Microbiology and Immunology 398 (2016) 147–183.
[70] O. Manor, et al., Health and disease markers correlate with gut microbiome composition across thousands of people, Nature Communications 11 (2020) 5206.
[71] D.G. Thanassi, J.B. Bliska, P.J. Christie, Surface organelles assembled by secretion systems of Gram-negative bacteria: diversity in structure and function, FEMS Microbiology Reviews 36 (2012) 1046–1082.

[72] I. Ofek, D.L. Hasty, N. Sharon, Anti-adhesion therapy of bacterial diseases: prospects and problems, FEMS Immunology and Medical Microbiology 38 (2003) 181–191.
[73] A.P. Hendrickx, J.M. Budzik, S.Y. Oh, O. Schneewind, Architects at the bacterial surface—sortases and the assembly of pili with isopeptide bonds, Nature Reviews Microbiology 9 (2011) 166–176.
[74] S.K. Mazmanian, G. Liu, E.R. Jensen, E. Lenoy, O. Schneewind, *Staphylococcus aureus* sortase mutants defective in the display of surface proteins and in the pathogenesis of animal infections, Proceedings of the National Academy of Sciences of the U S A 97 (2000) 5510–5515.
[75] N. Zrelovs, V. Kurbatska, Z. Rudevica, A. Leonchiks, D. Fridmanis, Sorting out the superbugs: potential of sortase A inhibitors among other antimicrobial strategies to tackle the problem of antibiotic resistance, Antibiotics 10 (2021).
[76] A.H. Chan, et al., Discovery of *Staphylococcus aureus* sortase A inhibitors using virtual screening and the relaxed complex scheme, Chemical Biology & Drug Design 82 (2013) 418–428.
[77] S. Cascioferro, et al., Pharmaceutical potential of synthetic and natural pyrrolomycins, Molecules 20 (2015) 21658–21671.
[78] J. Zhang, et al., Antiinfective therapy with a small molecule inhibitor of *Staphylococcus aureus sortase*, Proceedings of the National Academy of Sciences of the U S A 111 (2014) 13517–13522.
[79] G.P. Volynets, et al., Identification of novel small-molecular inhibitors of *Staphylococcus aureus* sortase A using hybrid virtual screening, Journal of Antibiotics 75 (2022) 321–332.
[80] G.T. Werneburg, D.G. Thanassi, Pili assembled by the chaperone/usher pathway in *Escherichia coli* and Salmonella, EcoSal Plus 8 (2018).
[81] H. Emtenas, L. Alderin, F. Almqvist, An enantioselective ketene-imine cycloaddition method for synthesis of substituted ring-fused 2-pyridinones, Journal of Organic Chemistry 66 (2001) 6756–6761.
[82] J.S. Pinkner, et al., Rationally designed small compounds inhibit pilus biogenesis in uropathogenic bacteria, Proceedings of the National Academy of Sciences of the U S A 103 (2006) 17897–17902.
[83] S.E. Greene, et al., Pilicide ec240 disrupts virulence circuits in uropathogenic *Escherichia coli*, mBio 5 (2014) e02038.
[84] L. Cegelski, et al., Small-molecule inhibitors target *Escherichia coli* amyloid biogenesis and biofilm formation, Nature Chemical Biology 5 (2009) 913–919.
[85] A.W. Lo, et al., Suppression of type 1 pilus assembly in uropathogenic *Escherichia coli* by chemical inhibition of subunit polymerization, Journal of Antimicrobial Chemotherapy 69 (2014) 1017–1026.
[86] T. Klein, et al., FimH antagonists for the oral treatment of urinary tract infections: from design and synthesis to in vitro and in vivo evaluation, Journal of Medicinal Chemistry 53 (2010) 8627–8641.
[87] A. Palmioli, P. Sperandeo, S. Bertuzzi, A. Polissi, C. Airoldi, On-cell saturation transfer difference NMR for the identification of FimH ligands and inhibitors, Bioorganic Chemistry 112 (2021) 104876.
[88] C.K. Cusumano, et al., Treatment and prevention of urinary tract infection with orally active FimH inhibitors, Science Translational Medicine 3 (2011) 109ra115.
[89] P.S. Guiton, et al., Combinatorial small-molecule therapy prevents uropathogenic *Escherichia coli* catheter-associated urinary tract infections in mice, Antimicrobial Agents and Chemotherapy 56 (2012) 4738–4745.

[90] A. Salminen, et al., Inhibition of P-fimbriated *Escherichia coli* adhesion by multivalent galabiose derivatives studied by a live-bacteria application of surface plasmon resonance, Journal of Antimicrobial Chemotherapy 60 (2007) 495–501.
[91] T. Defoirdt, Quorum-sensing systems as targets for antivirulence therapy, Trends in Microbiology 26 (2018) 313–328.
[92] B. LaSarre, M.J. Federle, Exploiting quorum sensing to confuse bacterial pathogens, Microbiology and Molecular Biology Reviews 77 (2013) 73–111.
[93] W.L. Ng, B.L. Bassler, Bacterial quorum-sensing network architectures, Annual Review of Genetics 43 (2009) 197–222.
[94] C.M. Waters, B.L. Bassler, Quorum sensing: cell-to-cell communication in bacteria, Annual Review of Cell and Developmental Biology 21 (2005) 319–346.
[95] K. Papenfort, B.L. Bassler, Quorum sensing signal-response systems in Gram-negative bacteria, Nature Reviews Microbiology 14 (2016) 576–588.
[96] A. Deep, U. Chaudhary, V. Gupta, Quorum sensing and bacterial pathogenicity: from molecules to disease, Journal of Lab Physicians 3 (2011) 4–11.
[97] B. Rémy, et al., Interference in bacterial quorum sensing: a biopharmaceutical perspective, Frontiers in Pharmacology 9 (2018) 203.
[98] M.I. More, et al., Enzymatic synthesis of a quorum-sensing autoinducer through use of defined substrates, Science 272 (1996) 1655–1658.
[99] M.R. Parsek, E.P. Greenberg, Quorum sensing signals in development of *Pseudomonas aeruginosa* biofilms, Methods in Enzymology 310 (1999) 43–55.
[100] J.A. Gutierrez, et al., Transition state analogs of 5'-methylthioadenosine nucleosidase disrupt quorum sensing, Nature Chemical Biology 5 (2009) 251–257.
[101] S. Fetzner, Quorum quenching enzymes, Journal of Biotechnology 201 (2015) 2–14.
[102] C. Reimmann, et al., Genetically programmed autoinducer destruction reduces virulence gene expression and swarming motility in *Pseudomonas aeruginosa* PAO1, Microbiology (Reading) 148 (2002) 923–932.
[103] Q. Jiang, J. Chen, C. Yang, Y. Yin, K. Yao, Quorum sensing: a prospective therapeutic target for bacterial diseases, BioMed Research International 2019 (2019) 2015978.
[104] P.D. Utari, R. Setroikromo, B.N. Melgert, W.J. Quax, PvdQ quorum quenching acylase attenuates *Pseudomonas aeruginosa* virulence in a mouse model of pulmonary infection, Frontiers in Cellular and Infection Microbiology 8 (2018) 119.
[105] S. Hraiech, et al., Inhaled lactonase reduces *Pseudomonas aeruginosa* quorum sensing and mortality in rat pneumonia, PLoS One 9 (2014) e107125.
[106] A.M. Stevens, Y. Queneau, L. Soulere, S. von Bodman, A. Doutheau, Mechanisms and synthetic modulators of AHL-dependent gene regulation, Chemistry Review 111 (2011) 4–27.
[107] N. Amara, et al., Fine-tuning covalent inhibition of bacterial quorum sensing, ChemBioChem 17 (2016) 825–835.
[108] B. Koch, et al., The LuxR receptor: the sites of interaction with quorum-sensing signals and inhibitors, Microbiology (Reading) 151 (2005) 3589–3602.

[109] J.E. Paczkowski, et al., Flavonoids suppress *Pseudomonas aeruginosa* virulence through allosteric inhibition of quorum-sensing receptors, Journal of Biological Chemistry 292 (2017) 4064–4076.
[110] D. Ren, J.J. Sims, T.K. Wood, Inhibition of biofilm formation and swarming of *Escherichia coli* by (5Z)-4-bromo-5-(bromomethylene)-3-butyl-2(5H)-furanone, Environmental Microbiology 3 (2001) 731–736.
[111] L.X. Weng, Y.X. Yang, Y.Q. Zhang, L.H. Wang, A new synthetic ligand that activates QscR and blocks antibiotic-tolerant biofilm formation in *Pseudomonas aeruginosa*, Applied Microbiology and Biotechnology 98 (2014) 2565–2572.
[112] Y.X. Yang, et al., A new quorum-sensing inhibitor attenuates virulence and decreases antibiotic resistance in *Pseudomonas aeruginosa*, Journal of Microbiology 50 (2012) 987–993.
[113] C.T. O'Loughlin, et al., A quorum-sensing inhibitor blocks *Pseudomonas aeruginosa* virulence and biofilm formation, Proceedings of the National Academy of Sciences of the U S A 110 (2013) 17981–17986.
[114] F.G. Glansdorp, et al., Synthesis and stability of small molecule probes for *Pseudomonas aeruginosa* quorum sensing modulation, Organic and Biomolecular Chemistry 2 (2004) 3329–3336.
[115] J.K. Vasquez, Y. Tal-Gan, G. Cornilescu, K.A. Tyler, H.E. Blackwell, Simplified AIP-II peptidomimetics are potent inhibitors of *Staphylococcus aureus* AgrC quorum sensing receptors, ChemBioChem 18 (2017) 413–423.
[116] T. Maeda, et al., Quorum quenching quandary: resistance to antivirulence compounds, ISME Journal 6 (2012) 493–501.
[117] C. Grandclement, M. Tannieres, S. Morera, Y. Dessaux, D. Faure, Quorum quenching: role in nature and applied developments, FEMS Microbiology Reviews 40 (2016) 86–116.
[118] D. Fleming, K.P. Rumbaugh, Approaches to dispersing medical biofilms, Microorganisms 5 (2017).
[119] C.W. Hall, T.F. Mah, Molecular mechanisms of biofilm-based antibiotic resistance and tolerance in pathogenic bacteria, FEMS Microbiology Reviews 41 (2017) 276–301.
[120] B.S. Tseng, et al., A biofilm matrix-associated protease inhibitor protects *Pseudomonas aeruginosa* from proteolytic attack, mBio 9 (2018).
[121] M. Rybtke, et al., The LapG protein plays a role in *Pseudomonas aeruginosa* biofilm formation by controlling the presence of the CdrA adhesin on the cell surface, Microbiologica 4 (2015) 917–930.
[122] C.H. Puga, E. Dahdouh, C. SanJose, B. Orgaz, Listeria monocytogenes colonizes *Pseudomonas fluorescens* biofilms and induces matrix over-production, Frontiers in Microbiology 9 (2018) 1706.
[123] X. Feng, et al., Inhibition of biofilm formation by chemical uncoupler, 3, 3′, 4′, 5-tetrachlorosalicylanilide (TCS): from the perspective of quorum sensing and biofilm related genes, Biochemical Engineering Journal 137 (2018) 95–99.
[124] J. Ranfaing, C. Dunyach-Remy, J.P. Lavigne, A. Sotto, Propolis potentiates the effect of cranberry (*Vaccinium macrocarpon*) in reducing the motility and the biofilm formation of uropathogenic *Escherichia coli*, PLoS One 13 (2018) e0202609.
[125] X. Liu, et al., Protein-mediated anti-adhesion surface against oral bacteria, Nanoscale 10 (2018) 2711–2714.

[126] J.B. Kaplan, et al., Recombinant human DNase I decreases biofilm and increases antimicrobial susceptibility in staphylococci, Journal of Antibiotics 65 (2012) 73–77.

[127] H.L. Brown, K. Hanman, M. Reuter, R.P. Betts, A.H. van Vliet, *Campylobacter jejuni* biofilms contain extracellular DNA and are sensitive to DNase I treatment, Frontiers in Microbiology 6 (2015) 699.

[128] F. Sivori, et al., Role of extracellular DNA in dalbavancin activity against methicillin-resistant *Staphylococcus aureus* (MRSA) biofilms in patients with skin and soft tissue infections, Microbiology Spectrum 10 (2) (2022) e0035122.

[129] J.H. Lee, et al., Coumarins reduce biofilm formation and the virulence of *Escherichia coli* O157:H7, Phytomedicine 21 (2014) 1037–1042.

[130] X. Feng, Q. Wu, L. Che, N. Ren, Analyzing the inhibitory effect of metabolic uncoupler on bacterial initial attachment and biofilm development and the underlying mechanism, Environmental Research 185 (2020) 109390.

[131] J.K. Rudkin, R.M. McLoughlin, A. Preston, R.C. Massey, Bacterial toxins: offensive, defensive, or something else altogether? PLoS Pathogens 13 (2017) e1006452.

[132] R.V. Ortines, et al., Neutralizing alpha-toxin accelerates healing of *Staphylococcus aureus*-infected wounds in nondiabetic and diabetic mice, Antimicrobial Agents and Chemotherapy 62 (2018).

[133] T.S. Migone, et al., Raxibacumab for the treatment of inhalational anthrax, New England Journal of Medicine 361 (2009) 135–144.

[134] M. Sakari, A. Laisi, A.T. Pulliainen, Exotoxin-targeted drug modalities as antibiotic alternatives, ACS Infectious Diseases 8 (2022) 433–456.

[135] K.O. Bender, et al., A small-molecule antivirulence agent for treating *Clostridium difficile* infection, Science Translational Medicine 7 (2015) 306ra148.

[136] M. Garland, et al., The clinical drug Ebselen attenuates inflammation and promotes microbiome recovery in mice after antibiotic treatment for CDI, Cell Rep Med 1 (2020).

[137] G.K. Azad, R.S. Tomar, Ebselen, a promising antioxidant drug: mechanisms of action and targets of biological pathways, Molecular Biology Reports 41 (2014) 4865–4879.

[138] B.D. Henry, et al., Engineered liposomes sequester bacterial exotoxins and protect from severe invasive infections in mice, Nature Biotechnology 33 (2015) 81–88.

[139] A. Filloux, Bacterial protein secretion systems: game of types, Microbiology (Reading) 168 (2022).

[140] J.A. Hotinger, H.A. Pendergrass, A.E. May, Molecular targets and strategies for inhibition of the bacterial type III secretion system (T3SS); inhibitors directly binding to T3SS components, Biomolecules 11 (2021).

[141] L.J. Mota, G.R. Cornelis, The bacterial injection kit: type III secretion systems, Annals of Medicine 37 (2005) 234–249.

[142] T.F. Moraes, T. Spreter, N.C. Strynadka, Piecing together the type III injectisome of bacterial pathogens, Current Opinion in Structural Biology 18 (2008) 258–266.

[143] J.A. Hotinger, A.E. May, Animal models of type III secretion system-mediated pathogenesis, Pathogens 8 (2019).

[144] J.A. Hotinger, A.E. May, Antibodies inhibiting the type III secretion system of gram-negative pathogenic bacteria, Antibodies 9 (2020).

[145] K. Kimura, et al., A small-molecule inhibitor of the bacterial type III secretion system protects against *in vivo* infection with *Citrobacter rodentium*, Journal of Antibiotics 64 (2011) 197–203.
[146] H.N. Le, et al., Treatment efficacy of MEDI3902 in *Pseudomonas aeruginosa* bloodstream infection and acute pneumonia rabbit models, Antimicrobial Agents and Chemotherapy 63 (2019).
[147] P. Casino, V. Rubio, A. Marina, Structural insight into partner specificity and phosphoryl transfer in two-component signal transduction, Cell 139 (2009) 325–336.
[148] N. Papon, A.M. Stock, Two-component systems, Current Biology 29 (2019) R724–r725.
[149] C. Van der Henst, et al., The histidine kinase PdhS controls cell cycle progression of the pathogenic alphaproteobacterium *Brucella abortus*, Journal of Bacteriology 194 (2012) 5305–5314.
[150] S.T. Cardona, M. Choy, A.M. Hogan, Essential two-component systems regulating cell envelope functions: opportunities for novel antibiotic therapies, Journal of Membrane Biology 251 (2018) 75–89.
[151] A.R. Tierney, P.N. Rather, Roles of two-component regulatory systems in antibiotic resistance, Future Microbiology 14 (2019) 533–552.
[152] S. Tiwari, et al., Two-component signal transduction systems of pathogenic bacteria as targets for antimicrobial therapy: an overview, Frontiers in Microbiology 8 (2017) 1878.
[153] R. Gao, A.M. Stock, Biological insights from structures of two-component proteins, Annual Review of Microbiology 63 (2009) 133–154.
[154] E.L. Hohmann, C.A. Oletta, K.P. Killeen, S.I. Miller, phoP/phoQ-deleted *Salmonella typhi* (Ty800) is a safe and immunogenic single-dose typhoid fever vaccine in volunteers, The Journal of Infectious Diseases 173 (1996) 1408–1414.
[155] C.A. Fihn, E.E. Carlson, Targeting a highly conserved domain in bacterial histidine kinases to generate inhibitors with broad spectrum activity, Current Opinion in Microbiology 61 (2021) 107–114.
[156] H. Hirakawa, J. Kurushima, Y. Hashimoto, H. Tomita, Progress overview of bacterial two-component regulatory systems as potential targets for antimicrobial chemotherapy, Antibiotics 9 (2020).
[157] H. Chen, et al., Recent advances in histidine kinase-targeted antimicrobial agents, Frontiers in Chemistry 10 (2022) 866392.
[158] M.T. Guarnieri, L. Zhang, J. Shen, R. Zhao, The Hsp90 inhibitor radicicol interacts with the ATP-binding pocket of bacterial sensor kinase PhoQ, Journal of Molecular Biology 379 (2008) 82–93.
[159] A. Kato, E.A. Groisman, Connecting two-component regulatory systems by a protein that protects a response regulator from dephosphorylation by its cognate sensor, Genes & Development 18 (2004) 2302–2313.
[160] A.P. Zavascki, L.Z. Goldani, J. Li, R.L. Nation, Polymyxin B for the treatment of multidrug-resistant pathogens: a critical review, Journal of Antimicrobial Chemotherapy 60 (2007) 1206–1215.
[161] V. Sperandio, A.G. Torres, B. Jarvis, J.P. Nataro, J.B. Kaper, Bacteria-host communication: the language of hormones, Proceedings of the National Academy of Sciences of the U S A 100 (2003) 8951–8956.
[162] M.B. Clarke, D.T. Hughes, C. Zhu, E.C. Boedeker, V. Sperandio, The QseC sensor kinase: a bacterial adrenergic receptor, Proceedings of the National Academy of Sciences of the U S A 103 (2006) 10420–10425.

[163] Y.H. Ho, T.C. Sung, C.S. Chen, Lactoferricin B inhibits the phosphorylation of the two-component system response regulators BasR and CreB, Molecular and Cellular Proteomics 11 (2012).
[164] A. González, et al., Identifying potential novel drugs against *Helicobacter pylori* by targeting the essential response regulator HsrA, Scientific Reports 9 (2019) 11294.
[165] B. Martin, et al., ComE/ComE ~ P interplay dictates activation or extinction status of pneumococcal X-state (competence), Molecular Microbiology 87 (2013) 394–411.
[166] A. Domenech, et al., Proton motive force disruptors block bacterial competence and horizontal gene transfer, Cell Host & Microbe 27 (2020) 544–555.
[167] A.M. Salam, C.L. Quave, Targeting virulence in *Staphylococcus aureus* by chemical inhibition of the accessory gene regulator system in vivo, mSphere 3 (2018).
[168] L.L. Ling, et al., A new antibiotic kills pathogens without detectable resistance, Nature 517 (2015) 455–459.
[169] C.G. Marshall, G. Broadhead, B.K. Leskiw, G.D. Wright, D-Ala-D-Ala ligases from glycopeptide antibiotic-producing organisms are highly homologous to the enterococcal vancomycin-resistance ligases VanA and VanB, Proceedings of the National Academy of Sciences of the U S A 94 (1997) 6480–6483.
[170] C.G. Marshall, I.A. Lessard, I. Park, G.D. Wright, Glycopeptide antibiotic resistance genes in glycopeptide-producing organisms, Antimicrobial Agents and Chemotherapy 42 (1998) 2215–2220.

9

Pre-clinical characterisation: Which animal model is best for infection?

Federico Fenaroli[1] **and Anna Griego**[2,3]
[1] *University of Stavanger, Stavanger, Norway;* [2] *Department of Pharmaceutical Science, University of Milan, Milan, Italy;* [3] *National Institute of Molecular Genetic (INGM), Milan, Italy*

1. Zebrafish, a tiny vertebrate star

Discovered in Indian rivers in 1822 by the Scottish physician Hamilton, few would have imagined that this tiny vertebrate would become an essential tool for modern biomedical research. The zebrafish belongs to teleost fish, evolutionary separated from humans for the past 400 million years. When George Streisinger started to work on this animal as a model system for developmental biology in Oregon in 1970, he met fierce scepticism regarding the value of an animal so distant from humans. The perseverance of this zebrafish pioneer, as often happens, paid off only 10 years later when a publication in the journal *Nature*, which made it to the cover page, started to lift this animal out of obscurity [1]. Since the 1980s, there has been an explosion of zebrafish research which now encompasses very diverse fields within biology such as development, genetics and biomedicine including, as we will see below, NP-based therapies. A further push for the use of the zebrafish came from the sequencing of the genome of this animal which showed how we humans share with this fish about 70% of our genes and, of the genes related to the disease this value goes up to 84% [2]. In addition to genetic similarity, the zebrafish shares with humans several organs strikingly similar to those of humans (i.e. heart, liver, kidney, brain, ear, intestine, pancreas eyes and muscles). These organs all develop in the first 24 h after fertilisation and have become important for the study of organ development. Finally, the zebrafish is

Nanotechnology Tools for Infection Control. https://doi.org/10.1016/B978-0-12-823994-0.00005-0

extremely cost- and time-effective compared to the mouse, the most popular animal model in medicine [3].

2. Why studying NPs in the zebrafish

The current strategy for the analysis of NPs is to conduct a hierarchical screen, starting with physical–chemical characterisation, then analysis in mammalian cell cultures and a few will reach the stage of preclinical testing in mice. Most of the NPs that are made will stop at the chemical assessment stage while fewer are studied in vitro and even fewer reach the in vivo studies. There is a large conceptual jump from simple cell culture studies to experiments in mice, as is the current strategy. Moreover, mice possess intrinsic disadvantages for imaging that complicate its use: (i) they are not transparent for imaging, and consequently, high-resolution microscopy methods at the whole-animal level are not possible to use. NPs localisation often employs an in vivo imaging system (IVIS), a low-resolution technology that allows one only to roughly locate NPs. (ii) Limited higher resolution imaging is theoretically possible using multiphoton microscopy, but this approach is invasive and restricted to exposed surfaces or thin slices of tissue [4]. The zebrafish can overcome many of these limitations and become an important intermediate model for bridging the gaps between cell culture and mice studies. Here we highlight a few areas where the zebrafish can give significant insights into NP behaviour in vivo.

NP interaction with innate immunity and endothelial cells. Innate immune cells, such as macrophages and neutrophils, are crucial for the study of NPs. These are the first line of defence against infections and, being naturally phagocytic, are responsible for the clearance of NPs from circulation. Within the zebrafish model, early developing leucocytes (i.e. macrophages and neutrophils) can be seen starting from 24 h post fertilisation (pf) where they colonise the whole body of the fish within 3 days pf [5,6]. The developing zebrafish embryo possesses ideal characteristics for studying innate immunity:

1. Transgenic zebrafish lines having fluorescently labelled leucocytes, such as macrophages (mpegl [7] and mfab4 [8]) and neutrophils (lyz [9] and mpx [10]), have been developed.
2. Zebrafish larvae are fully transparent for the first 36 h and the addition of the bathing water of phenythiourea (PTU) inhibits melanin production during the first days of development. Moreover, the transgenic line Casper is widely available in zebrafish labs and retains transparency until adulthood [11].

3. Innate immunity can be studied in the complete absence of adaptive immunity until about 21 days post-fertilisation. In this period the fish cannot reject foreign cells [12].

Macrophages and neutrophils arising within the first days post fertilisation are already able to phagocytose and eliminate injected bacteria such as *Escherichia coli* (Gram-negative) or *Bacillus subtilis* (Gram-positive) [5]. In several publications, these phagocytes have also been shown to engulf NPs when they are injected at different sites in the zebrafish [13,14]. Particularly, macrophages can devote a significant fraction of their volume to storing the sequestered NPs [15]. For blood-resident macrophages, we found that 25% of the volume of the cell is occupied by NPs after only 1 h of intravenous injection. Importantly, our group and others have shown how straightforward it is to quantify NPs uptake by phagocytes in zebrafish by analysing the fluorescence signal of NPs overlapping with that of macrophages and neutrophils [15,16]. This is a parameter that can help in deciding whether an NPs system is a good candidate for treating intracellular infections.

The endothelial cells that line the blood vessels are a very important cell type when NPs are injected systemically, and it is often overlooked when analysing NPs uptake. Only recently has the importance of endothelial interaction of NPs been realised by different research groups [17,18]. Unlike macrophages, which can be purified from the blood of sacrificed animals, these cells are very difficult to analyse in mammals and require chemical fixation and sectioning of tissues. In zebrafish, endothelial uptake, especially in the caudal region, occurs often and has been directly observed in numerous studies [19–21]. Using zebrafish, the group of Bussmann has recently shown the importance of the scavenger receptor stabilin-2 (stab2) for NPs uptake and demonstrated how this interaction can be blocked using the stab2-inhibitor dextran sulphate [20]. One important finding visualised in the zebrafish is that endothelial cells can internalise NPs and then transfer them into macrophages [22].

NPs–Drug toxicity. Zebrafish is an emerging animal model for studying drug toxicity and is widely regarded as a bridging platform between in vitro and in vivo studies [23]. Information on drug toxicity obtained from zebrafish larvae can greatly reduce the need for mice, an important aspect to consider given the principle of the 3Rs (Replacement, Reduction, Refinement).

The most common way to administer drugs is to add them directly to the water. Although drug addition within the water is an easy administration system, this approach has the limitation of not allowing proper control of the dose of the drug given to the zebrafish. A more precise method relies on the use of glass needles and performing drug(s) microinjections. This latter approach allows systemic drug distribution or local administration in selected sites – such as muscles, the yolk sac, the otic vesicle (ear) or in the brain region. Once in contact with the drug of interest, different parameters can be easily and rapidly analysed (i.e. lethality, heartbeat, presence of oedemas, swimming behaviour, body posture, and rate of development) to assess toxicity [24,25].

NPs circulation time. A fundamental NPs parameter that determines their suitability for drug delivery purposes is their circulation time after injection within the bloodstream. In mice, this often means that the animals must be sacrificed at the desired time point and blood extracted and analysed for the presence of NPs or their cargo. In zebrafish, NPs distribution in the blood can be monitored in real-time provided that the NPs are labelled with a fluorescent dye, either encapsulated or covalently attached. By following the decrease in fluorescence over time in the blood vessels, it is possible to rapidly estimate NP-circulation time in a reproducible manner. By injecting four different NPs solutions into the zebrafish and mice, Dal and colleagues have compared NPs circulation time between these two animal models. The results obtained in the zebrafish are predictive of the behaviour of the NPs circulation time in the murine model (Fig. 9.1), therefore providing an inexpensive and quick platform for this type of analysis [19].

Real-time visualisation of NP in vivo stability. The process of NPs degradation over time is also significantly easier to assess in zebrafish and has been performed via different methodologies. The simplest one has been via the visualisation of the decreased fluorescence over time within the macrophages [16]. Another, more elegant approach, exploit the Förster resonance energy transfer (FRET) technique [26,27]. This has been achieved by encapsulating two fluorescent dyes in the same NPs: a green fluorescent donor molecule (DIO) and a red fluorescent acceptor molecule (DIL). The close contact between the two molecules allows energy transfer upon irradiation with a 488 nm laser between the DIO to DIL only when NPs are still intact, resulting in red-emitting fluorescence. NPs that have been degraded are not capable of FRET and the DIL fails to emit red fluorescence. In another research study, the zebrafish has been employed to observe the loss of NPs stability using light at a specific wavelength. This was achieved by preparing liposomes with a photosensitive molecule that when exposed to light at 400 nm rapidly degrades and, consequently, allows control of the release of the

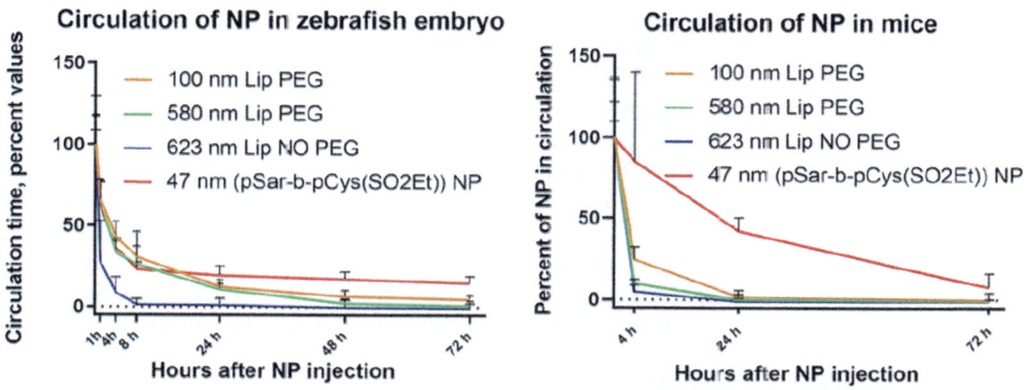

Figure 9.1 Nanoparticle circulation in zebrafish and mouse. Based on a fluorescence analysis, the presence in circulation of the same nanoparticles has been analysed in the zebrafish (*left*) and in mouse (*right*). The figure has been adapted without changes from an article published in the journal Small [19]. Link to the licence: CC BY 4.0.

drug cargo [21]. With this method, NPs degradation was readily observable and quantifiable in the blood of the animal system used. These techniques that employ light to observe NPs in vivo stability are simply not feasible in the murine system.

3. Zebrafish, nanoparticles and intracellular infections

The past 20 years have seen an explosion of newly established models of infection in the zebrafish, ranging from bacteria to viruses and fungi (for more information and complete lists of pathogens see Refs. [28–30]). When it comes to NPs studies, except individual papers on *Francisella noatunensis* ssb *orientalis* [31] (a fish pathogen), only two major intracellular human pathogens have been studied so far in the zebrafish: *Mycobacterium marinum* (*M. marinum*) and *Staphylococcus aureus* (*S. aureus*). Here below we highlight some of the evidence obtained with zebrafish infected by these two pathogens.

M. marinum is a close relative to *Mycobacterium tuberculosis* [32], the biggest bacterial killer worldwide and the causative agent of Tuberculosis (TB) in humans. The group of Ramakrishnan has pioneered the study of *M. marinum* in the zebrafish embryo, highlighting important crosstalk aspects of the interaction between mycobacteria and innate immunity. This is especially interesting because in humans *M. tuberculosis*'s infection is initially only restrained by innate immunity, while adaptive immunity intervenes only after about 3 weeks. Their first publication [13] has opened-up the use of zebrafish for studying intracellular infections. Once injected intravenously, mycobacteria are rapidly engulfed by macrophages that fail to sterilise the infection and aggregate in dynamic 'granuloma-like' structures reminiscent of human TB. A more recently established *M. marinum* infection system is obtained by injecting the bacteria into a closed compartment, namely the neural tube, that is located in the trunk of the zebrafish [33,34]. In this site, *M. marimum* forms much bigger, localised granulomas, that cause first angiogenesis and then angionecrosis leading to softening of tissues and spreading of mycobacteria. Importantly, these newly formed vessels are highly permeable, a factor that could help improve drug delivery into the granulomas [33–35].

Despite being found in about 30% of humans as part of our skin microbiota [36], *S. aureus* is the most dangerous among the Staphylococci species and can act as a facultative pathogen causing severe skin and respiratory infections. Initially considered purely an extracellular bacterium, *S. aureus* is, in reality, a facultative intracellular pathogen. A powerful *S. aureus* infection model has been developed in Renshaw's lab using the zebrafish embryo which helped clarify an important aspect of the interaction of this bacterium with innate immunity. *S. aureus* is rapidly taken up by macrophages and neutrophils which can initially restrict bacterial growth [14], employing autophagy [37,38]. While macrophages can completely eradicate bacteria, neutrophils allow *S. aureus* to slowly grow over time until the bacterium is able to overwhelm the zebrafish. In addition, Buchan and colleagues have shown how *S. aureus*-secreted toxins lead to reduced numbers of neutrophils at the infection site with consequent increased bacterial numbers and mortality [39].

Assessment of NPs in infected zebrafish embryos. Taken together, results coming from the zebrafish confirm the full potential of NPs for the treatment of intracellular infection with NPs containing rifampicin [15,40], the efflux pump inhibitor thioridazine [25] as well as gentamicin [41] and vancomycin [42]. The work of Anversa Dimer and colleagues on the delivery of Clarithromycin for the treatment of *S. aureus* also showed promising results although NPs were placed in the water rather than injected in the zebrafish larvae [43].

Different mechanisms have been shown to play a role in the efficacy of NPs over free drugs for eliminating intracellular infections, which will be hereby discussed.

1. The rationale put forward by many researchers for using NPs against intracellular infections is that NPs are naturally taken up by phagocytes such as macrophages and neutrophils which

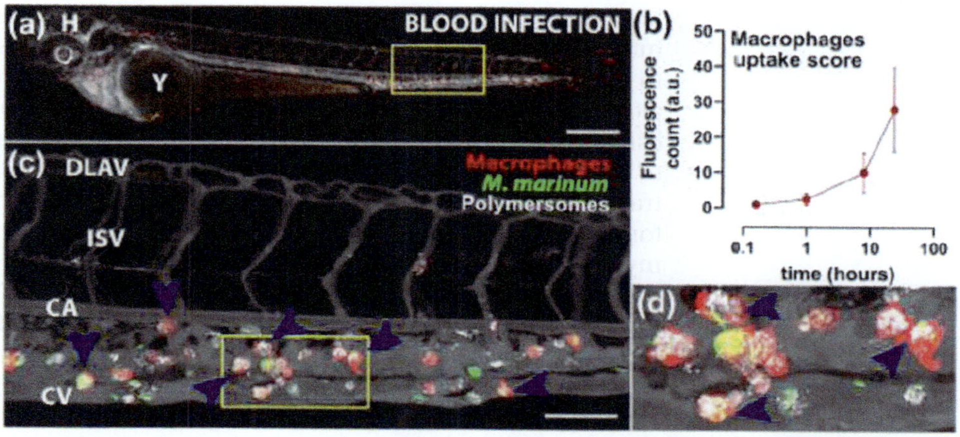

Figure 9.2 Nanoparticle uptake in zebrafish-infected macrophages. Polymersomes NP (in *white*) have been administered intravenously to *M. marinum*-infected (*green*) zebrafish embryos possessing macrophages fluorescently labelled (*red*). An overview of the whole zebrafish is shown in (A); the region in the *yellow square* in (A) is shown enlarged in (C) and the area in the *yellow square* in (C) is shown magnified in (D). In (D) is highlighted the presence of polymersomes NP into infected macrophages. A graph on time-dependent accumulation of polymersomes NP in macrophages is shown in (B). Adapted with permission from the journal ACS Nano [41]. Copyright 2020 American Chemical Society.

are the same cell types most intracellular pathogens (and certainly *M. marinum/M. tuberculosis* and *S. aureus*) able to infect. This way the drug concentrates in proximity to the infecting agent. While this is difficult to observe in mice, the zebrafish offers a perfect platform to evaluate such parameter. Indeed, all the studies of NPs against *M. marinum* or *S. aureus* have shown that drug-loaded NPs are found in the same bacteria-infected phagocytes (Fig. 9.2) and that this is one of the main reasons for the success of NPs-based drugs for treating infections [15,34,41].

2. Another mechanism has been described for TB [15]. Macrophages migrating to TB-infected areas is a hallmark of the disease and this process can be effectively exploited when using NPs to increase their share within the areas of infection. Fenaroli and colleagues showed that this could effectively be applied within a zebrafish TB model. *M. marinum* or PBS were injected in the hindbrain ventricle at 6 days post fertilisation, a time when the brain is already separated from the bloodstream via a blood–brain barrier. Consequently, NPs had no direct access to the hindbrain ventricle, and to reach this compartment they needed to be actively transported. When NPs were injected into the vasculature, these were found in the

hindbrain only in zebrafish infected with *M. marinum* into the hindbrain [15]. This argues strongly that NPs were transported to the infection site by macrophages that actively took up NPs along the vasculature of the zebrafish. It needs to be established whether this strategy would work in mammalian models of TB and in humans. It also needs to be assessed whether the transport of NPs by innate immune cells could be harnessed for fighting other intracellular pathogens other than mycobacteria.

3. A third process, involving increased accumulation of NPs via the vasculature into granulomas is described only for TB. The groups of Tobin and Jain have provided evidence that aggregates of infected macrophages (i.e. TB granulomas) cause local hypoxia and promote local angiogenesis. These groups also found that these vessels display increased permeability of small molecules [33,35]. On these premises, the group of Griffiths has shown that this is also happening when using NPs. When long-circulating liposomes bore polyethylene glycol (PEG, a molecule known to enhance NP circulation time), they accumulated at the diseased area by leaking from the diseased vessels into infected areas. These NPs fared better than NPs with short circulating times such as PLGA. Similar results were obtained in the mouse model [34]. This study shows that NPs designed to avoid macrophage clearance also end up in TB granulomas via a separate mechanism involving NPs crossing the endothelium adjacent to the infection locus.

In conclusion, the use of zebrafish for studying NPs and infections is rapidly expanding and is revealing how this transparent vertebrate is not simply an alternative animal model to mice but it is effectively another tool for expanding our knowledge of how NPs can help us fight a plethora of infectious agents.

4. Conventional models

Mouse. The simple handling, the reduced cost, and space requirement, the availability of immunological tools, and the possible generation of both inbred, outbred, and transgenic strains define mice as the preferred animal models. However, because humans are the natural host of *M. tuberculosis*, they cannot entirely mimic the immune process behind the latent infection.

The first two mice models employed to replicate *M. tuberculosis* infection are the Cornell and the low-dose chronic (or untreated) models [44,45]. The Cornell model was developed around the 1950s, and it is the first in vivo system to reproduce latent human tuberculosis [46]. To generate this model, mice are lengthily infected with a high dose of *M. tuberculosis*, and then antimycobacterial are administered to reduce the bacterial burden. This procedure determines the absence of detectable viable bacilli after the treatment, allowing then a spontaneous reactivation of the infection [46]. Contrarily, the low-dose or untreated mouse models are generated by infecting mouse with a low *M. tuberculosis* burden via aerosol or the intravenous route. After the infection, the mouse will develop an initial acute phase of the infection (e.g. bacterial multiplication), and *M. tuberculosis* spreading will be then only possibly contained by the mouse immune system,thus similarly recreating the human TB latency [45]. Overall, because of the simplicity and possibility of establishing a prolonged chronic tuberculosis infection, both the low-dose and Cornell mouse in vivo systems have been widely used.

Nevertheless, the low-dose and Cornell models use either BALB/c or C57BL/6 mouse strains, which are unable to mimic the complete spectrum of TB manifestations reported in infected humans. Particularly, mice infected with *M. tuberculosis* fail to assemble a hypoxic cellular, inflammatory granuloma, limiting the microenvironmental conditions favoring the generation of persistent and metabolically distinct mycobacteria subpopulations [47–49]. To overcome the lack of similarity in the immunological response between the mouse model and the humans, researchers have made considerable efforts to modulate the mice's immune system. In this regard, one of the most recently developed models, namely the Kramnik mouse model, uses the C3HeB/FeJ mouse strain, which can develop highly organised and necrotic granuloma following *M. tuberculosis* infection [50]. To recreate human-like granulomas, the Kramnik model is generated by infecting the mouse with a low *M. tuberculosis* burden (15–30 CFU via aerosol or 105 CFU through the intravenous route). Quickly after the inoculation, the mouse will show a rapid progression of the pathology in the lung, ending in the formation of necrotic microlesions after 2 weeks. Interestingly, the Kramnik mouse model appears to develop such highly organised encapsulated lesions primarily in the lung, while the spreading of the bacilli is better contained in other organs (e.g. spleen and liver) [51,52]. Thus, the Kramnik mouse model may represent a novel model for both preclinical screenings of new antimycobacterial molecules and the advancement of imaging techniques, such as positron emission tomography (PET).

Currently, a further improvement in mimicking *M. tuberculosis* infection using mice model is represented by an infection carried with an ultralow mycobacteria dose, which is sought to overcome the present limitation of this model and closely reproduce human TB [53]. Ultralow dose (1–3 CFU) *M. tuberculosis*-infected mice generally develop a highly heterogenous bacterial burden in several organs (i.e. lymph nodes and spleen), while developing single granuloma lesions within the lungs. Although such model exhibits a lower, but variable bacterial burden during the initial phase of the infection, 83 days post-*M. tuberculosis* infection a 10,000 CFU titer is reached with *M. tuberculosis* disseminated to the spleen [54]. In sum, although the ultralow dose mice model better mimics diverse aspects of human tuberculosis, still cannot fully reproduce LTBI and TB relapse.

An additional advancement in the employment of mice as a model in studying TB pathogenesis is the generation of humanised mice (hu-mice) models, which can recapitulate several aspects of human TB demonstrating their utility for TB infection studies [55,56]. To date, some of the most commonly used immunocompromised hu-mice include Rag1(2)nullIl2ngnull, NOD.Cg-PrkdcscidIl2rgtm1Sug (NOG), NOD.Cg-PrkdcscidIlrgtm1Wjl (NSG) and NOD.Cg.Rag1tm1Mo-MIl2rgtm1Wjl (NRG) mice engrafted with human hematopoietic stem cells. Although these mice strain can better reproduce immune response and show $CD45^+$ cell reconstitution (i.e. also including $CD4^+$ and $CD8^+$ T cells), B cells and limited myeloid cellular subsets, they are associated with only a 50% chance of successful engraftment, reflecting thus a limitation in their use to fully evaluate TB progression [57–60]. To overcome those limitations, during the last decades HLA-matched HSCs engraftment protocol has led to the generation of next-generation hu-mice (e.g. DRAGA, NSG-A2, BRGS-A2-DR2, NOG-DR4 and NOK-B51Tg mice strains), which have proved to be a potential excellent models to perform preclinical studies to gain more in-depth insights on *M. tuberculosis* infection establishment and progression [58].

Guinea pig. Guinea pigs are the second most used model to investigate both *M. tuberculosis* pathogenesis and validation of antimycobacterial drugs and vaccine efficacy. Differently from mice, they are highly susceptible to *M. tuberculosis*, and the progression of the infection recreates several aspects of the human TB [56,61]. To mimic a human-like granuloma, guinea pigs can be infected by exploiting different routes, ranging from the intranasal injection to the instillation of the lungs via the trachea.

However, to mimic a more physiological scenario, guinea pigs are generally infected via aerosol with a low dose of *M. tuberculosis*. By following mycobacterial exposure, this in vivo model first develops primary lesions, which are then substituted by secondary hematogenous lesions that depend on the onset of the acquired immunity [61,62].

Interestingly, guinea pigs are frequently employed to determine the immunological effect of mycobacterial components, making them a valuable model to evaluate diagnostic skin tests and vaccine efficacy [63]. Indeed, currently, the validation of a vaccine protective effect in guinea pigs remains the gold standard animal model for the advancement of the vaccine toward clinical trials. Guinea pigs have been demonstrating their utility also in the identification of putative TB antigens that can be exploited to create new vaccines. Moreover, their bigger size also helped the researchers to perform multiple analyses over the same animals [63–65]. Despite the above-listed advantages of using guinea pigs as a TB model, there are several limitations to consider in the use of this in vivo model. One of the major hurdles associated with this model is linked to guinea pig maintenance and the limited availability of immunological tools.

Lastly, although guinea pigs display an extensive similarity to humans' immune response with respect to *M. tuberculosis* infection, this animal model cannot still provide a direct comparison to all the features of the human TB [56,66].

Rabbit. Among all the hereby discussed TB animal models, the rabbit one is the most resistant to *M. tuberculosis* infection, partially reflecting human relative resistance towards TB active form of the infection [67]. The use of the rabbit to investigate *M. tuberculosis* infection was initially proposed by Lurie in 1928, who indeed demonstrate outbred market rabbit resistance to the pathogen [68]. After *M. tuberculosis* infection through the intravenous route, *M. tuberculosis* load peaks in the lung around 4 weeks post-infection. However, after this initial exponential bacilli dissemination, rabbits can reduce the bacteria burden around 10 weeks after infection [67]. Interestingly, rabbits can contain the persistent bacilli by mounting an effective human-like adaptive immune response, which leads to the formation of a caseous granuloma. Nonetheless, it is still unclear if and how closely such an immune response can replica human TB both in its active and latent form [56,67].

Although the rabbit model owns the unique possibility to investigate *M. tuberculosis* pathogenesis, this model is not widely used because of the rabbit size and advanced biocontainment (i.e. *M. tuberculosis* presence in the urine). Lastly, the lack of immunological reagents and TB clinical symptoms that are not obvious further limit the use of this animal model [56].

Non-human primates. The possibility of reproducing a human-like *M. tuberculosis* infection pushed by 1970 to use non-human primates (NHPs) as a robust and reproducible TB animal model [69]. The initial TB studies performed in NHP models utilised the Indian rhesus macaque (*Macaca mulatta*). However, in the last decades, TB NHP model investigations have primarily employed either cynomolgus macaque (*Macaca fascicularis*) of Philippine or Mauritian origin or captive bread of Indian or Chinese rhesus macaque (*Macaca mulatta*) [70–72]. Because NHPs show high immunological similarity with the human immune system, they are considered the most attractive models to study both active TB and LTBI [73–75]. Indeed, macaques, once infected with *M. tuberculosis*, can develop human-like granuloma structures, and mimic the clinical TB spectrum of the human host [69,76]. However, in spite of NHPs-human immune system parallelism, further studies are needed to confirm the human-like NHP response to the antitubercular treatment [77].

Rhesus macaques were initially infected with the H37Rv *M. tuberculosis* strain, causing the animal to develop active TB within 50–60 days post-infection. Then, to allow the establishment of the latent TB form, NHPs were infected with low and/or diverse *M. tuberculosis* strains [74]. Interestingly, NHPs studies using modified *M. tuberculosis* strains previously tested in the rodent model proved significant diversity in the pathology, bacterial load and immune response [78]. Thus, suggesting that the NHP model can be exploited to investigate the role of specific bacterial genes putatively relevant for the establishment/progression of the infection. Lastly, because within the NHPs each single mycobacterial can develop a single granuloma, one single animal can be assayed for mycobacterial persistence and pathogenicity and attenuation [69,79].

Moreover, NHPs are also a valuable model for settling new diagnostics and therapeutics technologies and preventing measures [74]. Among the developed technology, the fluorine-18 fluorodeoxyglucose (18F-FDG) positron emission tomography with computer tomography (PER/CT) emerged as a powerful tool to study and consistently analyse *M. tuberculosis*-mediated alveolar lesions (i.e. granuloma), and to track bacilli intrapulmonary spread, individual granuloma phenotypic variation and perturbation, and lastly TB progression [74].

Although NHP models allow the investigation of TB infection in an accurate preclinical model, the use of the NHP model presents diverse downsides. Still, diverse optimisations need to be

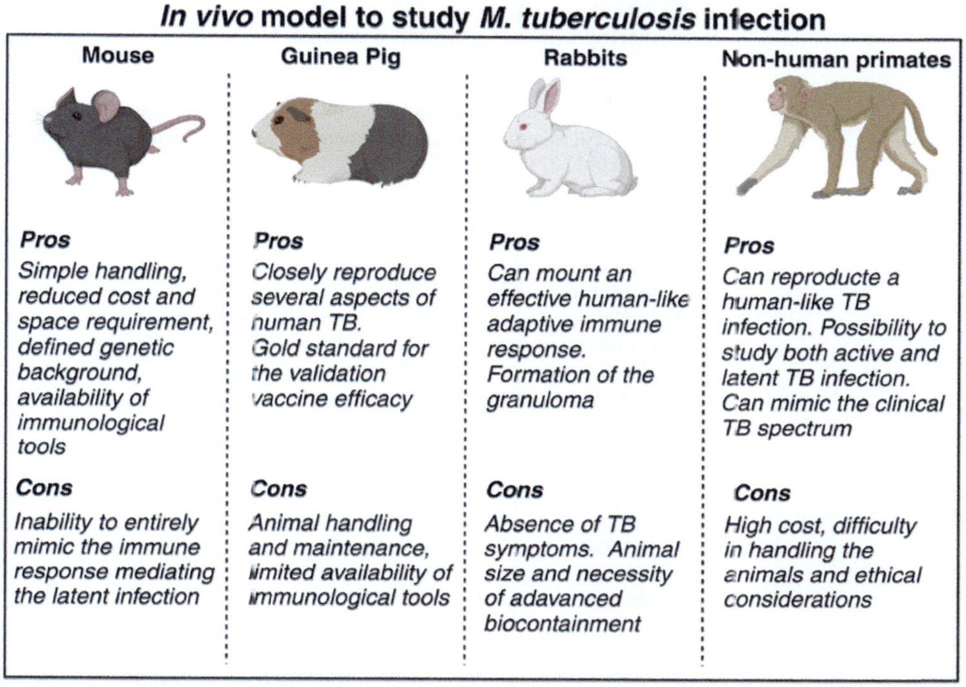

Figure 9.3 Advantages and limits of conventional organisms to model tuberculosis infection.

done to unveil the reported difference due to both the diverse species of NHPs and *M. tuberculosis* strains used, and the route of infection. Furthermore, the experimental use of the NHP model is also restricted by the limited number of possible experiments that can be performed, the reduced availability of reagents, the high cost, the difficulty in handling the animals and ethical considerations (Fig. 9.3).

References

[1] G. Streisinger, et al., Production of clones of homozygous diploid zebra fish (Brachydanio rerio), Nature 291 (5813) (1981) 293–296.
[2] K. Howe, et al., The zebrafish reference genome sequence and its relationship to the human genome, Nature 496 (7446) (2013) 498–503.
[3] A. Weintraub, All eyes on zebrafish, Laboratory Animals (NY) 46 (8) (2017) 323–326.
[4] R. Vaghela, et al., Actually seeing what is going on - intravital microscopy in tissue engineering, Frontiers in Bioengineering and Biotechnology 9 (2021) 627462.

[5] P. Herbomel, B. Thisse, C. Thisse, Ontogeny and behaviour of early macrophages in the zebrafish embryo, Development 126 (17) (1999) 3735–3745.

[6] P. Herbomel, B. Thisse, C. Thisse, Zebrafish early macrophages colonize cephalic mesenchyme and developing brain, retina, and epidermis through a M-CSF receptor-dependent invasive process, Developmental Biology 238 (2) (2001) 274–288.

[7] F. Ellett, et al., mpegl promoter transgenes direct macrophage-lineage expression in zebrafish, Blood 117 (4) (2011) e49–e56.

[8] E.M. Walton, et al., The macrophage-specific promoter mfap4 allows live, long-term analysis of macrophage behavior during mycobacterial infection in zebrafish, PLoS One 10 (10) (2015) e0138949.

[9] C. Hall, et al., The zebrafish lysozyme C promoter drives myeloid-specific expression in transgenic fish, BMC Developmental Biology 7 (2007) 42.

[10] G.J. Lieschke, et al., Morphologic and functional characterization of granulocytes and macrophages in embryonic and adult zebrafish, Blood 98 (10) (2001) 3087–3096.

[11] R.M. White, et al., Transparent adult zebrafish as a tool for in vivo transplantation analysis, Cell Stem Cell 2 (2) (2008) 183–189.

[12] A.H. Meijer, H.P. Spaink, Host-pathogen interactions made transparent with the zebrafish model, Current Drug Targets 12 (7) (2011) 1000–1017.

[13] J.M. Davis, et al., Real-time visualization of mycobacterium-macrophage interactions leading to initiation of granuloma formation in zebrafish embryos, Immunity 17 (6) (2002) 693–702.

[14] T.K. Prajsnar, et al., A novel vertebrate model of *Staphylococcus aureus* infection reveals phagocyte-dependent resistance of zebrafish to non-host specialized pathogens, Cellular Microbiology 10 (11) (2008) 2312–2325.

[15] F. Fenaroli, et al., Nanoparticles as drug delivery system against tuberculosis in zebrafish embryos: direct visualization and treatment, ACS Nano 8 (7) (2014) 7014–7026.

[16] S. Sieber, et al., Zebrafish as a predictive screening model to assess macrophage clearance of liposomes in vivo, Nanomedicine 17 (2019) 82–93.

[17] B.R. Kingston, et al., Specific endothelial cells govern nanoparticle entry into solid tumors, ACS Nano 15 (9) (2021) 14080–14094.

[18] Y. Sakurai, H. Akita, H. Harashima, Targeting tumor endothelial cells with nanoparticles, International Journal of Molecular Sciences 20 (23) (2019).

[19] N.K. Dal, et al., Zebrafish embryos allow prediction of nanoparticle circulation times in mice and facilitate quantification of nanoparticle-cell interactions, Small 16 (5) (2020) e1906719.

[20] F. Campbell, et al., Directing nanoparticle biodistribution through evasion and exploitation of stab2-dependent nanoparticle uptake, ACS Nano 12 (3) (2018) 2138–2150.

[21] G. Arias-Alpizar, et al., Light-triggered switching of liposome surface charge directs delivery of membrane impermeable payloads in vivo, Nature Communications 11 (1) (2020) 3638.

[22] J. Rességuier, et al., Biodistribution of surfactant-free poly(lactic-acid) nanoparticles and uptake by endothelial cells and phagocytes in zebrafish: evidence for endothelium to macrophage transfer, Journal of Controlled Release 331 (2021) 228–245.

[23] S. Cassar, et al., Use of zebrafish in drug discovery toxicology, Chemical Research in Toxicology 33 (1) (2020) 95–118.

[24] N. Palha, et al., Real-time whole-body visualization of Chikungunya Virus infection and host interferon response in zebrafish, PLoS Pathogens 9 (9) (2013) e1003619.
[25] C.B. Vibe, et al., Thioridazine in PLGA nanoparticles reduces toxicity and improves rifampicin therapy against mycobacterial infection in zebrafish, Nanotoxicology 10 (6) (2016) 680–688.
[26] J. Tao, et al., Toward understanding the prolonged circulation and elimination mechanism of crosslinked polymeric micelles in zebrafish model, Biomaterials 256 (2020) 120180.
[27] J. Tao, et al., Particle integrity and size effect on the journey of polymeric nanocarriers in zebrafish model and the correlation with mice, Small 17 (43) (2021) e2103584.
[28] V. Torraca, S. Mostowy, Zebrafish infection: from pathogenesis to cell biology, Trends in Cell Biology 28 (2) (2018) 143–156.
[29] C. Sullivan, et al., Modeling virus-induced inflammation in zebrafish: a balance between infection control and excessive inflammation, Frontiers in Immunology 12 (2021) 636623.
[30] E.E. Rosowski, et al., The zebrafish as a model host for invasive fungal infections, Journal of Fungi (Basel) 4 (4) (2018).
[31] L.S. Ulanova, et al., Treatment of Francisella infections via PLGA- and lipid-based nanoparticle delivery of antibiotics in a zebrafish model, Diseases of Aquatic Organisms 125 (1) (2017) 19–29.
[32] T. Tønjum, et al., Differentiation of Mycobacterium ulcerans, M. marinum, and M. haemophilum: mapping of their relationships to *M. tuberculosis* by fatty acid profile analysis, DNA-DNA hybridization, and 16S rRNA gene sequence analysis, Journal of Clinical Microbiology 36 (4) (1998) 918–925.
[33] S.H. Oehlers, et al., Interception of host angiogenic signalling limits mycobacterial growth, Nature 517 (7536) (2015) 612–615.
[34] F. Fenaroli, et al., Enhanced permeability and retention-like extravasation of nanoparticles from the vasculature into tuberculosis granulomas in zebrafish and mouse models, ACS Nano 12 (8) (2018) 8646–8661.
[35] M. Datta, et al., Anti-vascular endothelial growth factor treatment normalizes tuberculosis granuloma vasculature and improves small molecule delivery, Proceedings of the National Academy of Sciences of the U S A 112 (6) (2015) 1827–1832.
[36] S.Y. Tong, et al., *Staphylococcus aureus* infections: epidemiology, pathophysiology, clinical manifestations, and management, Clinical Microbiology Reviews 28 (3) (2015) 603–661.
[37] J.F. Gibson, et al., Neutrophils use selective autophagy receptor Sqstm1/p62 to target *Staphylococcus aureus* for degradation in vivo in zebrafish, Autophagy 17 (6) (2021) 1448–1457.
[38] T.K. Prajsnar, et al., The autophagic response to *Staphylococcus aureus* provides an intracellular niche in neutrophils, Autophagy 17 (4) (2021) 888–902.
[39] K.D. Buchan, et al., Human-specific staphylococcal virulence factors enhance pathogenicity in a humanised zebrafish C5a receptor model, Journal of Cell Science 134 (5) (2021).
[40] J. Trousil, et al., Rifampicin nanoformulation enhances treatment of tuberculosis in zebrafish, Biomacromolecules 20 (4) (2019) 1798–1815.
[41] F. Fenaroli, et al., Polymersomes eradicating intracellular bacteria, ACS Nano 14 (7) (2020) 8287–8298.

[42] X. Zhang, et al., Monitoring local delivery of vancomycin from gelatin nanospheres in zebrafish larvae, International Journal of Nanomedicine 13 (2018) 5377–5394.

[43] F. Anversa Dimer, et al., PLGA nanocapsules improve the delivery of clarithromycin to kill intracellular *Staphylococcus aureus* and Mycobacterium abscessus, Nanomedicine 24 (2020) 102125.

[44] R.M. Mccune, W. Mcdermott, R. Tompsett, The fate of *Mycobacterium tuberculosis* in mouse tissues as determined by the microbial enumeration technique. II. The conversion of tuberculous infection to the latent state by the administration of pyrazinamide and a companion drug, Journal of Experimental Medicine 104 (5) (November 1956) 763–802, https://doi.org/10.1084/jem.104.5.763.

[45] J.L. Sever, G.P. Youmans, Enumeration of viable tubercle bacilli from the organs of nonimmunized and immunized mice, American Review of Tuberculosis 76 (4) (October 1957) 616–635, https://doi.org/10.1164/artpd.1957.76.4.616.

[46] R.M. McCune, F.M. Feldmann, W. McDermott, Microbial persistence. II. Characteristics of the sterile state of tubercle bacilli, Journal of Experimental Medicine 123 (3) (March 1966) 469–486, https://doi.org/10.1084/jem.123.3.469.

[47] E.R. Driver, et al., Evaluation of a mouse model of necrotic granuloma formation using C3HeB/FeJ mice for testing of drugs against *Mycobacterium tuberculosis*, Antimicrobial Agents and Chemotherapy 56 (6) (June 2012) 3181–3195, https://doi.org/10.1128/AAC.00217-12.

[48] J. Harper, et al., Mouse model of necrotic tuberculosis granulomas develops hypoxic lesions, The Journal of Infectious Diseases 205 (4) (Febuary 2012) 595–602, https://doi.org/10.1093/infdis/jir786.

[49] S.M. Irwin, et al., Presence of multiple lesion types with vastly different microenvironments in C3HeB/FeJ mice following aerosol infection with *Mycobacterium tuberculosis*, Disease Models & Mechanisms 8 (6) (June 2015) 591–602, https://doi.org/10.1242/dmm.019570.

[50] I. Kramnik, P. Demant, B.B. Bloom, Susceptibility to tuberculosis as a complex genetic trait: analysis using recombinant congenic strains of mice, in: D.J. Chadwick, G. Cardew (Eds.), Novartis Foundation Symposia, John Wiley & Sons, Ltd, Chichester, UK, 1998, pp. 120–137, https://doi.org/10.1002/0470846526.ch9.

[51] I. Kramnik, Genetic dissection of host resistance to *Mycobacterium tuberculosis*: the sst1 locus and the Ipr1 gene, in: B. Beutler (Ed.), Immunology, Phenotype First: How Mutations Have Established New Principles and Pathways in Immunology, vol 321, Springer Berlin Heidelberg, Berlin, Heidelberg, 2008, pp. 123–148, https://doi.org/10.1007/978-3-540-75203-5_6.

[52] I. Kramnik, W.F. Dietrich, P. Demant, B.R. Bloom, Genetic control of resistance to experimental infection with virulent *Mycobacterium tuberculosis*, Proceedings of the National Academy of Sciences of the United States of America 97 (15) (July 2000) 8560–8565, https://doi.org/10.1073/pnas.150227197.

[53] C.R. Plumlee, et al., Ultra-low dose aerosol infection of mice with *Mycobacterium tuberculosis* more closely models human tuberculosis, Cell Host & Microbe 29 (1) (January 2021) 68–82, https://doi.org/10.1016/j.chom.2020.10.003.

[54] H. Su, et al., Genetic models of latent tuberculosis in mice reveal differential influence of adaptive immunity, Journal of Experimental Medicine 218 (9) (September 2021) e20210332, https://doi.org/10.1084/jem.20210332.
[55] L. Gonzalez, N. Strbo, E.R. Podack, Humanized mice: novel model for studying mechanisms of human immune-based therapies, Immunologic Research 57 (1–3) (December 2013) 326–334, https://doi.org/10.1007/s12026-013-8471-2.
[56] A. Singh, U. Gupta, Animal models of tuberculosis: lesson learnt, Indian Journal of Medical Research 147 (5) (2018) 456, https://doi.org/10.4103/ijmr.IJMR_554_18.
[57] M.A. Brehm, et al., Parameters for establishing humanized mouse models to study human immunity: analysis of human hematopoietic stem cell engraftment in three immunodeficient strains of mice bearing the IL2rγnull mutation, Clinical Immunology 135 (1) (April 2010) 84–98, https://doi.org/10.1016/j.clim.2009.12.008.
[58] M. Lepard, et al., Comparing current and next-generation humanized mouse models for advancing HIV and HIV/mtb Co-infection studies, Viruses 14 (9) (August 2022) 1927, https://doi.org/10.3390/v14091927.
[59] S.P. McDermott, K. Eppert, E.R. Lechman, M. Doedens, J.E. Dick, Comparison of human cord blood engraftment between immunocompromised mouse strains, Blood 116 (2) (July 2010) 193–200, https://doi.org/10.1182/blood-2010-02-271841.
[60] T. Pearson, et al., Non-obese diabetic–recombination activating gene-1 (NOD– Rag 1 null) interleukin (IL)-2 receptor common gamma chain (IL 2 rγ null) null mice: a radioresistant model for human lymphohaematopoietic engraftment, Clinical and Experimental Immunology 154 (2) (October 2008) 270–284, https://doi.org/10.1111/j.1365-2249.2008.03753.x.
[61] D. Dube, R. Sharma, N. Mody, M. Gupta, U. Agrawal, S.P. Vyas, Animal models of tuberculosis, in: Animal Biotechnology, Elsevier, 2020, pp. 21–41, https://doi.org/10.1016/B978-0-12-811710-1.00002-1.
[62] A.J. Lenaerts, et al., Location of persisting mycobacteria in a Guinea pig model of tuberculosis revealed by r207910, Antimicrobial Agents and Chemotherapy 51 (9) (September 2007) 3338–3345, https://doi.org/10.1128/AAC.00276-07.
[63] S. Clark, Y. Hall, A. Williams, Animal models of tuberculosis: Guinea pigs, Cold Spring Harbor Perspectives in Medicine 5 (5) (May 2015) a018572, https://doi.org/10.1101/cshperspect.a018572.
[64] I.M. Orme, D.N. McMurray, J.T. Belisle, Tuberculosis vaccine development: recent progress, Trends in Microbiology 9 (3) (March 2001) 115–118, https://doi.org/10.1016/S0966-842X(00)01949-1.
[65] A. Williams, et al., An assay to compare the infectivity of *Mycobacterium tuberculosis* isolates based on aerosol infection of Guinea pigs and assessment of bacteriology, Tuberculosis 85 (3) (May 2005) 177–184, https://doi.org/10.1016/j.tube.2004.11.001.
[66] J. Gao, et al., Guinea pig infected with *Mycobacterium tuberculosis* via oral consumption, Journal of Applied Animal Research 46 (1) (January 2018) 1323–1328, https://doi.org/10.1080/09712119.2018.1505622.
[67] Y.C. Manabe, et al., The aerosol rabbit model of TB latency, reactivation and immune reconstitution inflammatory syndrome, Tuberculosis 88 (3) (May 2008) 187–196, https://doi.org/10.1016/j.tube.2007.10.006.

[68] M.B. Lurie, The fate of human and bovine tubercle bacilli in various organs of the rabbit, Journal of Experimental Medicine 48 (2) (August 1928) 155–182, https://doi.org/10.1084/jem.48.2.155.
[69] D. Kaushal, S. Mehra, P.J. Didier, A.A. Lackner, The non-human primate model of tuberculosis: primate model of TB, Journal of Medical Primatology 41 (3) (June 2012) 191–201, https://doi.org/10.1111/j.1600-0684.2012.00536.x.
[70] P.L. Lin, et al., The multistage vaccine H56 boosts the effects of BCG to protect cynomolgus macaques against active tuberculosis and reactivation of latent *Mycobacterium tuberculosis* infection, Journal of Clinical Investigation 122 (1) (January 2012) 303–314, https://doi.org/10.1172/JCI46252.
[71] G.P. Walsh, et al., The Philippine cynomolgus monkey (Macaca fasicularis) provides a new nonhuman primate model of tuberculosis that resembles human disease, Nature Medicine 2 (4) (April 1996) 430–436, https://doi.org/10.1038/nm0496-430.
[72] J.A.M. Langermans, et al., Divergent effect of bacillus Calmette–Guérin (BCG) vaccination on *Mycobacterium tuberculosis* infection in highly related macaque species: implications for primate models in tuberculosis vaccine research, Proceedings of the National Academy of Sciences of the United States of America 98 (20) (September 2001) 11497–11502, https://doi.org/10.1073/pnas.201404898.
[73] T.W. Foreman, et al., CD4 + T-cell–independent mechanisms suppress reactivation of latent tuberculosis in a macaque model of HIV coinfection, Proceedings of the National Academy of Sciences of the United States of America 113 (38) (September 2016), https://doi.org/10.1073/pnas.1611987113.
[74] T.W. Foreman, S. Mehra, A.A. Lackner, D. Kaushal, Translational research in the nonhuman primate model of tuberculosis, ILAR Journal 58 (2) (December 2017) 151–159, https://doi.org/10.1093/ilar/ilx015.
[75] P.A. Darrah, et al., Aerosol vaccination with AERAS-402 elicits robust cellular immune responses in the lungs of rhesus macaques but fails to protect against high-dose *Mycobacterium tuberculosis* challenge, Journal of Illustration 193 (4) (August 2014) 1799–1811, https://doi.org/10.4049/jimmunol.1400676.
[76] S. Mehra, et al., Granuloma correlates of protection against tuberculosis and mechanisms of immune modulation by *Mycobacterium tuberculosis*, The Journal of Infectious Diseases 207 (7) (April 2013) 1115–1127, https://doi.org/10.1093/infdis/jis778.
[77] G. Magombedze, D. Dowdy, N. Mulder, Latent tuberculosis: models, computational efforts and the pathogen's regulatory mechanisms during dormancy, Frontiers in Bioengineering and Biotechnology 1 (2013), https://doi.org/10.3389/fbioe.2013.00004.
[78] S. Mehra, et al., The DosR regulon modulates adaptive immunity and is essential for *Mycobacterium tuberculosis* persistence, American Journal of Respiratory and Critical Care Medicine 191 (10) (May 2015) 1185–1196, https://doi.org/10.1164/rccm.201408-1502OC.
[79] R. Gopal, et al., S100A8/A9 proteins mediate neutrophilic inflammation and lung pathology during tuberculosis, American Journal of Respiratory and Critical Care Medicine 188 (9) (November 2013) 1137–1146, https://doi.org/10.1164/rccm.201304-0803OC.

10

Clinical translation and envisioned impact of nanotech for infection control: Economy, government policy and public awareness

Xiaohan Ma and Alessandro Poma
Division of Biomaterials and Tissue Engineering, UCL Eastman Dental Institute, Royal Free Hospital, UCL Medical School, London, United Kingdom

1. Introduction: Why nanotechnology against infections?

Infections constitute a significant portion of the global disease burden, with notable mortality rates linked to causes such as lower respiratory infections, diarrhoea, tuberculosis (TB), etc. (Fig. 10.1A). Particularly in developing countries, where resources like vaccines and anti-infectives may be constrained, mortality rates are notably elevated (Fig. 10.1B). Although the overall mortality is on a declining trajectory, a substantial gap persists between countries belonging to the high or low socio-demographic index, as evidenced by temporal trends in mortality (Fig. 10.1C). Regrettably, clinical trials for these infectious diseases trail behind those for conditions such as cancer and cardiovascular diseases (Fig. 10.1D). Therefore, there exists a pressing imperative to discern pragmatic and impactful strategies that facilitate enhanced treatment approaches for infectious diseases [1].

For treating these infections, antibiotics often serve as the primary choice. Under normal circumstances, antibiotics effectively inhibit the presence of various microbes, alleviating associated signs and symptoms. However, the amalgamation of antibiotics with other agents targeting specific bacterial resistance mechanisms is presently confronted with a significant surge in

Nanotechnology Tools for Infection Control. https://doi.org/10.1016/B978-0-12-823994-0.00004-9

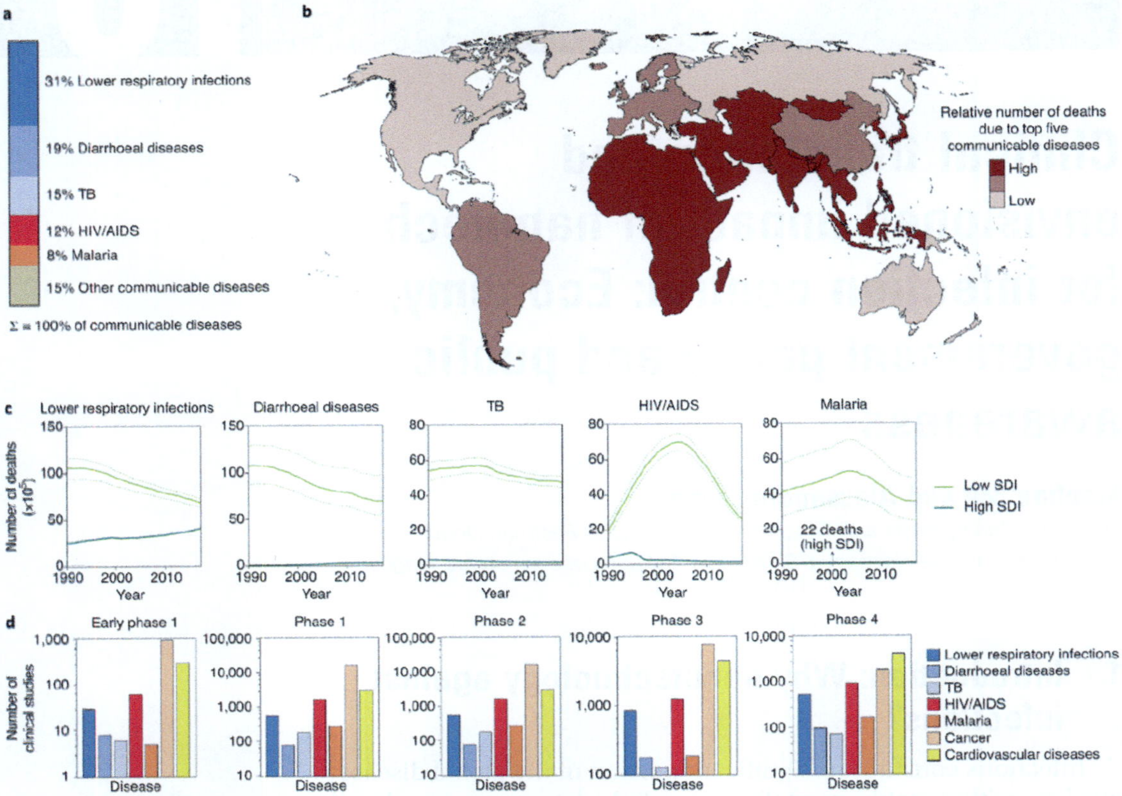

Figure 10.1 Global burden of infectious diseases. Reproduced with permission from Kirtane et al. [1].

resistance across numerous bacterial species, as reported by the European Antimicrobial Resistance Surveillance Network (EARS-Net) [2,3]. Since 1950, an escalating concern for governmental bodies and healthcare professionals revolves around the growing resistance of microbial strains to established therapeutic regimens. This dilemma is exacerbated by the scarcity of alternative treatments and strategies to overcome the challenges and barriers (such as biofilms), posed by these microbes during infection treatment [4,5]. Multidrug-resistant microorganisms pose a formidable and escalating global public health menace, complicating the successful treatment of various healthcare-associated infections with existing antibiotics [6]. Particularly vulnerable are patients in intensive care units or those undergoing surgery, transplantation, or cancer treatment [7]. As an illustrative case, over the past few decades, *Staphylococcus aureus* (*S. aureus*) has undergone multiple waves of antibiotic resistance and currently exhibits resistance to the entire β-lactam class of antibiotics, including penicillins, cephalosporins, and carbapenems [8]. These β-lactam antibiotic-resistant *S. aureus* strains are commonly referred to as methicillin-resistant *S. aureus* (MRSA) or superbugs. The proportion of healthcare-associated *S. aureus* infections attributed to MRSA has risen from 2% in 1974 to 64% in 2004 [9,10]. This predicament is partly attributed to the overuse and misuse of antibiotics, as well as the lack of novel therapies developed to address this pressing global health challenge [7].

As previously emphasised in this volume, the development of novel antibiotics demands substantial economic and labour investments, coupled with a time-intensive process [11]. The conventional application of oral or intravenous drugs to combat microbial infections presents several challenges. Current regimens, which often involve large doses to ensure adequate concentrations at the targeted organisms, are not universally effective and can lead to undesirable side effects, exacerbating drug resistance in microorganisms [5]. Moreover, in the case of multidrug-resistant infections, the administration of even higher antibiotic doses may result in intolerable toxic and adverse effects, therefore necessitating an urgent exploration of alternative strategies [12]. The poor availability of alternative treatments and strategies to address this issue is a matter of significant concern for governmental bodies and healthcare professionals, profoundly impacting global public health. One proposed avenue to tackle this challenge involves the utilisation of nanomaterials to augment and invigorate the antimicrobial effectiveness of both existing and emerging novel drug therapies [5].

In this context, nanomaterials introduce a wholly novel approach to combat microbial infections, as they are unfamiliar to bacteria and thus absent from the array of natural defences typically targeted by conventional antibiotic molecules. In an era marked by the alarming rise of multidrug resistance, the exploration of novel nanoantibiotics and the restructuring of existing antibiotics using nano-based drug delivery platforms emerge as critically significant areas. Undoubtedly, nanosystems pave the way for an entirely new antimicrobial frontier [13]. Nanostructures with effective functionality, however, while initially drawing inspiration from nature, transcend mere replication of observed phenomena. Rather, they are meticulously designed and engineered through a process that involves comprehending the fundamental principles governing optimised patterns in biological systems. Subsequently, constraints and boundary conditions associated with fabrication and the economic capabilities of synthetic materials are established to guide the design and construction of these nanostructures [13].

Mela and Kaminski in their paper titled *'Nano-vehicles to revitalise existing antimicrobials'* delve into the application of nanomaterials for precise and targeted drug delivery, as well as enhancing drug efficacy against bacteria [14]. They emphasise the significance of manipulating the surface properties of metallic, organic and DNA-based nanostructures to enable functionalisation with drugs and other molecules, particularly for targeted cell interactions. There is increasing supporting evidence for the success of this approach in experimental models, particularly in the case of potential of DNA nanostructures designed for precise patterns at the atomic level to deliver antimicrobials [5].

More in detail, the susceptibility of bacteria to nanoparticles (NPs) is contingent upon their biochemical composition, as various NPs target distinct biomolecules [15]. Additionally, rapidly proliferating bacteria exhibit greater susceptibility to both NPs and antibiotics compared to their slower-growing counterparts. This discrepancy may arise from the variable expression of stress-response genes observed between rapidly growing and slowly growing bacteria [15,16]. Notably, the antibacterial efficacy of NPs is more pronounced against Gram-positive bacteria than Gram-negative ones. This observation is likely tied to the nonporous nature of the cell walls in Gram-negative bacteria, which functions as a barrier hindering NPs entry [17]. Conversely, the relatively porous cell walls of Gram-positive bacteria, featuring covalent links with neighbouring proteins and components, facilitate the penetration of foreign molecules [17,18].

NPs with antibacterial properties have the potential to target multiple biomolecules and mitigate the evolution of multidrug-resistant microorganisms [19]. However, the translation of NPs into clinical use necessitates not only appropriate synthesis methods but also a comprehensive understanding of the physicochemical characteristics, in vitro and in vivo effects, biodistribution, pharmacokinetics and pharmacodynamics [18,20].

The distinct advantages of using NPs and other nanotechnologies as antibacterial agents, in contrast to traditional antibiotics, can be summarised as follows:

1. The large surface-area-to-volume ratio of NPs and, more broadly, of nanomaterials enhances the contact area with target organisms.
2. NPs with antimicrobial activity can overcome common resistance mechanisms, which normally result in evading the antibacterial activity of antimicrobial agents. These mechanisms include enzyme inactivation, reduced cell permeability,

modification of target sites/enzymes, biofilm formation and increased efflux through the overexpression of efflux pumps (Fig. 10.2, left) [18,21].

3. Employing multiple mechanisms simultaneously to combat microbes, such as interacting with bacterial cells, regulating cell membrane penetration and interfering with molecular pathways [22–25].
4. Serving as effective carriers of antibiotics [26,27]. NPs can act as vectors for drug transfer, enabling the delivery of higher doses of antimicrobial agents to infected sites [18,28].

The currently accepted mechanisms for the action of nanomaterials in combating bacterial infections include (1) direct interaction with the bacteria, leading to the disruption of membrane potential and integrity; (2) triggering host immune responses; (3) inhibition of biofilm formation; (4) generation of reactive oxygen species (ROS); and (5) inhibition of RNA and protein

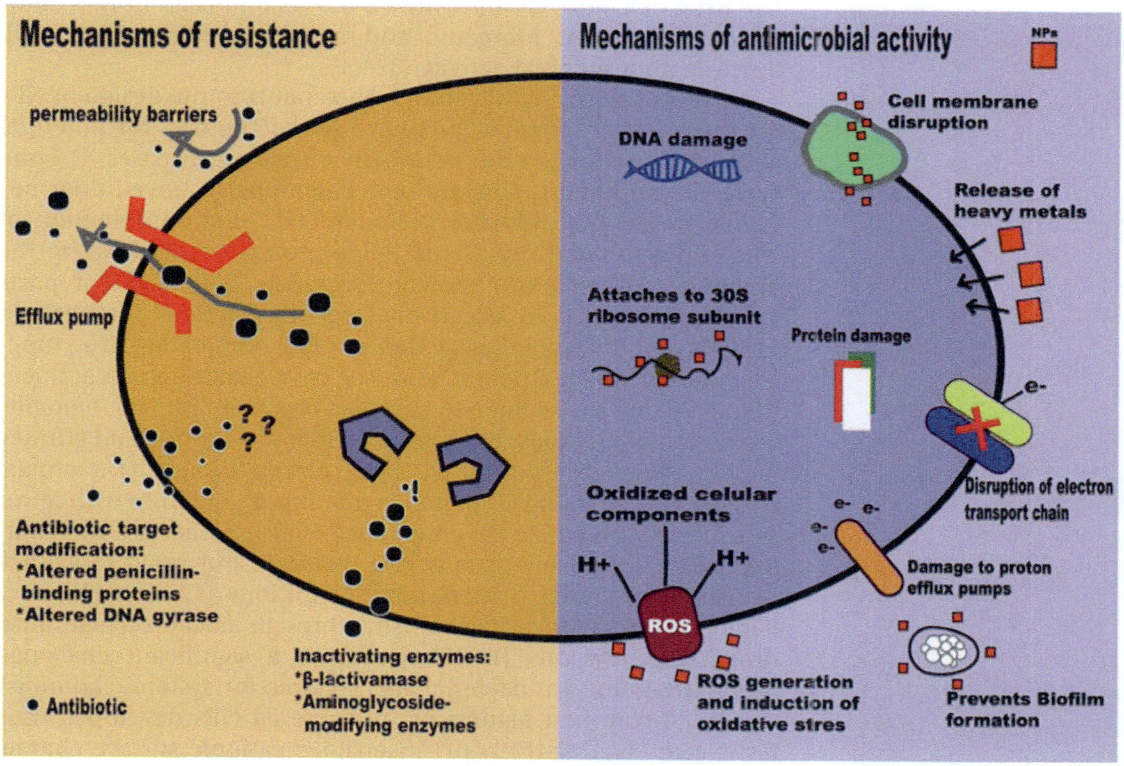

Figure 10.2 Mechanisms of antimicrobial resistance and actions of NPs. Reproduced with permission from Lee et al. [18].

synthesis through the induction of intracellular effects (Fig. 10.2, right) [18,28,29].

Furthermore, numerous studies have demonstrated a heightened accumulation of nanocarriers at infection sites as opposed to non-infected areas. In a specific investigation involving a unilateral bacterial infection in the calf muscle of rats, the animals received intravenous treatment with radiolabelled NPs, finding that the NPs concentration was approximately 40-fold higher (measured as the percentage of injected dose per gram of tissue) in the abscess compared to the muscle tissue [1].

Therefore, NPs are primarily harnessed through two antimicrobial mechanisms: either enhancing the efficacy of existing antibiotics (e.g. by serving as cargo-loading systems) or exerting entirely new bactericidal actions without antibiotics, acting as bioactives themselves [30,31]. Typically, the first class of NPs utilises their small size, large surface and unique surface chemistry to incorporate antimicrobials on the surface or within the core of biodegradable and/or biocompatible NPs, thus facilitating effective drug delivery [32]. In contrast, the second class of NPs comprises a range of inorganic and organic nanomaterials with intrinsic antimicrobial activity [32–35].

In recent years, significant advancements in the design of NPs for drug delivery applications have paved the way for potential strategies to enhance the treatment of various diseases. Despite these developments, NPs are only beginning to unveil their potential in treating infections. Nonetheless, the combination of NPs and antimicrobial agents holds promise in addressing the ongoing crisis of antimicrobial resistance [21]. Recent reports showcase progress in selectively targeting bacterial membranes for lysis [35], improving drug delivery [36], enhancing drug function [37–39] and the potential for selective accumulation at infection sites due to heightened vascular permeability [40]. Notably, the design of methods to improve antibiotic targeting and efficacy in vivo, such as through NP drug carrier design, is a crucial endeavour that could (1) enhance treatment outcomes with fewer side effects, (2) reduce the emergence of drug resistance by avoiding ineffective dosing or targeting that can spur rapid resistance development under unfavourable conditions [41] and (3) overcome drug resistance mechanisms through sustained high local drug concentrations [11,27]. However, a significant challenge lies in designing antibacterial NPs suitable for systemic administration. A common feature of antibacterial NPs developed thus far is a robust, relatively pH-insensitive cationic surface charge. While this charge exhibits potent bactericidal activity in vitro [42], it lacks specificity for bacteria and, in some cases, can adversely affect the blood circulation and biodistribution properties of NPs [43], potentially leading to toxicity [44]. Bacteria, being highly adaptable, have evolved to thrive in diverse environments, and low pH is particularly significant due to its association with serious infections and its implications for treatment. Certain antibiotics experience significant loss of activity in acidic conditions [45] and a reduction in localised pH often occurs as a consequence of worsening disease severity and prognosis, precisely when maximal efficacy is crucially important [46]. Bacteria may inhabit acidic environments in the body either due to natural prevailing conditions, such as in the stomach (pH 1.0–2.0), intestines (pH 5.0–8.0), vaginal tissue (pH 4.0–5.0), bladder (pH 4.5–8.0) and skin (pH 4.0–5.5) [47], or through a combination of bacterial activity and the resulting immune response. Infections associated with acidity result from poor oxygenation conditions, which trigger anaerobic fermentation in certain bacteria, thus producing organic acids like lactic and acetic acids [48]. Inflammation exacerbates acidity due to increased levels of acidic products, including lactic acid produced during phagocytosis [49]. These factors contribute to reducing the pH of infection sites, sometimes as low as pH 5.5 [50]. Clinical scenarios where pH-dependent loss of drug activity may be pertinent include pneumonias, particularly in cystic fibrosis patients [51], abscesses [52], and *Helicobacter pylori* (*H. Pylori*) infections, a major cause of peptic ulcers [53].

Taking the above into account, drugs carried by nanocarriers offer several distinctive characteristics in comparison with traditional drugs:

(1) Nanodrug carriers can traverse not only the bloodstream into capillaries but also navigate through endothelial cell gaps into lesions [54]. Drugs delivered by nanodrug carriers can be absorbed by cells through pinocytosis, significantly improving bioavailability.

(2) The substantial surface area of nano-sized carriers allows them to encapsulate hydrophobic drugs, enhancing drug solubility and reducing the need for co-solvents that are commonly used in conventional drugs, thereby minimising side effects.

(3) Drugs delivered by nanocarriers, as opposed to drug administration alone, enable targeted drug therapy with high bioavailability [55]. Nanodrug carriers, when modified with targeted tissue specificity (e.g. folic acid modification for drug-loading NPs and/or magnetic NPs), allow the facilitation of efficient drug delivery to specific tissues. This results not only in the overall reduction of the required administration dosage, which also exhibits a direct effect on the treatment costs, but also mitigates potential side effects of the drugs [56,57].

(4) Nanometre drug carriers can prolong the half-life of drug elimination, enhancing the duration and efficacy of drug concentration in the blood [58]. This leads to a reduction in the frequency of drug administration.

(5) Nanoscale drug carriers have the ability to traverse biological barriers in the human body, including the blood–brain barrier, blood–eye barrier and other cell biological membrane barriers. This enables drugs to reach lesion sites, thereby increasing overall efficacy [59–61].

Polymeric NPs emerge as compelling candidates for delivering antibiotics in bacterial infections. Typically, these carriers enable an increase in the maximal tolerated dose and the therapeutic index of encapsulated antibiotics [62,63]. This enhancement is attributed to modifications in the release and disposition of the antibiotic when encapsulated, as well as alterations in its biodistribution. Furthermore, intravenous administration of NPs holds promise for treating infections caused by intracellularly persisting microbes (e.g. *Brucella, Salmonella, Listeria* or *Mycobacterium*). In contrast, free drugs are cleared from the plasma within 12–24 h post-administration. Just to provide an example, the global impact of TB, claiming millions of lives, currently necessitates a comprehensive treatment involving multiple drug formulations over extended periods. However, challenges such as patient non-compliance with the treatment, as mentioned, can easily lead to multidrug resistance, escalating morbidity and mortality associated with mycobacterial TB. A recent paper has shed light on the current landscape of pulmonary TB treatment, emphasising the critical need for innovative approaches, and advocating for inhalation therapy utilising drug-loaded nano- and micron-sized materials, both organic and metallic, as vectors for delivering existing and novel TB drugs. In this respect, the authors also underscored the use of metallic NPs to augment the antimicrobial properties and efficacy of drug formulations [5]. Furthermore, it is also important to outline the works of Sharma et al. in this respect, where they elucidated that the treatment of *Mycobacterium tuberculosis*-infected mice with poly(lactic-*co*-glycolic acid) (PLGA) NPs formulations (five oral doses every 10 days) led to complete bacterial clearance from organs. Free drugs achieved bacterial clearance only after daily administration of 46 doses. Similar results were also obtained in guinea pigs [64]. The effectiveness of these PLGA NPs was further augmented by covalently attaching a lectin (a protein which binds to carbohydrates), wheat germ agglutinin [65]. Lectin-modified NPs achieved bacterial clearance in lungs, liver and spleen after three oral doses administered every 14 days (compared to 45 daily doses of free drugs). As proposed by the authors, the prolonged circulation of drugs encapsulated in lectin-decorated NPs may be attributed to the protein moieties enhancing prolonged adhesion of NPs to the intestinal surface [66].

Polymeric NPs, specifically those composed of alginate and pullulan, have been employed in the treatment of various microbial diseases caused by *Klebsiella pneumoniae* [67], *P. aeruginosa* [68] and *Diphtheria* [69]. These polymeric formulations showcase versatility in addressing a spectrum of infectious agents, demonstrating their potential in combating microbial diseases. Similarly, polymeric NPs composed of chitosan have found applications in diverse microbiological diseases caused by *Escherichia coli (E. coli)* [70] and *P. aeruginosa* [71], in addition to a number of viruses [72–75]. The adaptability of chitosan-based NPs across different pathogens highlights their broad utility in the field of antimicrobial therapy, showcasing their potential in addressing a range of infectious diseases [76].

NPs have also proven effective in shielding antibiotic agents from enzymatic degradation and reinstating their bactericidal effects against resistant bacteria (Fig. 10.3A). While initial results are promising, further validation through testing in animal biofilm

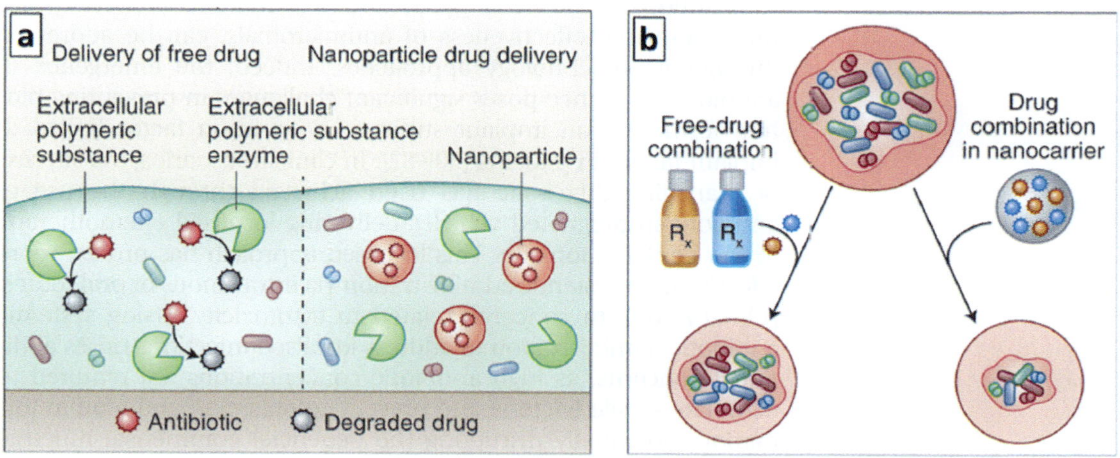

Figure 10.3 Nanocarrier systems can be designed to evade physical and chemical mechanisms for microbial drug resistance. (A) NPs can protect the cargo from drug-degrading enzymes present in the biofilm. (B) Simultaneous loading of a combination of drugs in NPs exhibited improved efficacy in comparison to the co-administration of the same free drugs. Adapted with permission from Kirtane et al. [1].

models and mechanistic confirmation is imperative to reliably showcase the ability of NPs to safeguard therapeutic payloads from enzymatic degradation. An innovative approach involves packaging multiple antimicrobial agents within the same NP (Fig. 10.3B). This strategy significantly enhances the likelihood of overcoming existing drug resistance mechanisms compared to using a single drug. Consequently, it allows for dose reduction and the treatment of drug-resistant infections. Notably, this approach dramatically reduces the number of administration events required to achieve efficacy, a particularly valuable feature in resource-limited settings [1].

Even triggered drug-release can be exploited by using tailored NPs. For example, nanocarriers designed to swiftly disintegrate upon exposure to bacterial phosphatase [77] [constructed from diblock copolymers of poly(phosphoesters) and polyethylene glycol, or PEG] and lipase [78] [constructed from triblock copolymers of poly(phosphoester), poly(caprolactone), and PEG] have been employed for the pathogen-triggered release of vancomycin [1]. More exotic applications include the combined use of natural antimicrobial products towards challenging bacteria, such as liposomal oleic acids against MRSA infections [9].

Based on the above, the delivery of antimicrobials through NPs-mediated methods certainly offers higher therapeutic efficacy compared to conventional therapies. This is achieved thanks also to the minimisation of off-target delivery and effective management of multidrug resistance [79].

Additionally, the challenge of biofilm formation, which hampers the therapeutic effectiveness of antimicrobials, can be addressed through nanotechnology approaches. Indeed, the emergence of antibiotic resistance poses significant challenges in preventing biofilm formation on implant surfaces, a common factor linked to implant failure in patients [80–82]. In clinical scenarios, the success of managing this issue has been achieved through the use of antibiotic-impregnated vehicles delivering localised chemotherapy to the implantation site. This localised approach has proven more effective than systemic administration via intravenous or oral routes, primarily due to concerns related to cytotoxicity. Using systemic antibiotic administration to address localised infections raises additional concerns, as high antibiotic concentrations are required to eliminate sessile bacteria and prevent colonisation and biofilm formation, potentially disrupting the beneficial commensal mucosal biota, such as the microbial community in the gut [83].

NPs immobilisation on implantable devices, wound dressings, bone cement or dental materials can serve as NPs-based antibacterial coating [84]. In the context of posing challenges to conventional therapeutic approaches, wound-associated biofilms harbouring a multitude of microorganisms, as mentioned before, not only present a physical barrier but also encompass various biological obstacles, including mediators produced by microorganisms, an unfavourable microenvironment, and a fraction of antibiotic-resistant organisms. Nano-sized materials are extremely suitable for penetrating biofilms, being extremely adaptable and modifiable to surmount natural barriers. This, in turn, enhances the transfer of nanomaterials, optimising both delivery and the effectiveness of drug cargo [5].

Particularly, metallic NPs demonstrate intrinsic antibiofilm formation potential, providing a valuable tool in overcoming this additional barrier to enhance therapeutic outcomes [79]. Nanotherapy appears to exert a substantial impact on bacterial and fungal biofilms through mechanisms that are not yet fully elucidated. Cremonini et al. reported the antibiofilm activity of biogenic selenium NPs, effectively impeding biofilm formation in Gram-negative *Pseudomonas aeruginosa* [85]. Similar results were observed for titanium oxide (TiO_2) NPs against fungal biofilms [86]. Certainly, metal and metal oxide NPs, such as silver, gold, copper, titanium, zinc, magnesium, cadmium and alumina, demonstrate multiple mechanisms of action, enabling them to simultaneously target various components of microorganisms [87].

Antimicrobial NPs for urinary tract infections (UTIs) primarily rely on gold, silver, titanium and metal-based oxides, such as zinc oxide [88–93]. NPs have also been specifically developed and successfully used for treating *H. pylori* infections [94].

Studies have revealed that NPs possessing characteristics such as high surface area, charge, ability to deliver a large number of antibiotics or other substances, size and shape make them ideal antimicrobial tools [95,96]. While the exact inhibitory mechanism employed by NPs is not fully assembled and explained, evidence suggests that induced oxidative stress [97–99], released metal ions [100–102] and other non-oxidative mechanisms are extensively involved in the process [103].

Silver ions exhibit the strongest bactericidal effect [12]. Silver-based compounds were once the primary agents in antimicrobial therapy until the 1940s when they were overshadowed by antibiotics. With the surge in antibiotic resistance, there has been a renewed interest in the antimicrobial properties of silver, particularly in the form of silver NPs (Ag NPs). While the precise mechanisms of action for their antimicrobial activity are not fully understood, and many have been investigated and are possibly involved to a certain extent (Fig. 10.4), studies suggest that Ag

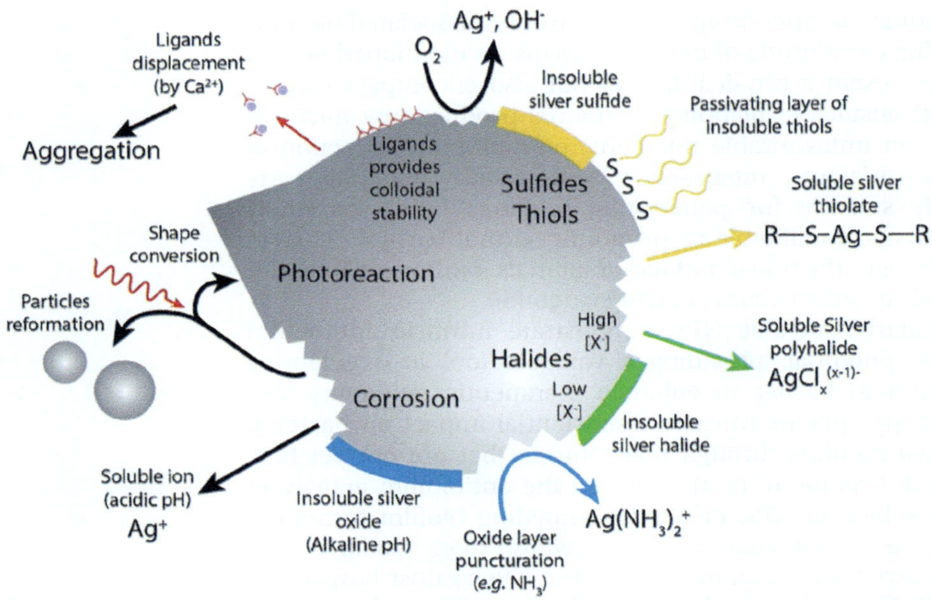

Figure 10.4 Different methods by which Ag NPs react for various physiochemical, biological and environmental conditions. Reproduced with permission from Le Ouay and Stellacci [105].

NPs exert a main direct toxic effect on bacterial cell walls and release silver ions (Ag^+) capable of disrupting the cell membrane and various intracellular functions [24]. These mechanisms provide both broad-spectrum activity and a high resistance barrier. Kim et al. have validated that the antimicrobial effect is also attributed to the production of free radicals from the surface of Ag NPs [104].

Despite attempts to incorporate Ag NPs on the surfaces of catheters and implantable medical devices to prevent biofilm formation and infections, universal success has not been achieved, making it an active area of investigation [106,107]. Indeed, Ag NPs effectiveness as antimicrobial agents would offer a degree of protection against healthcare-acquired infections associated with implanted biomedical devices [108,109]. As mentioned above, however, although the ionisation of Ag NPs in aqueous solution results in the generation of biologically active silver ions responsible for the observed antimicrobial effect [110], Ag NPs do have adverse effects on cells, including the production of reactive oxygen species that are toxic to both bacteria and eukaryotic cells [111,112]. In contrast, gold (Au) NPs exhibit low cytotoxicity and have found applications in medical imaging and serving as scaffolds for drug delivery [113].

Several studies have reported that metal NPs can be conjugated with different drugs to enhance their activities. As mentioned previously, the drug dosage often prescribed for a particular therapy is significantly high, leading to harmful effects. To counteract these and also maintain the cost-effectiveness of the therapy, the antibiotic dose should be reduced and the stability should be increased. In this respect, many examples in literature support the fact that metal (particularly Au and Ag) NPs have the potential to enhance the antimicrobial effects of the drug, reduce the dosages of the drug, combat its side effects and target the drug to the appropriate site of action [114]. Considering that multidrug-resistant bacteria have developed methods to inactivate or evade all classes of β-lactam antibiotics, investigations have explored whether attaching ampicillin to NPs could restore the efficacy of the antibiotic against β-lactam-resistant bacteria [113]. Recently, several studies have indicated that Ag NPs may strengthen the antibacterial effects of antibiotics against both susceptible and resistant bacteria, either additively or synergistically [2]. Furthermore, metal NPs conjugated with antibiotics exhibit synergistic effects against bacteria, hinder biofilm formation and have been employed to combat multidrug-resistant organisms [18,21]. Hongwei et al., for example, demonstrated the enhanced antimicrobial activity of vancomycin-capped Au NPs compared to plain vancomycin or cysteine-capped Au NPs [115]. In a study by Rai et al., significant antibacterial activity was demonstrated using Au NPs (52–22 nm) capped with cefaclor, a second-generation antibiotic [116]. The antimicrobial effectiveness was attributed to the presence of the β-lactam ring on the surface of the NPs. Studies have revealed that NPs possessing characteristics such as high surface area, charge, ability to deliver a large number of antibiotics or other substances, size and shape make them ideal antimicrobial tools [95,96].

Applications for therapeutic drugs often involve antibacterial nanodrugs, with Ag NPs demonstrating enhanced antibacterial efficiency due to their increased total surface area compared to traditional fine Ag particles [109]. Ag NPs of 10–100 nm in diameter can readily enter pathogens, bind with bacterial protein enzyme residues (e.g. thiols) and effectively eliminate bacteria. Metal-based NPs exhibit broad-spectrum antibacterial effects against both Gram-negative and Gram-positive bacteria, including antibiotic-resistant strains [117]. However, as previously mentioned, while Ag NPs alone are potent bactericidal agents, they can also be cytotoxic. Nonetheless, embedding them in a polymer matrix may mitigate their cytotoxicity [59,118].

The antimicrobial activity of Ag and copper (Cu) ions has been significantly enhanced by their incorporation in zeolite nanomaterials [119]. It has been demonstrated that the biological activity of Ag NPs is influenced by the capping or coating agent used, such as citrate or chitosan [120]. While Ag NPs can be challenging to functionalise with biomolecules and antibiotics, Ag–Au alloys offer an alternative avenue, combining the antimicrobial effects of Ag with the effectiveness of functionalisation and the stability of Au in the form of bimetallic NPs [21]. It is worth noting, though, that Ag NPs and Au NPs may exhibit reduced antibacterial activity when their surfaces are modified [23,25]. Additionally, Cu NPs with modified surfaces lose antimicrobial activity and fail to alter the morphology of microbial cells [121]. Biogenic synthetic strategies have also been employed for the preparation of Ag NPs [122], and Cu NPs have been used as well [123]. Other metal or metal compound NPs, such as zinc oxide (ZnO) NPs [124], TiO_2 nanotubes [125], Au-supported cerium oxide (CeO_2) NPs [126], also exhibit antibacterial activity [59]. It is essential to note that most research is based on in vitro experiments, necessitating additional in vivo and clinical studies to comprehensively understand the antibacterial activity of various NPs [59].

Certain nanoscale powder formulations, comprised of uncomplicated and harmless metal oxides like magnesium oxide (MgO) and calcium oxide (CaO) in nanocrystalline configuration, showcased robust antimicrobial characteristics. These formulations may harbour active forms of halogens, such as $MgO \cdot Cl_2$ and $MgO \cdot Br_2$. Upon interaction with vegetative cells of bacteria such as *E. coli, Bacillus cereus* (*B. cereus*) or *B. globigii*, more than 90% of the cells faced demise within a brief timeframe. Additionally, a distinct nanotube structure endowed with antimicrobial capabilities could be synthesised from a straightforward molecule originating from a hydrocarbon and an ammonium compound. This molecule, amalgamating the cell membrane-disrupting attributes of the quaternary ammonium compound with the colour-altering capabilities of the hydrocarbon diacetylene, served the dual role of a biosensor and a biocide [127].

Moreover, even magnetic NPs have been harnessed to devise innovative strategies for mitigating infections caused by various bacteria and addressing multidrug resistance, as well as eradicating biofilms. Core–shell magnetic NPs, in conjunction with human antibacterial peptides like cathelicidin LL-37, synthetic ceragenins CSA-13, CSA-131, and antibiotics such as colistin and vancomycin, have demonstrated the capability to annihilate MRSA and *P. aeruginosa*. This combination exhibited potent antibacterial properties, effectively overcoming bacterial drug resistance [128]. In a related investigation, positively charged magnetic NPs with a core of iron oxide (Fe_3O_4) and a shell of amino-silane entrapped multiple drug-resistant *S. aureus* and *E. coli*, resulting in complete elimination within 30 min upon exposure to radiofrequency. Remarkably, this strategy eradicated bacteria without inducing antibiotic resistance [129]. Furthermore, a nanocarrier incorporating superparamagnetic iron oxide NPs (SPIONs) and the antibiotic methicillin demonstrated the ability to prevent the biofilm formation by *S. epidermidis*. These NPs penetrated 20 μm thick biofilms in the presence of an external magnetic field, achieving complete eradication at SPION concentrations of 40 μg/mL and methicillin concentrations of 20 μg/mL [130]. Platinum (Pt) NPs were employed to inhibit oral bacteria (*S. mutans*) biofilms, successfully impeding their growth [131]. Another study screened 20 potent biofilm-forming strains of *P. aeruginosa*, exposing them to Fe_3O_4 NPs. Results indicated that at a concentration of 30 μg/mL, Fe_3O_4 reduced the biofilm biomass in most isolates, although in a few strains, it stimulated biofilm formation due to an iron source [132]. Similarly, Nichel (Ni) NPs demonstrated potential in preventing or eradicating biofilms produced by *Burkholderia cepacia* [133]. Hence, magnetic NPs, with their comprehensive antimicrobial activity, offer a promising avenue for eliminating bacterial biofilms and overcoming their inherent multiple drug resistance, presenting a distinct advantage over traditional antibiotics [134].

From the above and the previous chapters in this book, it is evident the increasing bulk of evidence in support of the development of nanotechnological tools for infection control. Going one step further, the developmental phase of nanoviricides, nanomedicines engineered for viral obliteration, is underway. These agents are designed to identify specific virus particles, engage with them at multiple junctures, nullify their potency and subsequently dismantle them. Promising targets for this approach encompass influenza, HIV, hepatitis C and rabies [127].

Nonetheless, there are still some significant hurdles to be discussed, including in terms of public awareness, toxicology and regulatory affairs as well as potential translation and impact. In the following sections, we hope to provide a reader with a suitable overview of these issues in relation of antimicrobial nanomaterials.

2. The background of the resistance problem and perception of nanotech

2.1 Resistance problem and antibiotic abuse

The problem of drug resistance has to be taken seriously. The WHO Global Antimicrobial Surveillance System sounded the alarm in 2017, declaring antibiotic resistance a formidable global challenge. The urgency to address this issue is underscored by the significant financial burden and health hazards it imposes on both individuals and societies worldwide [7]. The economic toll of combating antibiotic-resistant infections is staggering, with each individual case demanding an investment of approximately US$50,000. When considering the broader societal impact, the estimated annual cost levitates to a staggering US$20 billion. In Europe alone, infections caused by multidrug-resistant microorganisms result in approximately 25,000 deaths annually, incurring over 1.5 billion euros in healthcare expenses and productivity losses [135–139]. In addition, the report of the Centre for Disease Control and Prevention (CDC) also paints a dire picture, revealing that over 2.8 million cases of antibiotic-resistant bacterial infections afflict the United States annually, leading to a grim toll of more than 35,000 deaths [140]. The urgency of addressing this crisis is emphasised by prioritising the pathogens contributing to antibiotic resistance. These culprits, listed in order of priority, include *Acinetobacter baumannii, P. aeruginosa,* enterobacteria (such as *Klebsiella pneumoniae* and *Enterobacter cloacae*), *Enterococcus faecium, S. aureus, H. pylori,* several species of *Campylobacter* and *Salmonella, Neisseria gonorrhoeae, S. pneumoniae, Haemophilus influenzae,* and finally several species of *Shigella*. The need for effective strategies against these resistant pathogens is evident, given the significant public health impact [141,142].

It is now common knowledge that effective control and reduction of antibiotic use is a prerequisite for tackling the resistance problem. However, for a long time the dangers of antibiotic misuse were not sufficiently recognised, and as a result the majority of antibiotic usage extends beyond medical contexts and is notably pervasive in agriculture and aquaculture. The roots of this problem trace back to the early 20th century when farmers faced the challenge of meeting escalating consumer demands for meat and meat products. In 1950, an American Cyanamid study unveiled the growth-accelerating effects of antibiotics in livestock feed, revolutionising animal nutrition according to editors of *Successful Farming* magazine [4]. Following this revelation, antibiotics found broader application in promoting growth and routine disease prevention in livestock. Notably absent from discussions was a consideration of the potential impact on antibiotics crucial in human medicine. More than a decade into the nontherapeutic use of antibiotics in agriculture, a 1966 *New England Journal of Medicine* editorial warned of the looming threat of antibiotic resistance [5]. The 1969 Swann Report highlighted the potential dangers to the human population arising from antibiotic use in food animal production [7]. Over the years, accumulating data have established links between routine nontherapeutic antibiotic use in agriculture and antibiotic resistance. A pivotal moment came in 2010 when the US Food and Drug Administration (FDA), US Department of Agriculture (USDA) and the CDC testified before the US Congress, acknowledging a definitive association between nontherapeutic antibiotic use in food animal production and the antibiotic-resistance crisis in humans (Fig. 10.5) [9,143,144].

Nevertheless, there is still a long way to go to effectively control the use of antibiotics. Antibiotic use in aquaculture, the cultivation of aquatic organisms, is still widespread and subject to less stringent regulation compared to the use of antibiotics in animals raised for milk and meat. Furthermore, approximately 90% of the world's aquaculture production originates in Asia, where antibiotic use in aquaculture is not closely regulated [143,145]. Livestock, which plays a crucial role in the livelihoods of over 600 million farmers in developing countries by contributing significantly to about 30%–35% of agricultural gross domestic product, is equally hard hit by the abuse of antibiotics [146]. Even in the United States, over 50% of medically important antimicrobials sold in 2018 were designated for use in agricultural animals [147]. The good news is that recent legislation mandates veterinary feed directives when using medically important antimicrobials in animal feed, placing their use directly under the supervision of a licenced veterinarian. Furthermore, the European Union has implemented a ban on the routine use of antimicrobials in these animals and has imposed additional restrictions on their use for treating individual animals [148].

However, the use of antibiotics is like a double-edged sword, and stopping it completely will also bring new troubles. The emergence of new diseases and the resurgence of old infections in animals pose substantial economic losses for livestock keepers [149]. Swift detection and control of zoonoses are vital to prevent the spread of infections to entire herds and humans. Therefore, exploring innovative technologies to prevent and treat diseases caused by various microorganisms in veterinary animals is essential. Recent advancements in nanoscience and nanotechnology

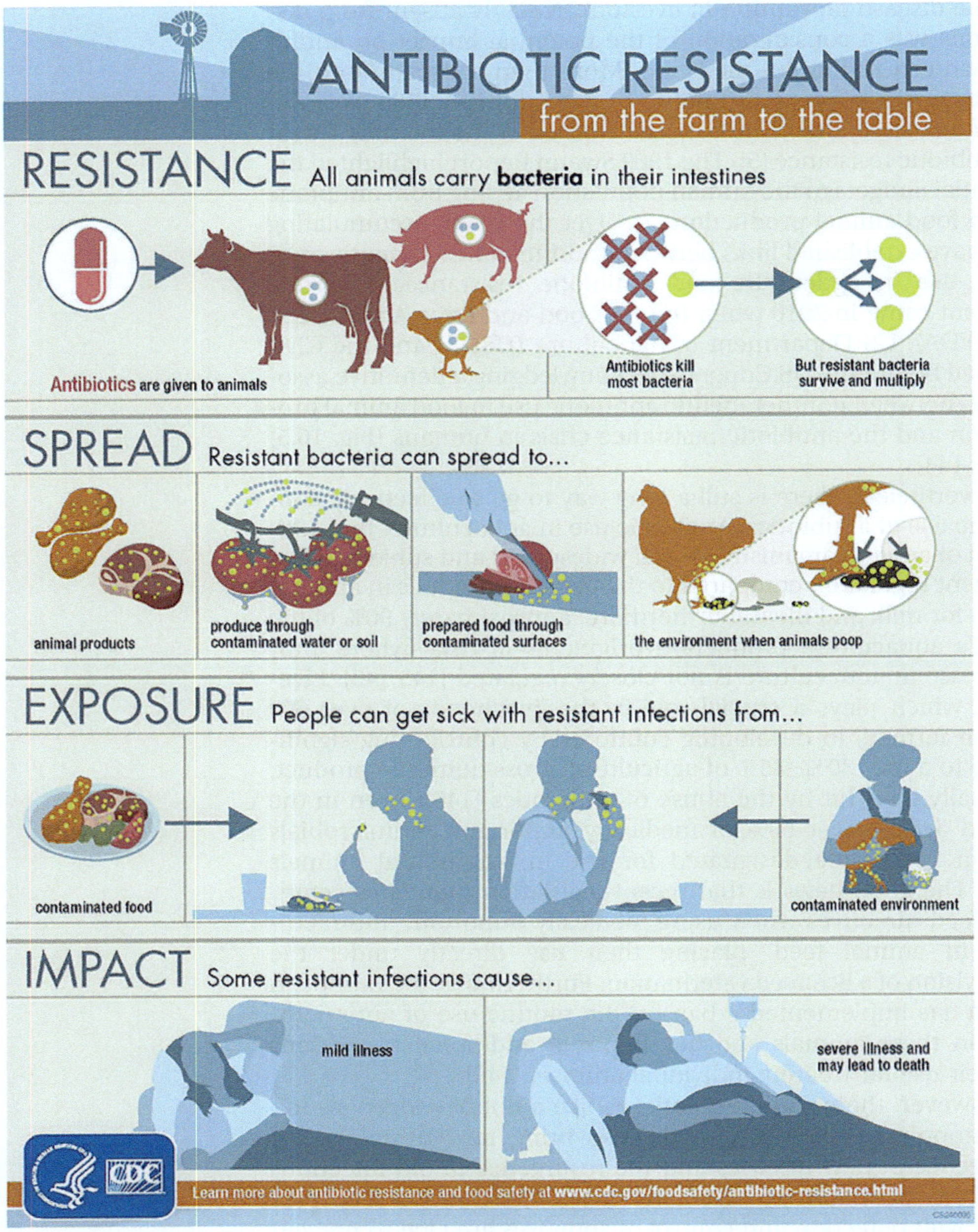

Figure 10.5 Origin of antibiotic resistance from nontherapeutic antibiotic use in food animal production. In the case of bacteria dwelling in farm animals developing resistance to antimicrobial drugs, the likeliness of them reaching humans is higher, through handling and eating raw or undercooked and contaminated meat, drinking or swimming in water contaminated with animal excrements and taking care of animals. Reproduced with permission from the Centre for Disease Control and Prevention (CDC) www.cdc.gov/foodsafety/antibiotic-resistance.html

have significantly impacted veterinary medicine, leading to the development of new diagnostic tools and treatments. These innovations aim to enhance the longevity and improve the quality of life for veterinary animals. While many studies on beneficial or cytotoxic effects have been conducted on rodents as in vivo models due to their biochemical and physiological similarities with human metabolism, limited research is available for veterinary animals [148,149].

2.2 Nanomedicine, promising or not?

Nanomedicine, a realm of cutting-edge technologies, embarked on significant research approximately a decade ago. The trajectory of nanomedicine's development aligns with the average timeline of 10–15 years for the maturation of high-tech innovations. The realm of nanomedicine has long held the promise of transforming treatment outcomes for countless patients. The question arises: has nanomedicine lived up to its initial expectations, delivering tangible benefits to patients, or does it still linger in the realm of 'lofty promises' with uncertain future outcomes? In an editorial for the *Journal of Controlled Release,* Prof. Park contends that nanomedicine has been excessively hyped, particularly in the context of cancer therapy, and its lofty promises may remain unfulfilled [150]. He suggests that redirecting the substantial resources, time and financial investments allocated to nanomedicine towards other priorities might be a prudent move. However, the reduction in publicly funded research investment in the field may not necessarily be a reflection of nanomedicine's failure. The US National Cancer Institute's decision to cease funding the Centres of Cancer Nanotechnology Excellence (CCNEs) after 15 years does not signal the demise of nanomedicine; rather, it indicates that nanomedicine has become resilient enough to compete in standard funding mechanisms. Prof. Grodzinski countered Park's perspective, highlighting the success of the CCNEs programme, which contributed to over 3400 nanomedicine publications, spawned more than 100 start-up companies, and initiated products entering over 30 clinical trials in the United States [151]. The Nanomedicine and Nanoscale Delivery (NND) focus group of the Controlled Release Society (CRS) also chimed in, advocating for the substantial progress made by nanomedicine [152]. The debate is ongoing: are we witnessing the wane of the nanomedicine hype, as Prof. Park suggests, or are we merely at the conclusion of the initial phase, ushering in a new, more mature era for nanomedicine? To address this question, the proposal is to adhere to the principle articulated by Prof. Park himself: '*Innovators who seek to revolutionise and disrupt an industry must tell investors the truth about what their technology can do today, not just what they hope it might do someday*' [153].

Despite these positive aspects, certain major corporations exhibit reluctance in channelling investments into nanomedicine research and development projects. This hesitation stems from existing uncertainties surrounding the regulatory framework governing these techniques (see following section). Additionally, the lukewarm social acceptance of nanotechnologies, coupled with opposition to inorganic NPs in certain countries, creates a less-than-ideal environment for substantial investment. It is noteworthy that, despite these challenges, nanomedicine enjoys a relatively higher level of acceptance from the general public compared to other applications of nanotechnologies in manufactured products. The French public debate on nanotechnology in 2009–2010 serves as a vivid illustration of these dynamics [154]. The augmentation of the surface-to-volume ratio leads to heightened particle surface energy, potentially induced by quantum effects. This phenomenon may render NPs more biologically reactive, as highlighted in discussions [155,156]. The escalated biological activity can manifest as either positive and desirable—exemplified by antioxidant activity, enhanced carrier capacity for therapeutics, and improved penetration of cellular barriers for drug delivery—or negative and undesirable, involving aspects such as toxicity, induction of oxidative stress, or disruption of cellular functions. It is essential to acknowledge that NPs can exhibit a combination of both positive and negative effects [157]. Therefore, by presenting these compounds differently, substances with identical chemical composition and formula to their bulk-sized counterparts may unveil properties that were previously unidentified [155]. And this is crucial for the further commercialisation of nanotechnology.

Indeed, despite the controversy surrounding advances in nanomedicine, it is undeniable that nanomedicine is improving our lives. Widely used nanotechnology has applications in various domains, including antimicrobial agents, drug delivery, diagnostics, vaccine formulation, feed additives, nutrient delivery, reproductive aids, animal growth, animal production and enhancing food quality [76]. These applications relate mainly to areas where antibiotic misuse is more serious, such as medicine, veterinary medicine, animal growth and production.

In addressing antibiotic resistance, the exploration of non-toxic antimicrobial agents is crucial, aiming to mitigate the devastating doses of antibiotics administered against various pathogens responsible for chronic infections in livestock, such as several species of *Brucella, Mycobacterium bovis, S. aureus* and *Rhodococcus equi* [158]. NPs are being employed as alternative antimicrobial agents to address the rising concerns about antibiotic usage. They contribute to the detection of pathogenic bacteria and serve as drug delivery agents for new drug and vaccine candidates, offering improved characteristics and performance. Various types of functionalised NPs, as illustrated before (such as liposomes, polymeric NPs, dendrimers, micelles and metal NPs), contribute to the success of nanotechnology in the animal growth promotion and production, as well as veterinary industry, providing cost-effective solutions and abundant resources to overcome economic losses [148].

Just to provide a few examples, in the realm of veterinary medicine, the bioavailability and pharmacokinetic parameters of tilmicosin, a semisynthetic antimicrobial agent, were enhanced in broiler chickens through oral administration using three distinct NPs. These included solid lipid NPs, nanostructured lipid carriers and lipid-core nanocapsules. Among the three nanoparticle types, tilmicosin formulated with lipid NPs exhibited superior improvements in drug bioavailability and pharmacokinetic parameters in broiler chickens [159]. Troncarelli et al. underscored the significance of micelles as antimicrobial agents in veterinary medicine, emphasising their potential applications and contributions to veterinary healthcare [76,160].

As highlighted in the introductory section and throughout this chapter, numerous studies have highlighted the potent antibacterial activity of Ag NPs against antibiotic-resistant strains in human medicine. However, the evaluation of antibacterial effects of combined therapy using Ag NPs and antibiotics against veterinary bacteria is limited. In a study involving *in ovo* administration of Ag NPs and/or amino acids, the impact on metabolism and immune responses in chicken embryos was investigated. The results indicated that Ag NPs, either alone or in combination with amino acids, did not affect embryonic growth but significantly improved immuno-competence. This suggests that Ag NPs and amino acid complexes hold potential as agents for enhancing innate and adaptive immunity in chickens [161]. In the realm of veterinary dermatology, nano-functionalised antimicrobial oils were incorporated into the formulation of shampoo, soap and ointment. These nano-functionalised oils exhibited remarkable antimicrobial activity against skin pathogens in animals. This underscores their value, safety, and specific role in controlling diseases in veterinary settings [76,162].

In addition to antimicrobials and related diagnostics, nanomaterials can be used as antiviral agents and enabling rapid and sensitive virus detection, contributing significantly to animal health and reproduction. Furthermore, the application of nanomaterials in food technology, particularly in ensuring the production of uncontaminated meat and meat products, marks a noteworthy advancement [76,163].

Before the advent of nanotechnology in medicine, treatments involving radiopharmaceuticals [164], liposomal drug carriers [164,165], antisense oligonucleotides, receptor-specific delivery of immunotherapy [166] and imaging contrast agents [167] were in use. However, nanomaterials have demonstrated superior effectiveness when appropriately applied. The 'first-generation' nanotherapeutics lacked specific biomolecular target recognition, encompassing clinically approved liposomes and albumin NPs. Current research concentrates on second-generation NPs, expected to go beyond the functions of the first generation. The primary emphasis is on 'active targeting', involving the biomolecular targeting of tissue/cell surface epitopes through *N*-surface-appended recognition moieties like peptides, antibodies or aptamers—a focus persisting for several years [168–172]. Nonetheless, be them targeted or pristine, organic or inorganic, any type of NPs development needs to navigate through the intricacies of the regulatory scenario, as detailed in the next section.

3. Nanotoxicology, environmental risks and regulatory policy

Nanomedicines face significant challenges related to biological safety, cost and large-scale production. When introduced into the body, nanomedicines interact with the biological environment, but the lack of standardised safety evaluation parameters complicates the assessment of their toxicity. Additionally, concerns arise regarding the stability and long-term storage of NPs-based products, emphasising the need for careful selection of lipids and polymers used in synthesis [173]. Achieving compliance with standard regulations for quality and safety remains a concern. Transitioning nanomedicine into a personalised drug entity requires large-scale synthesis with high reproducibility. While these drug-loaded nanocarriers are typically synthesised in small laboratory batches for preclinical and clinical investigations, scaling up production is challenging due to the complexities of different NP systems. Even slight alterations in the manufacturing process can lead to critical changes in nanomaterial properties. The development of nanomedicines is further hindered by the absence of standards and regulations in manufacturing practices, quality control and safety and efficacy evaluation (vide infra) [144,174].

Various factors, including particle type, size, surface charge, coating, protein binding, exposure route, dose and animal species, contribute to the pharmacokinetics of NPs. A comprehensive understanding of these pharmacokinetic parameters is crucial for assessing risks and ensuring biosafety in clinical applications [175]. The pharmacokinetic and pharmacodynamic characteristics of NPs are depicted in Fig. 10.6. The systemic or local effects and toxicity of NPs hinge on administration routes and physicochemical attributes, with chronic toxicity potentially linked to the intricate elimination pathways [176]. Generally, absorption through common administration routes (e.g. oral or pulmonary) is relatively low, typically below 5%, and there is a scarcity of long-term studies that offer a comprehensive interpretation of the toxicological implications of NPs absorption and penetration through tissues [175].

At the nanoscale, materials exhibit behaviours distinct from their larger counterparts. In nanomedicine, particles or nanotherapeutics with dimensions up to 1000 nm are commonly accepted [177]. Schütz et al. categorised medical NPs into three main types: soft, hard solid, and others. Soft particles typically comprise polymers, proteins or lipids, encompassing polymer NPs, micelles, vesicles, liposomes, core–shell systems, gels, polymeric drugs or polymer–drug conjugates. Hard solid-core NPs

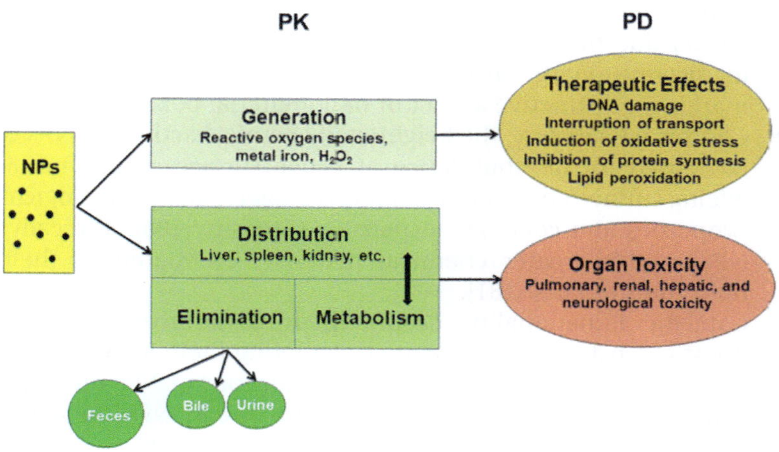

Figure 10.6 General pharmacokinetic (PK) and pharmacodynamic (PD) characteristics of NPs systems. Reproduced with permission from Lee et al. [18].

include metal and ceramic NPs like oxides, semiconductors or carbon nanotubes, along with nanocrystal drug formulations. Solid-core NPs with a polymer coating were also considered solid NPs. The dimensions of solid-core NPs are well-defined and less influenced by environmental parameters. However, the size and shape of soft nanoparticulate systems can largely depend on environmental factors such as temperature, pH, ionic strength or medium characteristics. Other particles, the third category, like antibody–drug conjugates and albumin particles, can also facilitate nanotype interactions due to their nanoscale size and construction [59].

The distinctive physical and chemical attributes of nanomaterials can be delineated across several dimensions [178]:

- Dimensionality: when reduced to the nanometre scale, properties exhibit size-dependent characteristics, encompassing (1) chemical attributes such as reactivity and catalysis; (2) thermal features, including melting temperature; (3) mechanical traits, like adhesion and capillary forces; (4) optical characteristics, involving absorption and light scattering; (5) electrical properties, typified by tunnelling current; and (6) magnetic attributes, exemplified by the superparamagnetic effect [178].
- Surface-to-Volume Ratio: the substantial surface-to-volume ratio of NPs stands as the pivotal determinant for the emergence of novel physical, chemical and mechanical properties relative to their bulk counterparts. Material in nanoparticulate form, despite an equivalent mass, displays heightened reactivity compared to larger particles [179].
- Quantum Confinement: a direct consequence of size reduction to the nanometre range is the manifestation of quantum effects due to electron movement confinement. This results in discrete energy levels contingent on the structural size, marking a distinctive aspect of nanomaterial behaviour [179].
- Chemical Reactivity: the heightened chemical activity of NPs is attributed to the abundance of active surface atoms, influencing surface adsorption, dispersion, aggregation, rheological properties and colloidal suspension viscosity [180]. Typically, NPs exhibit greater chemical reactivity compared to their bulk counterparts [181].
- Catalytic Functionality: despite their diminutive size, NPs boast a substantial surface area, rendering them ideal for catalytic activities [182]. The catalytic behaviour of NPs often diverges from traditional catalysts, with metal NPs on oxide supports showcasing superior activity compared to single-component NPs [183].

- Optical Characteristics: the optical properties of NPs (particularly metal ones) have long captivated the realm of physical chemistry. NPs frequently exhibit unexpected optical features, attributable to the confinement of electrons and the induction of quantum effects. For instance, gold NPs manifest as deep red to black in solution, showcasing the size-dependent nature of their optical behaviour [184].
- Additional Attributes: NPs also manifest enhanced hardness, plasticity, specific heat, thermal expansion, conductivity and diffusivity compared to larger counterparts. Unique features among NPs encompass surface plasmon resonance in certain metal particles and superparamagnetism in magnetic materials [185–188], rendering them desirable for medical applications as a magnetic targeting tool [178].

Attaining the requisite specificity, stability and compatibility for diverse applications necessitates the intricate modification and functionalisation of NPs through multiple steps. While augmented functionality brings numerous advantages, the concomitant rise in complexity raises pertinent concerns regarding reproducibility and scalability. This prompts the crucial question: to what extent must nanomaterials be complex for medical applications? According to Prof Weissleder, a prominent scientist and clinician with extensive experience in nanomedicine, the answer is straightforward: 'Just enough and no more'. In contrast, the functional complexity of nanomaterials in fundamental research has witnessed a substantial increase over the years. The field of nanomedicine witnesses the publication of thousands of research projects annually, showcasing intricate multicomponent architectures and sophisticated surface modifications driven by a relentless pursuit of innovation. Consequently, NPs exhibiting extraordinary properties have been documented, encompassing responsiveness to internal or external triggers, preferential accumulation in specific cell types, provision of enhanced contrast for multimodal imaging, superior stability, anti-fouling behaviour, and degradation into non-toxic clearable by-products over time [189,190].

While the utilisation of nanomaterials offers numerous advantages, it is essential to acknowledge certain drawbacks, with 'nano-toxicity' being a notable concern. The potential for NPs to accumulate in the bloodstream and organs raises apprehensions about their safety. For instance, Au NPs, typically considered biologically inert, may pose risks when employed in high doses or prolonged durations. Their relatively low clearance rate can lead to accumulation in tissues and the bloodstream, potentially inducing toxicity. A study conducted by Miller et al. exemplifies this concern, demonstrating that Au NPs persisted in the urine and blood of healthy individuals for a duration of 3 months following inhalation administration [191]. Although immediate adverse health effects were not observed, the cumulative presence of these particles in organs poses potential challenges, particularly in the context of long-term treatments [192]. Moreover, the elimination of metal NPs through urinary and biliary pathways is generally low, leading to their prolonged accumulation in the liver and spleen [175]. Additionally, depending on their composition, NPs do not undergo biodegradation into biologically benign components, resulting in extended tissue retention and amplified toxic effects [17,18]. Therefore, risks of bioaccumulation and redistribution from their site of disposition in organs and tissues are also suggested [155].

Selecting the optimal dose is a critical decision for therapeutic targeting and for minimising toxicity during medical translation [173]. Current in vitro doses causing cell damage are unrealistically high and impractical for human application [15]. Animal study data may not directly translate to humans, necessitating future research to identify appropriate and realistic doses [173]. Limited clinical studies on NPs dosing exist. Munger et al. reported two oral doses (10 ppm with a size ranging from 5 to 10 nm and 32 ppm with a size ranging from 25 to 40 nm) of a commercial solution of Ag NPs in healthy adult volunteers, which did not induce clinically significant changes in metabolic and haematologic profiles, urine, physical findings, or imaging morphology based on comprehensive assays and tests [193]. But based on what was mentioned in the previous sections and elsewhere in this book, more clinical studies are definitely needed before extensively applying NPs to patients.

To navigate this complexity, scientists encounter difficulties in establishing a singular, universal criterion for evaluation. Notably, the biocompatibility of Au NPs, traditionally viewed as benign, requires careful consideration [194]. In-depth studies on animal models have revealed that glycol-coated Au NPs with sizes of 10 and 60 nm exhibit toxicity levels deemed unsuitable for medical applications. In contrast, particles with sizes of 5 and 30 nm have demonstrated sufficient safety for such purposes. A noteworthy concern arising from these studies is the elevation of alanine and aspartate transaminase levels in biochemistry results, indicating mild liver damage [195]. As a precautionary measure, the development of methods targeting specific diseased cells and tissues is deemed essential before the widespread adoption of Au NPs in medicine [196].

The field of nanotoxicology currently grapples with a scarcity of comprehensive information. Semiconductor metals, commonly utilised in nanotechnology, are notably toxic, with even gold lacking proven safety in the quantities and formulations employed [197]. Although the diminutive size of NPs enhances their utility in medicine and industry, an increasing body of research indicates that benign bulk materials can become more toxic when transformed into ultra-fine particles [155]. These latter, irrespective of their chemical composition, serve as potent inducers of inflammatory lung injury. The unique toxicity associated with surface modifications is a notable concern, with enhanced endocytosis and potential inflammatory and pro-oxidant activity largely contingent on NPs surface chemistry and in vivo surface modifications [157]. Notable instances include increased pulmonary toxicity observed in carbon nanotubes compared to carbon black and carbonyl iron particles in mice and rats [198,199], respectively. Nanomaterials surface charge alteration influences uptake rates, as demonstrated by enhanced arterial uptake in an ex vivo dog femoral artery model [200]. Induction of cytotoxicity by nanomaterials, driven by oxidative stress from free radical generation, is also an area of concern. Modifying surface characteristics, such as converting insoluble carbon nanotubes to soluble forms, can mitigate cytotoxicity [155]. The interaction of NPs with the immune system and other body tissues remains unclear, with suggestions that their small sizes could act as haptens, modifying protein structures and potentially inducing autoimmune effects [201]. The large surface area of NPs enables protein absorption, influencing their handling by macrophages and activation of the complement system [202,203]. Adverse effects may not only be induced, but interactions with cell and subcellular structures, as well as distribution/biokinetics, are likely to differ significantly from larger-sized particles [157].

Concerns about the use of NPs include both local and systemic toxic complications, as well as potential deleterious effects on beneficial bacteria in humans [15,27]. The potential significant impact of NPs such as TiO_2 NPs on the human body also raises concerns, particularly considering the widespread use of these particles. Among the diverse group of NPs employed in various industries, TiO_2 NPs, owing to their white colour, are notably popular and find extensive use as a whitening food additive (E 171). Despite their prevalence, there is a scarcity of studies focussed on assessing the direct impact of TiO_2 NPs on bacteria, for example. Available data, however, suggest that TiO_2 NPs may have repercussions on the microbiota, potentially contributing to issues such as inflammatory bowel disease, obesity or immunological disorders. The concern extends to the possibility of TiO_2 NPs causing intestinal barrier impairment and dysbiosis of intestinal microbiota. Given the increasing use of TiO_2 NPs and their potential influence on human health, addressing these concerns becomes paramount, necessitating further research to elucidate the extent of their impact [204].

Another relevant example pertains reports documenting the elevations of liver enzymes and serum silver levels attributed to the absorption of Ag NPs from burn wound dressings [205]. The unregulated utilisation of Ag NPs in various household items, textiles, cosmetics and paints raises concerns regarding environmental contamination and the potential for human toxicity, emphasising the need for thorough and careful study [206,207].

Indeed, the utilisation of metallic NPs is subject to various limitations, including the generation of hazardous wastes, challenges in scaling up production, issues related to instability and aggregation and reliance on expensive organometallic NPs. These limitations highlight the need for addressing environmental concerns, optimising production processes and enhancing the stability of metallic NPs to maximise their efficacy and sustainability [208,209]. The release of nanomaterials into the environment and their potential impact on other species, indeed, has raised concerns, as highlighted by organisations such as the National Science Foundation (NSF) and the Environmental Protection Agency (EPA). This recognition underscores the need for careful consideration and assessment of the environmental implications associated with nanomaterials to ensure responsible and sustainable practices [155].

The exposure to ultrafine dust particles is undoubtedly known to pose health risks for humans, and this raises concerns about the potential health risks associated with engineered NPs. Engineered nanomaterials exhibit properties such as mobility across biological barriers, size-related chemical activity effects and the ability to penetrate cells, which could result in increased toxicity compared to bulk materials [210]. Nanomaterial sources include natural sources (e.g. salt spray from the ocean), unintentionally produced sources (e.g. cooking, material fabrication, diesel exhaust) and engineered NPs [211]. Two forms of NPs application, though, need to be distinguished concerning exposure and potential health risks: (i) NPs bound into a chemical matrix, such as a polymer or metal, are generally considered safe unless released due to chemical processes or wear; (ii) free NPs in the air or fluids that can be taken up by the body via the lung, skin or intestinal tract. Nanomaterials emissions, whether intentional or unintentional, can occur during various stages, including research and development, manufacturing, use, disposal and dispersion in the environment. Potentially exposed groups include staff in research and development, manufacturing, diagnosis and treatment, disposal, recycling, remediation and cleaning, transport and trade, as well as individuals involved in accidents, patients and the general population. Additionally, ecosystems might be affected. Toxicologists emphasise the need to investigate the health and environmental effects of NPs and the exposure of workers, as there is a consensus among stakeholders that the current level of knowledge is insufficient for risk assessments [211]. Key areas for further research and development include:

1. Developing harmonised nomenclature and criteria for nanomaterials characterisation.
2. Developing methodologies for routine measurements and equipment for determining the environmental fate of nanomaterials and detecting them in the environment, as well as for exposure assessment.
3. Understanding the toxicity and ecotoxicity of NPs.
4. Conducting epidemiological studies [211].

As discussed elsewhere in this volume in larger detail, the protein corona surrounding NPs also plays a pivotal role in dictating their biological fate. The components of the protein corona have the potential to influence both biodistribution and targeting, facilitating the desired therapeutic action. However, this same protein corona can also impact cellular uptake and toxicity, contributing to potential side effects. The ambivalent nature of the protein corona is a key factor limiting the efficacy of nanomaterials in current therapeutic approaches [212].

From the above, it is clear that the toxicity of NPs and other nanomaterials is a multifaceted phenomenon influenced by various factors. These factors encompass the intrinsic properties of the material, its stability in a biological milieu, the toxicity of potential degradation products, the potential for accumulation in clearance organs as well as systemic distribution and release of payloads. Furthermore, toxicological profiles exhibit a high degree of dependence on the anatomical environment, resulting in variations from one location to another. This variability complicates the translation of in vitro biocompatibility analyses to in vivo conditions [213]. Notably, long-term toxicity of NPs often arises due to their accumulation in the liver and spleen upon reticuloendothelial system (RES) clearance. To address this issue, the design of nanomaterials that undergo degradation over time, resulting in smaller particles subject to rapid renal elimination, is considered desirable. In this context, biodegradable polymers have gained popularity, as they can be readily excreted from the body upon degradation under physiological conditions [189,214,215].

The initial generation of nanomedicines, exemplified by liposomal preparations, received approval over a decade ago, predating a comprehensive awareness of safety concerns associated with nanomaterials. These early products, employed in cancer treatment, demonstrated efficacy without observable toxicity attributable to NPs. However, it is crucial to recognise that nanomaterials, such as phospholipids or biodegradable polymers, represent a distinct category from anticipated materials in the research pipeline. While in vitro use of NPs for diagnostics raises minimal concerns, introducing NPs into the human body for therapeutic purposes has prompted apprehensions about potential toxic effects. The small size of particles, particularly those below 50 nm, renders them versatile tools for drug delivery and cancer treatment but introduces the possibility of undesirable effects [216].

Since their first inception, the administration of liposomal nanotherapeutics intravenously for lung therapy has been extensively illustrated, revealing that nearly 75% of these NPs accumulate in organs such as the liver, spleen, kidney and heart, with minimal presence in the lungs—contrary to the intended target for lung disease treatment [217]. This phenomenon not only compromises treatment efficacy but also escalates the risk of systemic adverse side effects. As a result, the evaluation of nanoparticle biodistribution post-systemic administration through any route is imperative in both preclinical and clinical studies to address these concerns [218].

Various NPs exhibit diverse biological effects contingent on factors such as size, chemical composition, surface structure, solubility, shape and aggregation. For instance, quantum dots (QDs) may release potentially toxic cadmium and zinc ions, although their impact on cells is minimised due to protective coatings. Studies with 2-nm core Au NPs indicate that cationic particles possess moderate toxicity, while anionic particles are relatively nontoxic [219]. Additionally, research has explored the use of naturally occurring gum arabic as a nontoxic phytochemical excipient in the production of biocompatible Au NPs for diagnostic and therapeutic applications in nanomedicine [220]. Given the systemic administration of many nanoparticle formulations, evaluating compatibility of both NPs themselves and potentially toxic degradation products generated from NPs becomes essential, with a particular focus on possible interference with haemolytic activity, platelet function and blood coagulation pathways [127,221].

To provide an example, macrophages, which patrol the alveolar surfaces of the lung as part of the immune defence system, encounter difficulty in recognising particles smaller than 70 nm as 'foreign'. This limited recognition capability allows such particles to gain access to the pulmonary interstitium, which is a potentially vulnerable anatomical compartment. This observation raises concerns about the potential impact of NPs, particularly those below 70 nm, on the respiratory system and the ability of macrophages to effectively recognise and clear these particles [155,222]. Nonetheless, while the exact mechanism of toxic complications remains unclear, other observations might suggest that larger-sized NPs might pose a greater risk of adverse health effects [223]. Intravenously administered NPs have been found to accumulate in various organs, including the colon, lung, bone marrow, liver, spleen and lymphatic system [224]. Inhalation of NPs may induce cytotoxicity in the lungs [225]. Although some in vivo studies have reported no apparent life-threatening toxicity related to NPs [226,227], chronic toxicity, such as nephrotoxicity, hepatotoxicity or pulmonary toxicity, could result from the accumulation of NPs in these tissues [227–229].

From the above, potential toxicological effects might be related to the aspect ratio of the materials instead of the absolute size, particularly in case of pulmonary interactions. Indeed, there is compelling evidence indicating that high-aspect-ratio nanomaterials (HARNs) possessing the following characteristics: (i) thickness less than 3 μm; (ii) length exceeding 10–20 μm; (iii) biopersistence; and (iv) lack of dissolution or breakage into shorter fibres, have the potential to be retained within the narrow space surrounding the lungs, known as the 'pleural cavity', for extended periods. Long fibres retained in the pleural cavity have been associated with persistent inflammation, leading to irreversible diseases such as fibrosis and lung cancer [230].

The manufacturing process of NPs introduces an additional layer of complexity as chemicals employed in this process can adsorb onto the surface of the NPs, along with the intended drug or herb [231]. Recognising this, nanotechnology engineers are actively exploring eco-friendly manufacturing methods that reduce or eliminate dependence on toxic chemical processes [232]. The presence of adsorbed materials can significantly alter the properties, effects and/or toxicity of the NPs, underscoring the importance of mindful manufacturing practices [233].

Given these concerns and the related experimental variability, it is imperative to conduct comprehensive nanotoxicology studies, with a specific emphasis on the subcategory of toxicology [157,201]. The application of classical toxicological risk assessment categories becomes indispensable for evaluating the use of NPs. These categories encompass hazard identification, hazard characterisation, exposure assessment and risk calculation, as outlined by Luther in 2004 [234]. In summary, the incorporation of a robust risk management strategy is imperative for all medical products utilising NPs across diverse medical technology applications [76].

The application of nanotechnology and nanomaterials in drugs addresses a broad spectrum of health challenges, including enhanced bioavailability, altered biodistribution, increased drug efficacy, stabilisation of degradable drugs and targeted drug delivery. However, assessing the potential risks associated with these non-biological complex drugs proves to be a complex task, necessitating an integrative approach to effectively address the issue. It is not surprizing that in the realm of responsible research and innovation in nanomedicine, due emphasis is rightly placed on nanotoxicity and nanotoxicology. This research domain also provides a fertile ground for collaborative efforts, where scientists can engage with industry, regulators and governmental bodies. Such collaborations open avenues for multidisciplinary scientific research involving multiple stakeholders, contributing to ongoing debates on the regulation and safe use of nanomaterials [5]. In the year 2004, for example, the National Cancer Institute, the FDA and the National Institute of Standards and Technology collaboratively established the Nanotechnology Characterisation Laboratory. This initiative was devised to provide support for the preclinical characterisation of nanomedicines, standardise the procedures associated with the safety and efficacy analysis of nanomedicine, and enhance understanding of the health risks and safety considerations associated with nanoscale materials [235].

Since then, several influential bodies have undertaken risk assessments of nanotechnology, providing valuable perspectives on its potential impact. Notable entities include the National Nanotech Initiative (NNI), European Nanomedicine Technology (ENT), Innovation Medicines (IM) for Europe Platform and the International Life Sciences Institute (ILSI) Research Foundation/Risk Science Institute Nanomaterial Toxicity Screening Working Group. The NNI represents collaborative efforts involving the NSF, EPA and other US federal agencies, along with the United Kingdom Royal Society and the United Kingdom Health and Safety Executive Council [236]. The ENT, initiated in September 2005, aimed to bolster innovation in nanobiotechnologies for medical applications [155]. It stood as an industry-led initiative created in collaboration with the European

Commission. Focussed on harnessing nanotechnology for transformative advancements in healthcare, the ENT played a pivotal role in facilitating coordination among its members for joint research efforts. Additionally, it strived to enhance communication both within its member network and with the European Commission and member states, dedicated to fostering the growth of the nanomedicine industry in Europe and acting as a liaison between industry, academia and hospitals, working to seamlessly translate nanomedicine research 'from bench to bedside'. This role becomes particularly crucial in the context of open innovation, where collaborative efforts are essential for driving advancements in the field [154]. Similarly, the IM for the European Commission sought to enhance and expedite the development process of medicines, fostering efficient communication among the public sector, pharmaceutical industries and regulators. The ILSI nanomaterial toxicity screening working group focussed on developing a screening strategy for hazard identification of nanomaterials. The International Association of Nanotechnology's Nomenclature and Terminology Subcommittee, along with the American National Standards Institute Nanotechnology Standard Panel (ANSI-NSP), is actively involved in developing standard definitions for key terms in nanomaterial science [155].

To systematically identify, analyse and control factors that could impact the quality and safety of new drugs, the US FDA introduced a risk-based approach to drug engineering in 2000. This approach, eventually termed Quality-by-Design (QbD) in 2008 by the International Council for Harmonisation of technical requirements for pharmaceuticals for human use (ICH), represented a departure from traditional methods that solely focussed on testing product quality. QbD fundamentally sought to build quality and safety into the drug design process from its inception [237]. Despite its potential advantages, a comprehensive assessment of the major benefits and limitations of QbD in nanomedicine has not been conducted [238]. This gap in knowledge extends to specific deficiencies, including the absence of prior risk assessment, challenges related to production scale-up, the implementation of process analytical technology and the formulation of an effective control strategy [239].

The regulatory landscape for nanomedicines aligns with the standards applied to small traditional drugs. Regulatory agencies such as the FDA and the European Medicines Agency (EMA) scrutinise many nanodrugs as novel entities. Both the FDA and EMA require nanomedicines to meet identical criteria for safety, efficacy and pharmaceutical quality as other drug products. In adherence to the regulatory evaluation process, all nanoparticle submissions are required to showcase robust disease-related safety margins and elevated therapeutic efficacy. The aim is to deliver nanodevices that effectively address patient needs. However, the distinctive and hybrid nature of nanomedicines introduces significant analytical challenges during quality assessment, setting them apart from small molecular or biological drugs like antibodies [240]. A set of essential prerequisites has been outlined that serve as a go/no-go decision-making framework during the development process, guiding the transition towards an Investigational New Drug (IND) submission [241–243]. Navigating the regulatory landscape, however, and particularly the stringent evaluation processes of the FDA, poses a critical barrier to the translation of nanomedicine. Nanodrugs undergo rigorous scrutiny, adhering to strict FDA/EMA guideline approval protocols prior to progressing to Phase I clinical trials subsequent to IND acceptance (Table 10.1).

In 2010, the FDA published guidelines and reports, outlining crucial considerations for the evaluation of nanoformulation properties of NPs. In addition to the standard assessments for identity, strength, potency, stability and impurities, nanomedicine formulations demand the evaluation of specific physicochemical properties for the final drug product. These properties encompass particle size, size distribution, polydispersity, surface charge, drug loading, drug release profile and the intricate core–shell chemical and physical structure. Moreover, chemical and size stability during storage and interaction with biological media must also be assessed [244]. Adding to the complexity, classical characterisation methods may not be directly applicable to nanomaterials. More sophisticated methodologies are required to understand how nanomedicine properties impact safety and efficacy profiles. This involves a comprehensive exploration and evaluation of (1) their immunological effects, (2) pharmacokinetic profiles, (3) distribution to blood and tissues, (4) metabolism, (5) elimination, (6) accumulation in target tissues, (5) degradation profile and (7) toxicity [241,245–248]. Such detailed analyses are essential to determine the specific critical quality attributes (CQAs) of each nanomedicine system, ensuring regulatory compliance and successful translation into the market [249].

From the above, however, it is evident, that regional and national variations within regulatory authorities, particularly when conducting multi-centric international trials, pose a formidable challenge during the clinical trial phase [250]. Additionally, the patient acceptability of these nanosystems represents a crucial aspect that demands attention. Notably, in 2006, the International Centre for Technology Assessment and various consumer groups

Table 10.1 Major Requirements/Milestones for NPs from Preclinical Stage to Commercialisation.

Development stage	Objective	Major criteria to be analysed and critical outcomes
Discovery	Design and development of tunable and biocompatible NPs for optimal biological application	- Size [253] - Stability in biological conditions (in vitro and *in vivo*) - Chemical stability of dendrimers - Stability in manufacturing and drug storage process - Preliminary scale-up evaluation - Ease of manufacture based on the robust methodology for potential scale-up for cGMP - Encapsulation efficiency and adequate release kinetics - Physiochemical and biological characterisation - Quality control - Process design
Preclinical	Selection of the NPs with good druggability	- Stability studies - Preformulation analytical studies - Evaluation of degradation and elution for oral and *iv* administration. Specifically in the gastrointestinal (GI) system for oral administration - Evaluation of the conversion of the NPs to non-nanomedicines and remaining NPs in the administration sites - ADME profile - *In vitro* therapeutic profile (non-good laboratory practice, GLP): cellular assays, mechanism of cell uptake, therapeutic loading and release, and therapeutic effect compared to platform alone (if relevant). - *In vitro* demonstration of the specific mechanism of action of the encapsulated/conjugated drug (non-GLP) - *In vivo* therapeutic profile (non-GLP) - *In vivo* pharmacokinetics (non-GLP) showing adequate biodistribution, PK, PK/PD profiles, good efficacy and safety - Toxicity studies (acute dose limiting and chronic dosing, reach off-target effects (toxic levels) related to concentrations, genotoxicity) (non-GLP) and then toxicity studies using GLP standardised techniques - Toxicity of both dendrimers alone and dendrimer/drug - Selection of the route of administration as well the procedure of administration (e.g. daily dose) and to be stable in the selected formulation - Scale-up to GMP batch for clinical trials

Continued

Table 10.1 Major Requirements/Milestones for NPs from Preclinical Stage to Commercialisation.—*continued*

Development stage	Objective	Major criteria to be analysed and critical outcomes
		- Complexity of the manufacturing process and industrialisation standpoint
	Studies under good laboratory practice (GLP)	- To be performed during the clinical trials: - *In vivo* toxicokinetics, in vivo safety pharmacology, and in vivo reproductive toxicology
IND application	Needs to be approved by the regulatory agencies (e.g. FDA, EMA)	Information from - Preclinical toxicity (FDA/EMA) - Formulation for the selected route of administration - Animal pharmacology and toxicity (from preclinical studies) - Manufacturing information related to composition and stability For additional studies to be done, see ref [254] Nontoxic with minimal side effects, no significant drug interactions At least as effective as current standard or best alternative
Clinical trials		
Phase I	Assess dosing, acute toxicity, and NPs excretion in healthy humans but in some cases with humans with the disease	Testing for therapeutic specific side effects identified in preclinical studies
Phase II	Evaluation of the safety and efficacy of NPs in patients	Multiple patient groups and at multiple sites
Phase III	Large, randomised placebo-controlled trials to demonstrate further safety and efficacy and compare the investigational platform to the gold standard	Drug safety and efficacy relative to the gold standard of care
NDA application	Needs to be approved by the regulatory agencies (e.g. FDA, EMA)	Information from - NPs - Results of animals' studies - Clinical trial outcomes - NPs behaviour in the body - NPs manufacturing, processing and packaging - Phase IV strategy studies

lodged a legal petition against the FDA, citing a perceived lack of proactivity in regulating products containing nanomaterials within its purview. In response to these concerns, the FDA established a Nano Task Force [251]. To realise the successful translation of nanomedicines, a collaborative network of stakeholders must coalesce. This collective effort involves the active participation of academics, industry investors, government entities and contract research and manufacturing organisations. Given that nanotechnology is an interdisciplinary domain, the formulation of effective intellectual property and commercialisation strategies becomes imperative for sustained growth [1,252].

Current considerations in nanomaterial regulations draw from established standards for conventional materials. From the above, it is clear that the toxicology of NPs is a multifactorial domain, spanning exposure assessments, impacts on immune responses (influenced by both core and surface composition), and the fate, transport and deposition of nanomaterials. Key elements encompass physicochemical characteristics (both core and composition), in vitro models for studies on absorption, target binding/receptor screening, cellular uptake, and cytotoxicity, as well as in vivo models for efficacy/proof of concept, imaging studies, functional assessments and investigations into mechanisms of tissue uptake and clearance. These multifaceted studies contribute to a comprehensive understanding of the biokinetics and toxicity profile of nanomaterials in animals and humans [155,156].

The government, in collaboration with academia and commercial organisations, is urged to take a leading role in establishing the necessary infrastructure for clearly and uniquely identifying and assessing the potential risks associated with nanomaterials. This involves several key initiatives, including:

1. Identification of 'representative or model' nanomaterials, considering their structure, size, properties and activities.
2. Development of comprehensive toxicity testing protocols covering various exposure routes such as inhalation, dermal contact, ingestion and injection. These protocols aim to characterise the full spectrum of nanomaterials in relation to their properties, proposed uses, potential impact on predisposed or susceptible individuals and ultimate clinical applications.
3. Strengthening manufacturing processes under Good Manufacturing Practice (GMP) standards, particularly in the realm of nanomedicine. This entails focussing on fabrication, shipping, handling and storage to maintain the stability and quality of the final nanomedicine products.

4. Implementation of measures to detect and monitor exposure levels in workplaces, air/waterborne releases, humans, other organisms and environmental media.
5. Proactive risk management through the assessment of the impact of nanotechnology products on the environment.

These strategic actions are crucial for ensuring the responsible development and utilisation of nanomaterials, particularly in the context of nanomedicine, where considerations of safety and quality are paramount [155].

To secure FDA approval for human use, careful consideration of certain limitations is paramount to prevent potential regulatory obstacles. Notably, the shape and size of NPs are critical factors that demand close attention. For successful NPs administration, hydrodynamic diameters should exceed 5–6 nm to avoid removal by renal clearance systems, yet remain below 200 nm to evade clearance by the liver and spleen [255]. Diverse studies have demonstrated the significant impact of size and shape on the biodistribution and properties of NPs in biological environments. For instance, studies on short interfering RNA (siRNA) conjugated to Au NPs revealed that 50 nm spheres and 40 nm stars exhibited higher uptake efficiency compared to 13 nm spheres. While all three forms were initially localised in endosomes, after 24 h, 50 nm spheres and 40 nm stars were no longer detected in endosomes or lysosomes, whereas 13 nm spheres remained in endosomes [256]. In-depth investigations into the morphological characteristics of NPs may provide effective regulatory control over their cellular properties [257]. Surface chemistry and charge also play pivotal roles in the biodistribution, pharmacokinetic properties and cytotoxicity of NPs. Generally, NPs with a near-neutral charge are preferred, and surface modification, such as PEGylation, is commonly employed to achieve a neutral charge and prolong circulation time, preventing phagocytosis by reticuloendothelial cells [258]. For specific targeting and effects, various targeting moieties, including antibodies, aptamers and small molecules, have been widely exploited [259,260]. Monoclonal antibodies, with their two epitope binding sites, high selectivity and binding affinity, are extensively used for protein recognition and targeting. Aptamers, folded single-strand oligonucleotides, are utilised for selective binding to molecular targets through high-throughput screening methods [261]. Small molecules such as folic acid, transferrin and the RGD peptide sequence are also commonly employed for surface modification of NPs. Particularly, the cyclic RGD peptide, a component of the extracellular matrix protein fibronectin, is known for its high affinity to integrins, making it a valuable modification for NPs to enable targeted interventions [262,263].

Despite the numerous advantages of nanoparticle-based systems discussed in this book, continuous efforts are needed to further improve this field. Nanotechnology indeed comes with its share of uncertainties and concerns. The risks associated with nanomaterials are not fully understood, making it challenging to predict their impact accurately. Initial studies have indicated potential negative effects on living organisms and have raised concerns about environmental contamination and nanowaste disposal. A major concern remains the toxicity of nanoparticle carriers when used in real patients. Addressing this issue involves reducing the dosage of nanocarriers and enhancing their biodegradability in vivo. For instance, in the case of mesoporous silica nanoparticle (MSNP)-based nanocarriers, one potential method is to introduce zinc or iron elements into the silica network, which may facilitate the excretion of NPs from the body after drug release [264].

The scientific community is particularly focussed on understanding the toxicity, proper characterisation and exposure pathways of nanomaterials. Ethical and societal concerns also play a significant role, encompassing issues such as potential health risks, intellectual property rights and broader societal impacts. In the pursuit of economic competition and innovation, there is a cautionary note about prioritising scientific prudence and public health. Striking a balance between reaping the benefits of nanomedicine and ensuring the safety of these technologies is crucial. It is an evolving field, and ongoing research and regulatory efforts are essential to mitigate potential risks and maximise the positive impact of nanotechnology [12]. Given the substantial research efforts dedicated to the field, however, it is anticipated that nanomedicine will continue to advance, offering significant benefits to humanity in the near future.

4. Economical perspective towards clinical translation

The realm of nanomedicine is experiencing rapid evolution, recently catapulted into global prominence by the US FDA emergency use authorisation of two NPs-based vaccines developed by BioNtech/Pfizer and Moderna in the battle against the acute respiratory syndrome coronavirus 2 (SARS-CoV-2) [265]. In this context, nanoencapsulation serves a pivotal role by safeguarding the messenger RNA (mRNA), which is susceptible to enzymatic degradation. The unprecedented deployment of these mRNA-based vaccines, marking a milestone in the ongoing fight against the COVID-19 pandemic, also signifies a monumental accomplishment in the domain of nanomedicine. This underscores the vast, untapped potential within the field [189,266].

Nanomedicine has evolved from a theoretical concept to a thriving industrial sector, with a market reality characterised by approved products and devices. This burgeoning industry engages over 200 companies worldwide, offering a diverse array of products. Notably, significant investments are being made each year to drive nanotechnology research and development, with cumulative investments in the United States alone reaching US$40 billion over the last 20 years [267]. The exponential growth of this industry positions it as a potent force in shaping the global economy. The landscape of nanomedicine applications is vast, with drug delivery reigning as the largest sector. Biomaterials emerge as the fastest-growing segment, underscoring the dynamic nature of the field. Despite the fragmentation of the market, a cohort of key players commands attention. Nanosphere Inc., Par Pharmaceutical Companies Inc., AMAG Pharmaceutical Inc., Elan Corporation PLC, Life Technologies Corporation, Abraxis BioScience Inc. (now CelGene), Flamel Technologies S.A., Oxonica Plc, Wyeth Pharmaceuticals Inc, MagForce GmbH, NanoBiotix, Arrowhead Research Corporation and others contribute significantly to the vibrancy of the sector.

The intricate dynamics of the nanomedicine market underline its potential to reshape the future of healthcare, with diverse applications driving innovation and economic impact [154]. Riding on a trajectory of continuous growth, the global nanomedicine market is poised to reach new heights, as indicated by the Grand View Research report of 2023–2030 [268]. The market size of US$174.13 billion in 2022 is projected to soar to an impressive US$410.15 billion by 2030, driven by a robust compound annual growth rate (CAGR) of 11.57%. This forecast underscores the expanding influence of nanomedicine across diverse applications, cementing its role as a transformative force in healthcare and technology [241].

The horizon of nanodrugs continues to broaden, with a steady surge anticipated in their numbers. This concerted effort aims not only to enhance treatment modalities but also to elevate the quality of life for patients [242,243]. Despite commendable global endeavours spanning 3 decades, the regulatory nod from authorities such as the FDA and the EMA has been granted to only a select few NPs. Up until 2022, the FDA and EMA had greenlit a total of approximately 100 nanomedicine-based formulations (Table 10.2) [269].

Table 10.2 Representative list of FDA/EMA-approved and globally marketed nanomedicine-based formulations from Thapa et al. [270].

Type of formulation	Nanosystem type	Product name	Active ingredient(s)	Company	Approving organisation and approval date	Indication(s)
Lipid-based nanomedicine	Liposome	Doxil	Doxorubicin hydrochloride	Johnson and Johnson	FDA (1995) EMA (1996)	Metastatic ovarian cancer, HIV-associated Kaposi's sarcoma, multiple myeloma
	Lipid complex	Abelcet	Amphotericin B	Liposome Co	FDA (1995)	Aspergillosis in patients refractory to or intolerant of conventional amphotericin B and for invasive fungal infections
	Liposome	DaunoXome	Daunorubicin citrate	Galen Ltd	FDA (1996) EMA (1996)	HIV-associated Kaposi's sarcoma
	PEGylated liposome	Caelyx	Doxorubicin hydrochloride	Janssen Pharmaceutica NV	EMA (1996)	Metastatic breast cancer, ovarian cancer, AIDS-related Kaposi's sarcoma
	Unilamellar liposome	AmBiosome	Amphotericin B	NeXstar Pharmaceuticals	FDA (1997) EMA (2006)	Fungal infections in febrile neutropenic patients; Aspergillosis, candidiasis and cryptococcosis infections refractory to amphotericin B
	Liposome	Inflexal V	Inactivated influenza virus vaccine	Crucell (former Berna Biotech Ltd.)	EMA (1997)	Prevents influenza infection
	Lipid surfactant	Curosurf	Pulmonary surfactant	Chiesi Farmaceutici	FDA (1999)	Respiratory distress syndrome (RDS)
	Liposome	Myocet	Doxorubicin hydrochloride and an anthracycline cytotoxic agent	Teva Pharmaceutical Industries Ltd	EMA (2000)	Metastatic breast cancer
	Liposome	Visudyne	Verteporfin	QLT PhotoTherapeutics	FDA and EMA (2000)	Severe eye conditions like macular degeneration, decreased vision, ocular histoplasmosis, pathologic myopia
	Liposome	Depocyt	Cytarabine	Pacira Pharmaceuticals	FDA (1999) EMA (2001	Intrathecal treatment of lymphomatous meningitis

Continued

Table 10.2 Representative list of FDA/EMA-approved and globally marketed nanomedicine-based formulations from Thapa et al. [270].—*continued*

Type of formulation	Nanosystem type	Product name	Active ingredient(s)	Company	Approving organisation and approval date	Indication(s)
	Liposome	DepoDur	Morphine sulphate	Endo Pharmaceuticals	FDA (2004) Disc.* EMA (2006)	Postoperative analgesia
	Liposome	Mepact	Mifamurtide	Takeda France SAS	FDA (2001) EMA (2009)	High grade non-metastatic osteosarcoma and myosarcoma
	Liposome	Marqibo	Vincristine	Talon Therapeutics	FDA (2012) Disc.* EMA (2012)	Philadelphia chromosome-negative acute lymphoblastic leukaemia in adult patients
	Liposome	Lipodox	Doxorubicin hydrochloride	Sun Pharmaceutical Industries Ltd. (SPIL)	FDA (2013)	Kaposi's sarcoma, ovarian cancer, multiple myeloma
	Liposome	Onivyde	Irinotecan	Merrimack Pharmaceuticals	FDA (2015)	Metastatic pancreatic cancer
	Liposome	Lipusu	Paclitaxel	Luye Pgarna	FDA (2016)	Lung squamous cell carcinoma
	Liposome	Onpattro	Patisiran sodium	Alnylam Pharmaceuticals, Inc	FDA and EMA (2018)	Polyneuropathy of hereditary transthyretin-mediated amyloidosis in adults
	Liposome	Pfizer-BioNTech vaccine	mRNA vaccine	Pfizer Pharmaceuticals	FDA (2020)	Prevention of COVID-19 infection
	Liposome	Moderna vaccine	mRNA vaccine	ModernaTx Inc	FDA (2020)	Prevention of COVID-19 infection

Polymer-based nanomedicine	Nanoemulsion	Diprivan	Propofol	AstraZeneca LP	FDA (1989) EMA (2001)	Anaesthetic agent for induction and maintenance of anaesthesia. For sedation of patient under critical care and those requiring mechanical ventilator
	Polymer-protein conjugate	Adagen	Adenosine deaminase	Enzon Pharmaceuticals Inc	FDA (1990)	Adenosine deaminase-severe combined immunodeficiency disorder
	Polymer-based	Oncaspar	L-asparaginase	Enzon Pharmaceuticals Inc	FDA (1994) EMA (2016)	Acute lymphoblastic leukaemia
	Micelle	PegIntron	PEGylated interferon alpha-2B	Merck & Co. Inc	EMA (2000) FDA (2001)Disc.*	Hepatitis
	Polymer-protein conjugate	Neulasta	Filgrastim	Amgen, Inc	FDA (2002)	Neutropenia
	Polymer-protein conjugate	Pegasys	PEGylated interferon alpha-2A	Genentech, Inc	FDA and EMA (2002)	Hepatitis B and hepatitis C
	Polymer-protein conjugate	Somavert	Recombinant human growth hormone receptor antagonist	Pfizer, Inc	EMA (2002) FDA (2003)	Acromegaly
	Nanoemulsion	Restasis	Cyclosporine	Allergan	FDA (2003)	Chronic dry eye
	Nanoemulsion	Estrasorb	Estradiol	Novavax, Inc	FDA (2003)	Treatment of moderate to severe vasomotor symptoms in postmenopausal women
	Polymer-protein conjugate	Macugen	Pegaptanib sodium	Pfizer, Inc	FDA (2004)	Wet age-related macular degeneration
	Micelle	Genexol-PM	Paclitaxel	Lupin Ltd	FDA (2007)	Breast cancer
	Polymer-protein conjugate	Mircera	Epoetin beta	Vifor pharma	EMA and FDA (2007)	Renal anaemia
	Polymer-peptide conjugate	Cimzia	Certolizumab pegol	UCB	FDA (2008) EMA (2009)	Rheumatoid arthritis, Crohn's disease, psoriatic arthritis, ankylosing spondylitis
	Polymer-protein conjugate	Krystexxa	Pegloticase	Savient Pharmaceuticals	FDA (2010)	Severe and treatment-refractory chronic gout
	Polymer-protein conjugate	Plegridy	Peginterferon beta-1a	Biogene	FDA (2014)	Relapsing remitting multiple sclerosis in adults

Continued

Table 10.2 Representative list of FDA/EMA-approved and globally marketed nanomedicine-based formulations from Thapa et al. [270].—*continued*

Type of formulation	Nanosystem type	Product name	Active ingredient(s)	Company	Approving organisation and approval date	Indication(s)
	Polymer-protein conjugate	Adynovate	Recombinant antihaemophilic factor	Baxalta US Inc	FDA (2015)	Haemophilia A
	Polymer-protein conjugate	Rebinyn	Recombinant coagulation factor IX	Novo Nordisk Inc	FDA (2017)	Haemophilia B
	Polymer steroid mixture	Zilretta	Triamcinolone acetonide	Flexion Therapeutics	FDA (2017)	Knee osteoarthritis
	Micelle	Apealea	Paclitaxel	Oasmia Pharmaceutical AB	FDA (2018)	Ovarian cancer, peritoneal cancer, fallopian tube cancer
Nanocrystals	Nanocrystal	Avinza	Morphine	King Pharma	FDA (2002)	Chronic pain
	Nanocrystal	Ritalin LA	Methylphenidate hydrochloride	Novartis	FDA (2002)	Attention deficit hyperactivity disorder in children
	Nanocrystal	Zanaflex	Tizanidine hydrochloride	Acorda	FDA (2002)	Muscle relaxant
	Nanocrystal	Emend	Aprepitant	Merck & Co. Inc	FDA (2003)	Antiemetic
	Nanocrystal	Tricor	Fenofibric aid	Abott Laboratories	FDA (2004)	Antihyperlipidaemia
	Nanocrystal	NanOss	Hydroxyapatite	RTI Surgical	FDA (2005)	Bone substitute
	Nanocrystal	Megace ES	Megestrol acetate	Par Pharmaceuticals	FDA (2005)	Anorexia, cachexia and AIDS-related weight loss
	Nanocrystal	IVEmend	Fosaprepitant dimeglumine	Merck & Co. Inc	FDA and EMA (2008)	Antiemetic

	Nanocrystal	Focalin XR	Dexmethylphenidate hydrochloride	Novartis	FDA (2008)	Attention deficit hyperactivity disorder in children
	Nanocrystal	Invega	Paliperidone palmitate	Janssen Pharmaceuticals	FDA (2009)	Schizophrenia
Inorganic nanoparticles	Iron nanoparticles	Dexferrum	Iron dextran	American Regent	FDA (1996)	Iron deficiency in chronic kidney disease
	Iron nanoparticles	Venofer	Iron sucrose	Lutipold Pharmaceuticals, Inc	FDA (2000)	Iron deficiency in chronic kidney disease
	Hafnium oxide nanoparticles	Hensify	Hafnium oxide	Nanobiotix	EMA (2019)	Locally advanced squamous cell carcinoma
Protein based nanoparticles	Engineered fusion protein nanoparticle	Ontak	Denileukin diftitox	Eisai Co., Ltd	FDA (1999)	Leukaemia, T cell lymphoma
	Albumin nanoparticle	Abraxane	Paclitaxel	Eli Lilly	FDA (2005) EMA (2008)	Metastatic breast cancer

*Disc.** Discontinued.

It is not uncommon for the transition from promising preclinical studies to actual applications in patients to be accompanied by challenges and sometimes disappointment. The complexities of real-world medical contexts, patient variability and unexpected factors can contribute to outcomes that differ from early expectations. The journey from preclinical research to clinical application involves numerous steps, including regulatory hurdles, safety assessments and the adaptation of technologies to the intricacies of human biology. Despite the challenges, each step in this process contributes valuable insights that help refine and improve nanomedicines for future use. The acknowledgement of such challenges is essential for the scientific community to learn, adapt and continue refining approaches to ensure the successful translation of promising preclinical findings into effective and safe clinical applications [59,271].

In its inception, nanomedicine emerged with the primary aim of advancing cancer treatment [272]. In more recent times, the scope of nanomedicine has expanded, giving rise to a diverse array of products designed for the diagnosis and treatment of various diseases. Despite the extensive body of research published, though, the current repertoire of nanomedicines either sanctioned by the FDA and/or EMA or undergoing clinical trials remains disproportionately diminutive [273]. A comprehensive search on PubMed yields (January 2024) a staggering 48,031 articles on 'nanomedicines', juxtaposed against only 100 nanomedicines are already being marketed [270].

Noteworthy is the composition of FDA-approved nanomedicines, predominantly comprising liposomes, polymers, micelles, polymer-conjugated proteins and nanocrystals. A modest fraction encompasses metal-containing NPs, such as hydroxyapatite, calcium phosphate and IO [245,274]. Within this category, IONPs are present in six approved products primarily intended for addressing iron deficiency. However, a notable caveat arises as four of these products were withdrawn from the market due to safety concerns, leaving only two, Ferumoxytol and Resovist, currently in use [235,275]. The high success rate of approved nanoformulations is underscored by the fact that only these four have been discontinued [243,246,276,277]. This reflects the ongoing progress and potential within the nanomedicine landscape [278].

The discrepancy between the substantial volume of scientific literature published annually on NPs formulations and those approved for clinical use is attributed to both experimental and regulatory barriers. On the experimental front, challenges arise from the need for a comprehensive characterisation scheme and an extended toxicity profile for tested NPs. Conversely, regulatory obstacles stem from the absence of well-defined international guidelines and the necessity to articulate the cost-benefit considerations associated with nanomedicine formulations (as discussed in the previous section). Realistic expectations for the nanomedicine field are contingent upon a thorough comprehension of nanoformulations and their interactions within the human body [274]. While acknowledging these challenges, efforts to gain a more precise understanding of nanomedicine are imperative. This involves the meticulous characterisation of existing approved nanomedicines to grasp their intrinsic properties and biological effects fully. Such insights will pave the way for the development of intelligent novel nanomedicines tailored to precisely target diseases and personalised nanotherapies. A retrospective review of nanoformulation clinical trials since the 2000s reveals a consistent increase, notably peaking in the years 2013–15 (Figure 10.7) [173,274].

While the current number of nanotech-based medicines may seem limited, there is a significant presence of clinical trials involving NPs, with precisely 636 listed in the US NIH database ClinicalTrials.gov as of January 2024, particularly in phase I (223) and phase II (264). Anticipated advancements in these trials may lead to approvals and subsequent market availability in the coming years, thereby contributing to the growing number of successful nanopharmaceuticals.

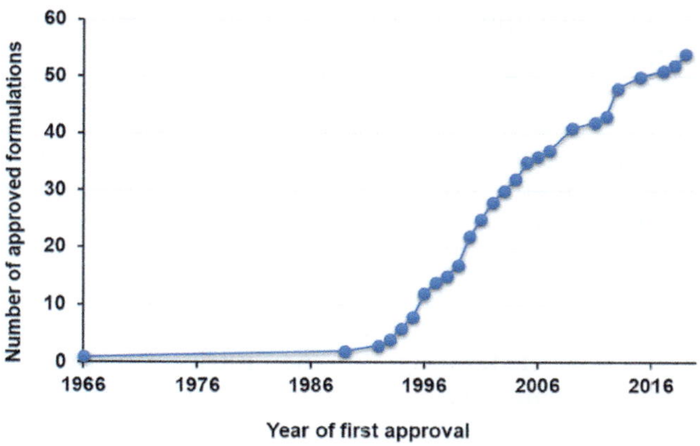

Figure 10.7 Evolution of the approved nanomedicine formulations (cumulative number/year). First year of approval reported for formulations approved by multiple agencies (e.g. EMA and FDA). Reproduced with permission from Germain et al. [153].

The prevailing model in the innovation chain of nanobiotech often involves discoveries originating in academic laboratories, followed by the transfer of these breakthroughs to spin-offs or high-tech small- and medium-sized enterprise (SMEs) that cater to niche markets. These entities play a crucial role in validating concepts and initiating early clinical trials, sometimes progressing up to stage IIa. Subsequently, larger companies acquire these SMEs, bringing innovative and validated devices, molecules or concepts into their portfolio. This collaborative and evolving model underscores the dynamic nature of the nanopharmaceutical landscape [154]. These processes and steps are schematised in Fig. 10.8.

It is worth noting that the average approval rate of nanomedicines compared to classical drugs varies across different fields, with notable distinctions observed in oncology versus other clinical applications. He et al. conducted an analysis of the success rates of nanomedicine formulations in oncology across various clinical phases. In this context, the success rate for nano-enabled cancer drugs in phase 1 was found to be 94%, a statistic attributed to their favourable safety profile and improved pharmacokinetics. However, as drugs progress to phase 2 and 3, the success rates decrease to 48% and 14%, respectively, with an estimated total success rate from phase 1 to approval standing at 6%. This indicates that nanomedicines in oncology perform comparatively better than conventional drugs, which exhibit a success rate of 3.4% [279]. Nevertheless, it is correct to state that nanomedicine has predominantly focussed on cancer, and that the clinical outcomes for other applications have been less promising. The reasons behind the limited success of nanomedicines outside of oncology in reaching clinical trials and market approval are multifaceted and may involve challenges related to formulation, manufacturing and specific biological interactions. Further research and development efforts are essential to address these challenges and broaden the impact of nanomedicine across a wider spectrum of clinical applications [153]. The complexity of NPs stands out as a critical aspect, requiring thorough analysis. This complexity poses a significant challenge for the design and development of NPs, extending to the intricacies of the manufacturing process. Addressing this complexity is paramount for achieving scale-up manufacture reproducibility essential for clinical use. Importantly, it represents a major barrier that hinders adoption by the pharmaceutical industry, underscoring the need for innovative solutions and strategies to overcome these challenges [241].

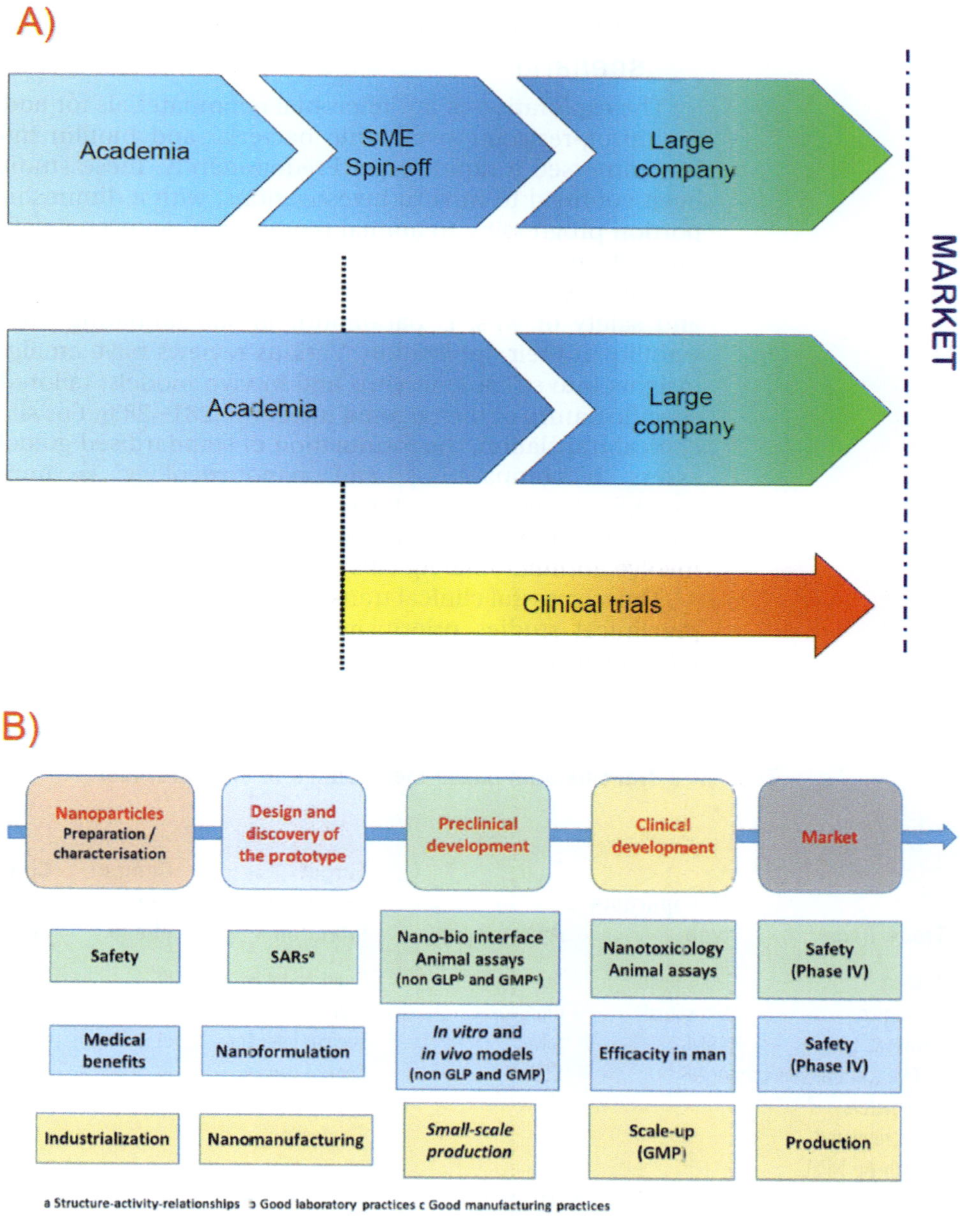

Figure 10.8 Innovation chain of nanomedicine (A) and overview of critical paths to clinical applications of NPs (B). Adapted with permission from Mignan et al. [241] Copyright 2020 American Chemical Society.

4.1 Antimicrobial nanoparticles translational scenario

The exploration of antimicrobial nanomaterials for addressing multidrug-resistant planktonic bacterial and biofilm infections has witnessed a rapid surge. Predominantly, these studies have been confined to in vitro investigations, with a diminishing proportion progressing to animal models, and an even smaller fraction advancing to human trials [274,280]. The establishment of appropriate in vitro and in vivo models, elucidating both efficacy and safety of NPs, is paramount in substantiating the clinical viability of their application. Various reviews have amalgamated insights into suitable in vitro and in vivo models, tailored to the specific nature of the targeted infection [281–283]. For successful clinical translation, the formulation of standardised guidelines to assess biocompatibility and nanotoxicology is imperative. Notably, the majority of formulations undergoing clinical testing either pertain to nanocarriers designed for antibiotic delivery or involve antimicrobial Ag NPs (Table 10.3) [7].

The successful clinical translation of nanomedicines hinges on preclinical studies prioritising therapeutic efficacy parameters relevant to clinical trials, coupled with a meticulous evaluation

Table 10.3 Nanomaterial-based therapeutics in clinical trials.

Trade name	Nanoparticle type	Active agent	Target pathogens or infection	Clinical trial phase	Clinical trial number
Arikace	Liposomal	Amikacin	Gram negative	III	NCT01315691
Pulmaquin	Liposomal	Ciprofloxacin	Gram negative	III	NCT02104245
Silvasorb	AgNP	Silver	Topical infection	III	NCT00659204
AgTive (central venous catheters impregnated with Ag NPs)	AgNP	Silver	Central venous catheter-related infection	IV	NCT00337714
NA	Polymeric nanoparticle	Doxycycline	Chronic periodontitis	II	NCT02726646
NA	Polymeric nanoparticle	Ammonium polyethyleneimine	Oral infection	II	NCT01167985

Ag NP, silver nanoparticle; *NA*, not applicable.
Adapted with permission from Makabenta et al. [7].

of the safety aspects of the nanoparticle system, encompassing both material and drug concentrations within tissues. The bulk of research in this domain, along with filed patents, emanates from the endeavours of academic researchers [177,284], often backed by governmental nanotechnology funding programmes, such as those in the United States, Germany or Japan [176]. While substantial strides have been made in research, the realisation of the commercial success of nanomedicines faces hurdles without robust support from industry for clinical trial development and the absence of comprehensive national and international regulations. This predicament is evident in the relatively modest number of clinical trials—only 35—exploring the use of NPs in infectious diseases (data from ClinicalTrials.gov, as of January 2024), despite the plethora of research papers published. These trials encompass diverse systems and applications, ranging from ciprofloxacin liposomes (NCT01515007) to the use of amikacin liposomes in bronchiectasis (NCT00775138), cystic fibrosis (NCT00558844) or chronic infection (NCT01315691); and in other populations, such as newborns (NCT00815516) [285]. There are also clinical trials addressing their use antimicrobial agents in medical devices, such as Ag NPs in central venous catheters (NCT00337714) [285].

4.1.1 Liposomal NPs

Among all the nanomedicines accessible in the market or in various stages of clinical translations, liposome or lipid-based NPs are the most prevalent category (33%) [269]. The first FDA-approved liposomal formulation was Doxil, an encapsulated doxorubicin formulation within liposomes, securing its initial FDA approval in 1995 and exhibiting enhanced cardiac safety in comparison to traditional doxorubicin [272]. Subsequently, several other FDA-approved drug delivery methodologies have emerged, encompassing DaunoXome (liposomal daunorubicin), Myocet (liposomal doxorubicin), Onivyde MM-398 (liposomal irinotecan) and Abraxane (albumin-bound paclitaxel), among others. The success of these carriers is attributed to various factors, including their high biocompatibility, capacity to transport both hydrophilic and hydrophobic drugs, and their propensity to accumulate in tumour tissues [286,287]. Beyond enhancing therapeutic safety, NPs serve the purpose of mitigating peak toxicities through the gradual release or transport of inherently unstable compounds, such as RNA vulnerable to rapid extracellular degradation by RNases [288]. A pivotal milestone was the 2018 FDA approval of Onpattro, the inaugural siRNA drug utilising lipid NPs for encapsulation and delivery [289]. This ground-breaking translation has spurred further exploration of RNA interference (RNAi) for diverse disease treatments and the development of mRNA-based vaccines [189,290].

Various antimicrobials designed for the treatment of airway infections can be effectively delivered through liposomal carriers. In the realm of controlled antibiotic delivery, two liposomal nanoformulations have progressed to advanced clinical trials or received approval for some applications. Arikace, presenting a liposomal rendition of the antibiotic amikacin, has been intricately engineered to enhance therapeutic efficacy and half-life while concurrently mitigating renal and neurological toxicity associated with amikacin [291]. In parallel, Pulmaquin, a nanoliposome-based formulation, is designed to facilitate both rapid and delayed release of ciprofloxacin [292]. Despite the persistent challenges, it is foreseeable that these innovative therapeutics will eventually offer solutions to currently unmet clinical demands (vide infra) [7,274,280]. The realm of liposomal formulations in addressing bacterial diseases, extensively discussed by Sallovitz et al. [293], spans both human and veterinary medicine. Various bacteria, including *S. aureus*, as well as several species of *Salmonella*, *Brucella* and *Mycobacteria* have been subjects of investigation concerning liposomal formulations [294].

Amikacin is a semisynthetic aminoglycoside antibiotic derived from kanamycin A, and employed against a broad spectrum of Gram-negative organisms and is particularly effective in treating severe chronic lung infections with multidrug-resistant organisms, including *P. aeruginosa* in both cystic fibrosis and non-cystic fibrosis clinical patients [295]. In its liposomal formulation, the encapsulation process offers advantages such as sustained release, rapid delivery times and protection from charged sputum compared to free amikacin [296]. The resulting liposomal amikacin for inhalation, Arikace, is administered through aerosolised delivery—an approach recognised for maximising pulmonary drug concentration while minimising systemic toxicity risks [296–298]. Arikace has shown promising progress in combating lung infections caused by multidrug-resistant organisms, with its nanoformulation providing prolonged and sustained drug release, as well as efficient penetration into bacterial biofilms. Notably, Zhang et al. [299] delved into the efficacy of liposomal amikacin against nontuberculous mycobacteria in both in *in vivo* (rat model) and in vitro settings. Their findings highlighted the ability of the nanoformulated drug to effectively penetrate bacterial biofilms, enhance cellular uptake of amikacin in macrophages and restrict the distribution of amikacin to other tissues.

Further in vitro studies have demonstrated the ability of Arikace to effectively penetrate *M. avium* complex biofilms, the most common non-tuberculous mycobacteria species found in cystic fibrosis patients. The incorporation of amikacin into liposomes has led to a fourfold increase in drug uptake in pulmonary macrophages compared to free amikacin [218,299]. Another study determined that Arikace exhibits activity against both *P. aeruginosa* and *Mycobacterium abscessus (M. abscessus)* [300]. A double-blind, randomised phase II clinical trial conducted by Olivier et al. [301] investigated the application of inhaled liposomal amikacin for the treatment of non-tuberculous mycobacterial lung disease. The results of the trial demonstrated that the liposomal formulation facilitated the negative conversion of sputum and exhibited lower toxicity in comparison to parenteral amikacin. Furthermore, Okusanya et al. [302], through a randomised controlled clinical trial, reported that liposomal amikacin contributed to improved lung function and reduced bacterial density in the lungs of patients afflicted with chronic *Pseudomonas* infection [303]. In a recent development, the FDA has granted approval for the use of liposomal amikacin via inhalation as a treatment for refractory *M. avium* complex [304]. Concurrently, this nanoparticulate formulation is undergoing advanced clinical trials for its efficacy in addressing *P. aeruginosa* infection in cystic fibrosis patients [305]. This innovative approach facilitates a targeted and localised drug administration, thereby diminishing the systemic exposure of antibiotics with potential toxicity. Furthermore, the inherent ability of liposomes to infiltrate biofilms and be assimilated by alveolar macrophages suggests additional pharmacological advantages [32,306]. Local delivery to the site of infection offers several advantages, especially in terms of optimising drug exposure. By directly targeting the infected area, this approach allows for higher concentrations of the drug to be delivered precisely where it is needed most, minimising exposure to healthy tissues and reducing off-target effects. This strategy is particularly effective for localised infections, where systemic administration might result in lower drug concentrations at the infection site. However, for systemic infections that affect multiple sites or organs, local delivery may have limitations, and systemic administration might be more appropriate [1].

Ciprofloxacin, a widely utilised antibiotic for treating various acute and chronic lung infections [307], has been subject to preclinical assessments highlighting the favourable pharmacokinetic attributes of aerosolised liposomal ciprofloxacin. This nanostructured liquid vesicle, composed of lipids encapsulating ciprofloxacin, demonstrated heightened efficacy in *in vitro* studies involving

M. avium and *M. abscessus* strains when compared to free ciprofloxacin [308]. Additionally, findings from preclinical mouse models indicated that aerosolised nanoliposomal ciprofloxacin boasted an extended elimination half-life of up to 10 h, with detectable ciprofloxacin levels in the lungs even 24 h post-aerosol therapy—a notable contrast to the approximately 2-hour half-life of free ciprofloxacin [309]. Noteworthy superiority in antibacterial efficacy was confirmed for liposomally encapsulated ciprofloxacin relative to its unencapsulated counterpart [310]. Based on these results, the formulation Pulmaquin (Linhaliq) represents a dual-release composition, constituting a 1:1 blend of nanoliposomal ciprofloxacin and free ciprofloxacin, featuring an antibiotic slow-release feature [308]. In a phase II study, non-cystic fibrosis patients with bronchiectasis treated with Pulmaquin experienced a substantial reduction of 4.2 log colony-forming units (CFU) in *P. aeruginosa* density in sputum by day 28. Considering these encouraging results, two parallel phase III studies (NCT01515007 and NCT02104245) were conducted to assess the efficacy of Pulmaquin in non-cystic fibrosis patients with bronchiectasis infected with *P. aeruginosa.* The outcomes demonstrated a significant decline in annual exacerbation frequency and sputum *P. aeruginosa* density compared to the placebo group, with the treatment proving safe and well-tolerated [218,311].

Other noteworthy contributions to the antimicrobial liposomal scenario include the work of MacLeod and Prescott, who demonstrated the efficacy of liposomal entrapped gentamicin in eradicating *S. aureus* mastitis in bovines [312]. Specific liposomal compositions have exhibited substantial antibacterial effects against both Gram-positive and Gram-negative bacteria. For instance, liposomes incorporating dipalmitoyl phosphatidylcholine and dimyristoylphosphatidyl glycerol, encapsulating tobramycin, demonstrated considerable antibacterial efficacy [313,314]. These findings underscore the potential of liposomal formulations as versatile tools in combatting bacterial infections across diverse bacterial species [76].

Another innovative approach for topical drug delivery involves a novel liposome formulation stabilised by chitosan-modified Au NPs (AuChi) for the differential release of the model antibiotic vancomycin, with the aim of inhibiting the growth of *S. aureus* bacteria for the topical treatment of skin bacterial infections. The working principle revolves around toxin-triggered antibiotic release from Au NPs-stabilised liposomes, specifically designed to combat bacteria secreting toxins. In this system, cationic AuChi binds to the negatively charged surfaces of liposomes through electrostatic attraction, thereby stabilising the liposomes and preventing fusion with one another, thus avoiding undesirable antibiotic leakage. When these stabilised liposomes are in proximity to *S. aureus* bacteria, the toxins secreted by the bacteria insert into the liposome membrane, creating pores through which the encapsulated antibiotic is released. The released vancomycin, situated in close proximity to the bacteria, promptly exerts its antimicrobial activity in a rapid and localised manner. The optimisation of liposome composition and chitosan-modified Au NPs coverage on the liposome surface ensures that liposome fusion activity and undesired drug leakage are prevented under normal storage conditions. Simultaneously, the liposomes remain susceptible to pore-forming toxins secreted by bacteria. Upon incubation with toxins, the liposomes become permeable, leading to the rapid release of encapsulated antibiotic payloads through the pores formed by the toxins. The effectiveness of this antimicrobial drug delivery approach is underscored by the demonstration that, in the presence of toxin-secreting bacteria, 100% of the encapsulated antibiotics are released from the Au NPs-stabilised liposomes, resulting in the effective inhibition of bacterial growth within 24 h. This method introduces a groundbreaking paradigm for the treatment of bacterial infections, allowing for the specific release of drugs at infectious sites while minimising potential off-target effects [315].

4.1.2 Inorganic NPs

In the face of escalating antibiotic resistance in bacteria, inorganic nanomaterials have emerged as promising candidates. Inorganic NPs undergoing or with a promising potential clinical translation mainly include metal NPs, metal oxide NPs and carbon NPs.

As extensively highlighted in the previous sections, metal NPs play a crucial role in the biomedical field, particularly in their ability to bind with drugs, antibodies and ligands, making them highly valuable in various applications [316]. Their advantages include greater durability, lower toxicity and higher stability and selectivity compared to organic alternatives [317]. Metal NPs can be conjugated with various functional groups, resulting in stable NPs within the size range of 1–100 nm. This adaptability positions metal NPs as versatile tools in addressing critical challenges in the biomedical field, offering innovative solutions for diagnostics, imaging, and therapeutic interventions [76,318]. Biologically synthesised Ag NPs with an average size of 60 nm were utilised in concentrations of 15 and 20 mg/kg in an Ag NPs-loaded vaccine, which was administered in vivo. The in vivo toxicity assessment demonstrated the safety of Ag NPs and the Ag NPs-loaded vaccine in both animal models tested (mice and dogs).

Given the escalating threat of antibiotic-resistant bacteria in both human and veterinary medicine, there is a growing need for innovative therapeutic approaches. The development of combined therapy incorporating low levels of antibiotics and Ag NPs presents a novel strategy to enhance antibacterial effects [319,320]. An example is the integration of Ag NPs into wound care formulations, exemplified by Acticoat bandages (Smith & Nephew), incorporating nanocrystal silver highly lethal to pathogens in wounds, therefore adding another dimension to this antimicrobial arsenal [127]. Another product containing Ag NPs is Silvasorb, an antimicrobial gel that also can be used to treat infected wounds [321]. In addition, AgTive is a marketed silver-impregnated central venous catheter with improved bactericidal activity. Comprising polyurethanes impregnated with Ag NPs, these catheters interact with body fluids and intravenous solutions, resulting in the release of significantly larger amounts of silver ions from the catheter therefore reducing bloodstream infection [21,322].

Among metal oxide NPs, ZnO NPs have garnered significant interest for their potential commercial applications, being extensively employed in diverse fields such as catalysis, sensors, environmental remediation and personal care products. More recently, the application of ZnO NPs has extended into various realms of veterinary sciences, leveraging their antibacterial, antineoplastic, wound healing, and angiogenic properties. ZnO NPs have been utilised in tissue repair, serving as a food preservative, and incorporated as a feed additive in veterinary applications. This multifaceted utilisation underscores the versatility of ZnO NPs [76]. Furthermore, recent example shows that the combination of noble metals and ZnO NPs can enhance antimicrobial activity and demonstrate potential for multifunctional applications. ZnO NPs are also used in photocatalysis and solar-energy conversion. However, the inherent limitations of pure ZnO NPs, such as fast electron/hole recombination and low charge separation efficiency, hinder their energy-conversion efficiency [323]. To address this, the deposition of gold (Au) onto the surface of ZnO, even at a low Au/ZnO molar ratio of 0.2%, has been found to substantially enhance the generation of ROS [324]. Comparative analysis revealed that the antibacterial activity was significantly enhanced (approximately threefold increase) against two representative bacterial strains (*S. aureus* and *E. coli*), when bacteria were treated with ZnO/Au hybrid nanosystems under simulated sunlight irradiation, in contrast to pure ZnO NPs. This improvement is attributed to the high charge separation efficiency and enhanced ROS generation facilitated by the unique ZnO/Au hybrid structures. This example introduces an alternative approach to enhance the photocatalytic and antibacterial activity of metal oxides through integration with noble metals, showcasing the potential of hybrid nanosystems for multifunctional applications [325,326].

Despite the extensive research efforts in the realm of metal oxide NPs formulations for antimicrobial applications, iron oxide NPs (IO NPs) stand as the sole representative of metal oxide NPs with FDA approval, featuring applications in both imaging and the treatment of iron deficiency [245,327,328]. However, it is pertinent to acknowledge that many IO NPs formulations have been withdrawn from clinical use, possibly due to associated side effects such as severe lower back pain and life-threatening hypersensitivity reactions, or inferior imaging efficacy compared to alternative MRI agents [275]. The FDA approval process for these IO NPs formulations involved rigorous physicochemical and biological assessments at preclinical and clinical stages, yet these measures did not entirely assure biological safety and efficacy, suggesting the need for additional tests in the future. This could potentially impede the progress of other metal oxide NPs in antimicrobial applications. Nonetheless, there are promising avenues to explore, such as Ferumoxytol, incorporating IO NPs coated with polyglucose sorbitol carboxymethylether, which is currently deemed extremely safe for clinical use [327,329,330]. Given the demonstrated antibacterial, antiviral and antiparasitic activity of IO NPs, investigating the antimicrobial potential of Ferumoxytol appears to be a worthwhile pursuit. The limited representation of metal oxide NPs in FDA approval may stem from inadequate attention to crucial biological and technical considerations essential for the translation to preclinical and clinical stages. Key biological challenges encompass stability in blood plasma, traversing biological barriers, selective targeting to infected organs/cells, potential initiation of immune responses, safe elimination from humans post-treatment, and assessment of potential biotoxicities associated with long-term administration. Additionally, technical questions related to large-scale production issues and requisite physicochemical property tests for reproducible metal oxide NPs production must be addressed [87].

Carbon NPs, including nanodiamond, graphite, graphene oxide, fullerenes, carbon nanotubes, carbon nanohorns and more, have been extensively researched and applied in biomedical fields for diagnostic and therapeutic purposes, owing to their biocompatibility and low toxicity. These NPs find utility as drug carriers, showcasing their versatility in various biomedical applications [331]. Despite their promising applications, it is crucial to note that the impact of carbon NPs on organisms with prolonged exposure and higher concentrations remains unclear, as highlighted previously. Single-walled carbon nanotubes, for instance, have been shown to trigger oxidative stress and exhibit cytotoxicity in cultured cell lines [332]. Furthermore, concerns about the toxicity and biodegradability of carbon nanomaterials pose significant challenges in their clinical application [333,334]. As such, careful consideration and further research are necessary to fully understand and address the potential risks associated with the extended and concentrated use of carbon NPs in biomedical contexts [76]. However, due to the excellent properties of carbon NPs, such as high aspect ratio, high sensitivity, high conductivity and excellent stability, they may have a greater potential for applications involving ex vivo diagnosis of infections.

4.2 Issues to focus on in clinical translation

The challenges associated with the clinical translation of nanomedicine are indeed numerous and intricate. Several key difficulties include:

(i) Lack of Education in Business Management: there is a deficiency in education, particularly at the academic level, regarding business management. Bridging this gap is crucial for researchers to navigate the complexities of translating nanomedicine innovations into viable commercial entities;

(ii) Pre-clinical Characterisation and Safety Assessment: performing pre-clinical characterisation and safety assessments at early stages is challenging. This is often attributed to the absence of standardised protocols and limited access to specialised characterisation facilities, hindering robust evaluation and understanding of nanomedicine formulations;

(iii) Scale-Up and GMP Manufacturing: scaling up the production of nanomedicines and adhering to Good Manufacturing Practices (GMP) pose significant challenges. The transition from laboratory-scale production to large-scale manufacturing is a critical step, and challenges in achieving consistency and quality can arise;

(iv) Regulatory Framework Uncertainty and Fragmentation: as extensively discussed previously, the regulatory landscape for nanomedicines is characterised by uncertainty and fragmentation, especially for complex borderline products that integrate multiple technologies. The lack of clear and harmonised regulations complicates the regulatory pathway for these innovative products. Addressing these challenges necessitates collaborative efforts across academia, industry and regulatory bodies to establish comprehensive education, standardised protocols and a more cohesive regulatory framework for the successful clinical translation of nanomedicine [152,153,335].

As mentioned earlier, nanotechnology stands as a significant and burgeoning industry, and this transformative field engenders the creation of novel materials endowed with diverse and beneficial functions in the realm of medicine. Therefore, the toxicology of NPs and nanostructures in medical applications is a paramount aspect when considering clinical translation [76]. Potential toxic effects have a direct impact on the success or failure of clinical translation, and there are already examples of what is at stake.

Significant safety insights are surfacing in the context of COVID-19 vaccines. Notably, severe allergic reactions, including instances of anaphylactic shock, have been reported following the administration of both Pfizer/BioNT and Moderna vaccines [336]. The suspected culprit behind these allergic reactions is the PEG content found in the solid lipid NPs [336]. However, it remains plausible that the adverse reactions may stem from other components within the formulations, such as ionic condensing lipids, which have not undergone prior human testing. The US FDA Centre for Biologics Evaluation and Research is actively investigating not only PEG but also four other ingredients in this regard [336,337]. Identifying the specific component responsible for these reactions holds the key to refining future vaccine formulations to mitigate immunogenicity or screen for potential immune responses. For instance, if PEG is pinpointed as the immunogenic element, pre-administration screening for anti-PEG antibodies could effectively identify individuals prone to adverse allergic reactions. This underscores the imperative for concurrent advancements in research and development, particularly in the realms of patient screening and monitoring [235].

A pivotal factor in preclinical studies lies in comprehending the toxicity of nanomaterials, as extensively discussed in the previous sections. Nanostructures hold allure in the field of medicine not only due to their chemical and biological activity but also because they possess the capability to access regions inaccessible through traditional methods. These structures can be inhaled, ingested, translocate through the skin, and, once inside the body, penetrate tissues, cells and physical barriers, such as traversing from the lungs to the bloodstream or crossing the blood–brain barrier to reach vital organs. However, the potential benefits of these nanostructures coexist with the risk of unintended harm, which acts like a broad-spectrum property. Over 2 decades of nanotoxicology research has elucidated the intricate interactions of nanomaterials with cells, animals, humans and the environment. These interactions are notably complex and have been associated with various adverse effects, including cell apoptosis, inflammation, exacerbation of asthma, fibrosis, the onset of chronic inflammatory lung diseases and carcinogenesis [338]. The broad spectrum of NPs, each characterised by distinct materials used in their production, results in variations in structure, surface area, solubility, cytotoxicity, and physical and chemical properties [339].

In addition to toxicity, the clinical apprehension surrounding resistance to NPs remains a pertinent concern [340]. Although infrequent, instances of bacteria exhibiting resistance to Ag, Au or Cu NPs have been documented, even following exposure to a single dose of NPs [176,340,341]. Mechanisms underlying this resistance may involve alterations in outer membrane permeability and heightened expression of efflux pumps [340,341]. The expanding clinical use of Ag NPs has heightened anxieties regarding bacterial resistance to these NPs [342]. Notably, resistance to Ag NPs attributed to sil genes has been observed in clinical isolates of *K. pneumoniae* and *Enterobacter cloacae* derived from burn cases [341]. Genetic modifications in bacteria can lead to the swift evolution of resistance to Ag NPs [343], while Al_2O_3 NPs have been implicated in promoting the increased expression of conjugation-promoting genes and facilitating the horizontal transfer of antibiotic resistance genes [25]. Further complicating matters, the phenotypic shift in flagellin production in *E. coli* isolates resistant to Ag NPs has been identified as a factor inducing NP aggregation and diminishing the antimicrobial efficacy of Ag NPs [341,344]. The emergence of resistance to NPs underscores the importance of ongoing vigilance and comprehensive understanding to navigate potential challenges in their clinical application [18].

For the nanomaterials discussed in this chapter, their efficacious antibacterial mechanisms may encounter challenges when transitioning into the in vivo environment. Firstly, the in vivo milieu is characterised by a polyanionic system [345], where metal cations originating from metal NPs may be attracted by other host molecules. This phenomenon has the potential to divert these NPs from their intended antimicrobial path at a systemic level or reduce the cation concentration in the immediate environment of the infection site. Secondly, ROS generated by NPs can face substantial diminishment or neutralisation in vivo, as biomolecules such as ascorbic acid (vitamin C), uric acid, bilirubin, albumin, glutathione, γ-tocopherol (vitamin E), or ubiquinol of blood lipoproteins have the capacity to intercept them [346]. Additionally, metal NPs, as previously highlighted may induce immunotoxicity, cytotoxicity and genotoxicity in both pathogenic bacteria and healthy human cells [347]. Considering these factors, the most plausible clinical application of metal NPs against bacterial infections may be confined to topical or local use (with the limitation explored in the previous section). This approach accounts for the intricate in vivo dynamics that could potentially compromise the efficacy and safety of systemic administration [141].

In general, it is paramount to perform animal studies to understand the underlying mechanisms as well as potential therapeutic activity of antimicrobial substances. The zebrafish has emerged as an increasingly important in vivo model for studying infectious diseases [348]. Animal studies, including those utilising zebrafish, play a crucial role in unravelling the underlying mechanisms and evaluating the potential therapeutic activity of antimicrobial substances [349]. Leveraging in vivo models allows researchers to gain insights into the complex interactions between pathogens and the host organism, facilitating a deeper understanding of disease processes and aiding the development of effective treatment strategies. The use of zebrafish as a model organism provides unique advantages, including optical transparency during early developmental stages and genetic tractability, making it a valuable tool in infectious disease research. Rodents are also often used as animal models. The translation of findings from rodent models to humans is indeed a critical step in drug development, however the process has complexities. Enhanced permeability observed in rodent models may not necessarily translate directly to humans due to physiological and anatomical differences. Additionally, the correlation between the degree of targeting and the severity of infection raises important questions about the applicability of nanoencapsulation across different infection scenarios [350]. The choice of disease models and the relevance of the bacterial load used in rodent models compared to human infections are crucial factors to consider. If the numbers used in rodents are not representative of the human context, the interpretation of the data may need adjustment. Moreover, the balance between on-target accumulation and potential off-target effects is a key consideration. If a substantial fraction of the drug accumulates at non-target sites, especially if these sites are associated with toxicity, it could impact the overall therapeutic benefit. These challenges underscore the importance of rigorous preclinical testing and thoughtful consideration during the transition from animal models to human clinical trials. It is a complex process that requires a thorough understanding of both the disease and the potential impact of the nanomaterial (e.g. drug delivery nanosystems) in human patients [1].

For preclinical testing, organoids indeed hold great promise as ex vivo models for studying infectious diseases. However, challenges persist in the absence of widely accepted standardised protocols and guidelines for generating and maintaining organoid cultures. Additionally, genetic variations among individuals from whom cultures are derived contribute to inherent variability in each generated culture. This variability introduces heterogeneity into the system, complicating data analysis and the interpretation of results obtained with each culture. Questions linger regarding the optimal methods for assessing both the quality and validity of these cultures. As researchers work towards refining and standardising organoid culture protocols, addressing these challenges will be crucial to enhance the reliability and reproducibility of findings in infectious disease research using organoids [351,352].

In addition, the market success necessitates a favourable cost-effectiveness ratio, an aspect where current nanotechnology systems face challenges due to their relatively high prices. The cost of treatments is a significant factor in determining their accessibility and feasibility, especially in low-resource countries. If nanosystems incorporate expensive excipients or require specific synthesis and storage conditions that are not easily met in such settings, it could limit the widespread adoption of these treatments. Addressing these challenges might involve exploring alternative excipients that are more cost-effective or developing formulations that are more stable under varied storage conditions. Finding ways to simplify the synthesis process, perhaps through scalable and cost-efficient methods, could also contribute to reducing the overall cost of nanosystems. The goal is to make these innovative treatments not only effective but also practical and affordable, ensuring that they can benefit a broad range of populations, including those in low-resource settings. It requires a multidisciplinary approach that considers economic, logistical, and healthcare infrastructure factors alongside the technical aspects of nanomedicine development [353].

While polymeric and liposomal formulations have their drawbacks in terms of requiring large excipient quantities, the emergence of aqueous dispersions of nano-milled drug crystals presents a promising alternative [354]. The physicochemical properties of the drug and the size of drug crystals become critical factors in determining drug release kinetics following subcutaneous or intramuscular injection. By carefully manipulating these factors, researchers aim to achieve controlled and sustained drug release, optimising therapeutic outcomes [355]. However, a potential concern with sustained release systems is the risk of prolonged exposure to sub-therapeutic drug concentrations, which could contribute to the development of drug resistance. Balancing the advantages of extended drug release with the need for maintaining therapeutic efficacy remains a key consideration in the development of such formulations [356].

Cost-effectiveness studies in various countries often favour conventional treatments [357–359], yet nanotechnology treatments may find a niche in specific situations, such as Ambisome for disseminated histoplasmosis and AIDS patients [360]. The pharmaceutical landscape in recent years has grappled with escalating costs and a stagnation in approval rates, prompting major pharmaceutical companies to assume risk-averse stances in research and development precisely when innovative approaches are most crucial [361]. Despite their higher costs, nanotechnology treatments can potentially optimise resource utilisation and enhance the quality of patients' lives by mitigating adverse effects [176,362]. Nanomedicines, by introducing new functionalities, emerge as a compelling solution that not only broadens the scope of therapeutic strategies but also presents the opportunity for broad-spectrum therapies. Whether through novel drug discovery, repurposing, or a multi-purposing approach, the development of broad-spectrum strategies not only diversifies business risk but also holds the potential for increased revenue with prorated expenses. In this context, nanomedicines uniquely offer opportunities to enhance the therapeutic potential of clinically approved drugs through various means, including heightened selectivity and localised delivery. Consequently, nanomedicines are poised to catalyse breakthroughs in broad-spectrum antimicrobial treatments. As the development of lead nanomedicines progresses, positioning them for market entry becomes crucial, especially at a juncture when the pharmaceutical industry is actively seeking new avenues for disruptive innovations. The continued advancement of nanomedicines holds the promise of transforming the landscape of infectious disease treatment and contributing to the much-needed paradigm shift in pharmaceutical research and development [363].

5. Conclusions

In conclusion, nanomaterials represent an innovative and unconventional approach for addressing challenging multidrug-resistant planktonic as well as biofilm bacterial infections. The adjustable properties of nanomaterials, particularly their surface functionalities, offer a versatile design space that can be finely tuned to optimise therapeutic efficacy while minimising host toxicity. This chapter has outlined instances where NPs exhibit efficacy against bacteria in both planktonic and biofilm forms through a diverse array of mechanisms. The potential of nanomaterials extends from topical to systemic treatments of planktonic as well as biofilm-associated infections in a plethora of therapeutic contexts. Crucially, the multifaceted antibacterial mechanisms of nanomaterials introduce novel strategies that can impede or halt the development of drug resistance. As an example, the combination of bactericidal effects with biofilm dispersion strategies emerges as an ideal approach for ensuring the comprehensive eradication of biofilms. Stimuli-responsive NPs, capitalising on unique microenvironments at infection sites such as pH variations and pathogen-derived metabolites, exemplify one avenue for targeting multidrug-resistant bacteria [141].

While the conceptual foundation supporting the application of nanomedicines for antimicrobial therapy (and not only) is solidified, the translation of these concepts into practical implementation necessitates the resolution of critical considerations. Safety, regulation, and manufacturing emerge as paramount challenges that demand attention. In our opinion, pivotal questions during the developmental phase of a nanomedicine include:

(i) How does the nanomedicine offer a superior solution to the clinical problem?

(ii) Is it feasible to manufacture the nanomedicine on a sufficiently large scale?

(iii) Does the justification for additional costs associated with nanomedicine production, including rigorous quality control, exist?

Addressing these questions not only ensures the effective translation of nanomedicine concepts into real-world applications but also establishes a robust foundation for their safe and scalable integration into medical practices [363].

Transitioning from laboratory success to clinical application indeed poses a unique set of challenges. The complexities of biological interactions and potential toxicological implications from chronic administration require thorough investigation and understanding. The shift from controlled experimental conditions to the dynamic and diverse environment of the human body introduces new variables and considerations. To bridge the gap between laboratory research and clinical implementation, it is crucial to conduct comprehensive preclinical studies that closely mimic human physiology and pathology. This involves refining the understanding of how nanomaterials interact with biological systems over extended periods, including their biodistribution, pharmacokinetics and long-term effects. Ongoing studies are actively investigating the pharmacokinetic profiles of NPs to enhance our understanding of their fate within the body. Certainly, significant barriers to clinical use remain, chiefly concerning systemic safety and the long-term effects of NPs on the body, in addition to some issues with current public perception and worry as well as with associated costs and regulatory process [66].

Without the shadow of a doubt, interdisciplinary collaboration stands as the linchpin for ensuring the genuine success of nanomedicine. An interdisciplinary team facilitates the identification of key factors for the clinical translation of nanoparticle systems, encompassing safety, loading capacity, controlled release in specific milieus and targeted biodistribution. The selection of NPs is intricately tied to disease targets and the characteristics of the loaded drugs. Through this collaborative approach, nanomedicine systems are poised to revolutionise the design of patient-friendly dose regimens, concurrently enhancing effectiveness. The collective expertise of diverse disciplines converges to unlock the full potential of nanomedicine, offering innovative solutions that have the potential to significantly impact healthcare outcomes [176]. The development of effective antimicrobial nanomaterials therefore necessitates synergistic and collaborative efforts across a variety of fields, involving chemists, physicists, engineers, healthcare and biomedical researchers (biologists, microbiologists, pharmacists, physicians, etc.), and clinical researchers in the health field. All of these figures are indispensable in in realising the full potential of nanomedicine, each responsible for specific tasks such as developing robust materials and chemical entities, as well as quantitative techniques providing the foundation for accurate measurements and assessments, designing and developing effective therapeutic agents and also the design and execution of clinical trials to bridge the gap between laboratory discoveries and real-world applications [141,176].

Moreover, industry funding is paramount in guaranteeing that the promising products born out of interdisciplinary collaborations make their way to the market, ultimately benefiting patients. Continuous interaction among scientists, clinicians, regulatory bodies and industry partners is essential. Partnerships spanning fundamental, translational and industrial sectors will play a pivotal role in advancing antimicrobial nanomaterials into clinical applications. The feedback loop between these stakeholders can help refine research directions, improve methodologies and address safety concerns. In summary, strategies based on nanomaterials present a promising and alternative avenue to traditional antibiotics for treating challenging infections, thereby addressing the complexities faced in the post-antibiotic era [141]. Rigorous clinical assessment, coupled with ongoing monitoring and post-market surveillance, are paramount in ensuring the safety and efficacy of antimicrobial nanomedicine in real-world scenarios. As technology advances, interdisciplinary efforts and a commitment to understanding both the potential benefits and risks of nanomaterial-based antimicrobial treatments will be instrumental in overcoming the challenges and successfully translating innovations from the lab to the clinic [66].

References

[1] A.R. Kirtane, M. Verma, P. Karandikar, J. Furin, R. Langer, G. Traverso, Nanotechnology approaches for global infectious diseases, Nature Nanotechnology 16 (4) (2021) 369–384, https://doi.org/10.1038/s41565-021-00866-8. From NLM Medline).

[2] P. Aleš, S. Monika, K. Martina, P. Robert, B. Kateřina, V. Renata, K. Milan, H. Markéta, P. Grażyna, C. Joanna, et al., Strong and nonspecific synergistic antibacterial efficiency of antibiotics combined with silver nanoparticles at very low concentrations showing No cytotoxic effect, Molecules (2015), https://doi.org/10.3390/molecules21010026.

[3] Prevention, E. C. f. D.; Control, Antimicrobial Resistance Surveillance in Europe 2015. Annual Report of the European Antimicrobial Resistance Surveillance Network (EARS-Net), ECDC, 2015.

[4] C.L. Ventola, The antibiotic resistance crisis: part 1: causes and threats, P and T 40 (4) (2015) 277–283 (From NLM PubMed-not-MEDLINE).

[5] S. Contera, J. Bernardino de la Serna, T.D. Tetley, Biotechnology, nanotechnology and medicine, articles, Emerging Topics in Life Sciences 4 (6) (2020) 551–554, https://doi.org/10.1042/ETLS20200350. From NLM Medline).

[6] A.Y. Peleg, D.C. Hooper, Hospital-acquired infections due to gram-negative bacteria, New England Journal of Medicine 362 (19) (2010) 1804–1813, https://doi.org/10.1056/NEJMra0904124. From NLM Medline).

[7] J.M.V. Makabenta, A. Nabawy, C.H. Li, S. Schmidt-Malan, R. Patel, V.M. Rotello, Nanomaterial-based therapeutics for antibiotic-resistant bacterial infections, Nature Reviews Microbiology 19 (1) (2021) 23–36, https://doi.org/10.1038/s41579-020-0420-1. From NLM Medline).

[8] H.F. Chambers, F.R. Deleo, Waves of resistance: *Staphylococcus aureus* in the antibiotic era, Nature Reviews Microbiology 7 (9) (2009) 629–641, https://doi.org/10.1038/nrmicro2200. From NLM Medline).

[9] C.M. Huang, C.H. Chen, D. Pornpattananangkul, L. Zhang, M. Chan, M.F. Hsieh, L. Zhang, Eradication of drug resistant *Staphylococcus aureus* by liposomal oleic acids, Biomaterials 32 (1) (2011) 214–221, https://doi.org/10.1016/j.biomaterials.2010.08.076. From NLM Medline).

[10] R.M. Klevens, J.R. Edwards, F.C. Tenover, L.C. McDonald, T. Horan, R. Gaynes, S. National Nosocomial Infections Surveillance, Changes in the epidemiology of methicillin-resistant *Staphylococcus aureus* in intensive care units in US hospitals, 1992-2003, Article, Clinical Infectious Diseases 42 (3) (2006) 389–391, https://doi.org/10.1086/499367. From NLM Medline).

[11] A.J. Huh, Y.J. Kwon, Nanoantibiotics: a new paradigm for treating infectious diseases using nanomaterials in the antibiotics resistant era, Journal of Controlled Release 156 (2) (2011) 128–145, https://doi.org/10.1016/j.jconrel.2011.07.002. From NLM Medline).

[12] V. Taleski, D. Bosnakovski, M. Zdravkovska, V. Markovski, Z. Stojanovska, S. Jovevska, Where Nanotechnology and Nanomedicine Meet\ud–Applications and Potential Risks\ud, 2015 (Articles).

[13] W. Gao, L. Zhang, Nanomaterials arising amid antibiotic resistance, Nature Reviews Microbiology 19 (1) (2021) 5–6, https://doi.org/10.1038/s41579-020-00469-5.

[14] I. Mela, C.F. Kaminski, Nano-vehicles give new lease of life to existing antimicrobials, Emerging Topics in Life Sciences 4 (6) (2020) 555–566, https://doi.org/10.1042/ETLS20200153. From NLM Medline).

[15] S.T. Khan, J. Musarrat, A.A. Al-Khedhairy, Countering drug resistance, infectious diseases, and sepsis using metal and metal oxides nanoparticles: current status, Colloids and Surfaces B: Biointerfaces 146 (2016) 70–83, https://doi.org/10.1016/j.colsurfb.2016.05.046. From NLM Medline).

[16] P.S. Stewart, Mechanisms of antibiotic resistance in bacterial biofilms, International Journal of Medical Microbiology 292 (2) (2002) 107–113, https://doi.org/10.1078/1438-4221-00196. From NLM Medline).

[17] S. Zaidi, L. Misba, A.U. Khan, Nano-therapeutics: a revolution in infection control in post antibiotic era, Nanomedicine 13 (7) (2017) 2281–2301, https://doi.org/10.1016/j.nano.2017.06.015. From NLM Medline).

[18] N.-Y. Lee, W.-C. Ko, P.-R. Hsueh, Nanoparticles in the treatment of infections caused by multidrug-resistant organisms, Frontiers in Pharmacology 10 (2019) Review, https://doi.org/10.3389/fphar.2019.01153.

[19] Y.N. Slavin, J. Asnis, U.O. Hafeli, H. Bach, Metal nanoparticles: understanding the mechanisms behind antibacterial activity, Journal of Nanobiotechnology 15 (1) (2017) 65, https://doi.org/10.1186/s12951-017-0308-z. From NLM Medline).

[20] A.C. Burdusel, O. Gherasim, A.M. Grumezescu, L. Mogoanta, A. Ficai, E. Andronescu, Biomedical applications of silver nanoparticles: an up-to-date overview, Nanomaterials 8 (9) (2018), https://doi.org/10.3390/nano8090681. From NLM PubMed-not-MEDLINE).

[21] P.V. Baptista, M.P. McCusker, A. Carvalho, D.A. Ferreira, N.M. Mohan, M. Martins, A.R. Fernandes, Nano-strategies to fight multidrug resistant bacteria-A battle of the titans, Frontiers in Microbiology 9 (2018) 1441, https://doi.org/10.3389/fmicb.2018.01441 (From NLM PubMed-not-MEDLINE).

[22] M.K. Rai, S.D. Deshmukh, A.P. Ingle, A.K. Gade, Silver nanoparticles: the powerful nanoweapon against multidrug-resistant bacteria, Journal of Applied Microbiology 112 (5) (2012) 841–852, https://doi.org/10.1111/j.1365-2672.2012.05253.x. From NLM Medline).

[23] T.C. Dakal, A. Kumar, R.S. Majumdar, V. Yadav, Mechanistic basis of antimicrobial actions of silver nanoparticles, Frontiers in Microbiology 7 (2016) 1831, https://doi.org/10.3389/fmicb.2016.01831. From NLM PubMed-not-MEDLINE).

[24] N. Duran, M. Duran, M.B. de Jesus, A.B. Seabra, W.J. Favaro, G. Nakazato, Silver nanoparticles: a new view on mechanistic aspects on antimicrobial activity, Nanomedicine 12 (3) (2016) 789–799, https://doi.org/10.1016/j.nano.2015.11.016. From NLM Medline).

[25] H.A. Hemeg, Nanomaterials for alternative antibacterial therapy, International Journal of Nanomedicine 12 (2017) 8211–8225, https://doi.org/10.2147/IJN.S132163. From NLM Medline).

[26] K.M. Varier, M. Gudeppu, A. Chinnasamy, S. Thangarajan, J. Balasubramanian, Y. Li, B. Gajendran, Nanoparticles: antimicrobial applications and its prospects, in: M. Naushad, S. Rajendran, F. Gracia (Eds.), Advanced Nanostructured Materials for Environmental Remediation, Springer International Publishing, 2019, pp. 321–355.

[27] L. Zhang, D. Pornpattananangku, C.M. Hu, C.M. Huang, Development of nanoparticles for antimicrobial drug delivery, Current Medicinal Chemistry 17 (6) (2010) 585–594, https://doi.org/10.2174/092986710790416290. From NLM Medline).

[28] R.Y. Pelgrift, A.J. Friedman, Nanotechnology as a therapeutic tool to combat microbial resistance, Advanced Drug Delivery Reviews 65 (13–14) (2013) 1803–1815, https://doi.org/10.1016/j.addr.2013.07.011. From NLM Medline).

[29] B. Nurit, H.-H. Yael, D. Avi, K. Wahid, H. Ronen, Alternative antimicrobial approach: nano-antimicrobial materials, Evidence-based Complementary and Alternative Medicine (2015), https://doi.org/10.1155/2015/246012.

[30] L.S. Wang, A. Gupta, V.M. Rotello, Nanomaterials for the treatment of bacterial biofilms, ACS Infectious Diseases 2 (1) (2016) 3–4, https://doi.org/10.1021/acsinfecdis.5b00116. From NLM Medline).

[31] A. Gupta, R.F. Landis, V.M. Rotello, Nanoparticle-based antimicrobials: surface functionality is critical, F1000Res 5 (2016), https://doi.org/10.12688/f1000research.7595.1. From NLM PubMed-not-MEDLINE).

[32] E. Tobin, S. Brenner, Nanotechnology fundamentals applied to clinical infectious diseases and public health, Open Forum Infectious Diseases 8 (12) (2021) ofab583, https://doi.org/10.1093/ofid/ofab583. (Accessed 24 April 2023).

[33] K. Blecher, A. Nasir, A. Friedman, The growing role of nanotechnology in combating infectious disease, Virulence 2 (5) (2011) 395–401, https://doi.org/10.4161/viru.2.5.17035. From NLM Medline).

[34] A.A. El-Sharif, M.H. Hussain, Chitosan-EDTA new combination is a promising candidate for treatment of bacterial and fungal infections, Current Microbiology 62 (3) (2011) 739–745, https://doi.org/10.1007/s00284-010-9777-0. From NLM Medline).

[35] F. Nederberg, Y. Zhang, J.P. Tan, K. Xu, H. Wang, C. Yang, S. Gao, X.D. Guo, K. Fukushima, L. Li, et al., Biodegradable nanostructures with selective lysis of microbial membranes, Nature Chemistry 3 (5) (2011) 409–414, https://doi.org/10.1038/nchem.1012. From NLM Medline).

[36] M. Moogooee, H. Ramezanzadeh, S. Jasoori, Y. Omidi, S. Davaran, Synthesis and in vitro studies of cross-linked hydrogel nanoparticles containing amoxicillin, Journal of Pharmaceutical Sciences 100 (3) (2011) 1057–1066, https://doi.org/10.1002/jps.22351. From NLM Medline).

[37] J.L. Italia, A. Sharp, K.C. Carter, P. Warn, M.N. Kumar, Peroral amphotericin B polymer nanoparticles lead to comparable or superior in vivo antifungal activity to that of intravenous Ambisome(R) or Fungizone, PLoS One 6 (10) (2011) e25744, https://doi.org/10.1371/journal.pone.0025744. From NLM Medline).

[38] G. Griffiths, B. Nystrom, S.B. Sable, G.K. Khuller, Nanobead-based interventions for the treatment and prevention of tuberculosis, Nature Reviews Microbiology 8 (11) (2010) 827–834, https://doi.org/10.1038/nrmicro2437. From NLM Medline).
[39] G. Mohammadi, H. Valizadeh, M. Barzegar-Jalali, F. Lotfipour, K. Adibkia, M. Milani, M. Azhdarzadeh, F. Kiafar, A. Nokhodchi, Development of azithromycin-PLGA nanoparticles: physicochemical characterization and antibacterial effect against *Salmonella typhi*, Colloids and Surfaces B: Biointerfaces 80 (1) (2010) 34–39, https://doi.org/10.1016/j.colsurfb.2010.05.027. From NLM Medline).
[40] H. Maeda, Tumor-selective delivery of macromolecular drugs via the EPR effect: background and future prospects, Bioconjugate Chemistry 21 (5) (2010) 797–802, https://doi.org/10.1021/bc100070g. From NLM Medline).
[41] M.A. Kohanski, M.A. DePristo, J.J. Collins, Sublethal antibiotic treatment leads to multidrug resistance via radical-induced mutagenesis, Molecular Cell 37 (3) (2010) 311–320, https://doi.org/10.1016/j.molcel.2010.01.003. From NLM Medline).
[42] A.I. Lopez, R.Y. Reins, A.M. McDermott, B.W. Trautner, C. Cai, Antibacterial activity and cytotoxicity of PEGylated poly(amidoamine) dendrimers, Molecular BioSystems 5 (10) (2009) 1148–1156, https://doi.org/10.1039/b904746h. From NLM Medline).
[43] J. Wang, J.D. Byrne, M.E. Napier, J.M. DeSimone, More effective nanomedicines through particle design, Small 7 (14) (2011) 1919–1931, https://doi.org/10.1002/smll.201100442. From NLM Medline).
[44] C. He, Y. Hu, L. Yin, C. Tang, C. Yin, Effects of particle size and surface charge on cellular uptake and biodistribution of polymeric nanoparticles, Biomaterials 31 (13) (2010) 3657–3666, https://doi.org/10.1016/j.biomaterials.2010.01.065. From NLM Medline).
[45] R.C. Mercier, C. Stumpo, M.J. Rybak, Effect of growth phase and pH on the in vitro activity of a new glycopeptide, oritavancin (LY333328), against *Staphylococcus aureus* and Enterococcus faecium, Journal of Antimicrobial Chemotherapy 50 (1) (2002) 19–24, https://doi.org/10.1093/jac/dkf058. From NLM Medline).
[46] H.P. Simmen, H. Battaglia, P. Giovanoli, J. Blaser, Analysis of pH, pO_2 and pCO_2 in drainage fluid allows for rapid detection of infectious complications during the follow-up period after abdominal surgery, Infection 22 (6) (1994) 386–389, https://doi.org/10.1007/BF01715494. From NLM Medline).
[47] K.E. Barrett, Ganong's Review of Medical Physiology, 2010.
[48] S. Fuchs, J. Pane-Farre, C. Kohler, M. Hecker, S. Engelmann, Anaerobic gene expression in *Staphylococcus aureus*, Journal of Bacteriology 189 (11) (2007) 4275–4289, https://doi.org/10.1128/JB.00081-07. From NLM Medline).
[49] A.S. Trevani, G. Andonegui, M. Giordano, D.H. Lopez, R. Gamberale, F. Minucci, J.R. Geffner, Extracellular acidification induces human neutrophil activation, Journal of Immunology 162 (8) (1999) 4849–4857 (From NLM Medline).
[50] M. Vermeulen, M. Giordano, A.S. Trevani, C. Sedlik, R. Gamberale, P. Fernandez-Calotti, G. Salamone, S. Raiden, J. Sanjurjo, J.R. Geffner, Acidosis improves uptake of antigens and MHC class I-restricted presentation by dendritic cells, Journal of Immunology 172 (5) (2004) 3196–3204, https://doi.org/10.4049/jimmunol.172.5.3196. From NLM Medline).

[51] S. Tate, G. MacGregor, M. Davis, J.A. Innes, A.P. Greening, Airways in cystic fibrosis are acidified: detection by exhaled breath condensate, Thorax 57 (11) (2002) 926–929, https://doi.org/10.1136/thorax.57.11.926. From NLM Medline).
[52] H.P. Simmen, J. Blaser, Analysis of pH and pO2 in abscesses, peritoneal fluid, and drainage fluid in the presence or absence of bacterial infection during and after abdominal surgery, Americas Journal of Surgery 166 (1) (1993) 24–27, https://doi.org/10.1016/s0002-9610(05)80576-8. From NLM Medline).
[53] F.R.-M. Aleksandar, K.L. Timothy, A.P. Vlad, J.Y. Christopher, L. Robert, C.F. Omid, Surface charge-switching polymeric nanoparticles for bacterial cell wall-targeted delivery of antibiotics, ACS Nano (2012), https://doi.org/10.1021/nn3008383.
[54] J.W. Nichols, Y.H. Bae, Odyssey of a cancer nanoparticle: from injection site to site of action, Nano Today 7 (6) (2012) 606–618, https://doi.org/10.1016/j.nantod.2012.10.010 (From NLM PubMed-not-MEDLINE).
[55] R. Pandey, Z. Ahmad, S. Sharma, G.K. Khuller, Nano-encapsulation of azole antifungals: potential applications to improve oral drug delivery, International Journal of Pharmacy 301 (1–2) (2005) 268–276, https://doi.org/10.1016/j.ijpharm.2005.05.027. From NLM Medline).
[56] K.B. Sutradhar, M.L. Amin, Nanotechnology in cancer drug delivery and selective targeting, International Scholarly Research Notices 2014 (2014).
[57] A.M. Master, A. Sen Gupta, EGF receptor-targeted nanocarriers for enhanced cancer treatment, Nanomedicine 7 (12) (2012) 1895–1906, https://doi.org/10.2217/nnm.12.160. From NLM Medline).
[58] X. Wang, S. Wang, Y. Zhang, Advance of the application of nano-controlled release system in ophthalmic drug delivery, Drug Delivery 23 (8) (2016) 2897–2901, https://doi.org/10.3109/10717544.2015.1116025. From NLM Medline).
[59] H. Su, Y. Wang, Y. Gu, L. Bowman, J. Zhao, M. Ding, Potential applications and human biosafety of nanomaterials used in nanomedicine, Journal of Applied Toxicology: JAT (2017), https://doi.org/10.1002/jat.3476. Articles.
[60] V.B. Patravale, A.A. Date, R.M. Kulkarni, Nanosuspensions: a promising drug delivery strategy, Journal of Pharmacy and Pharmacology 56 (7) (2004) 827–840, https://doi.org/10.1211/0022357023691. From NLM Medline).
[61] T.R. Stowe, C.J. Wilkinson, A. Iqbal, T. Stearns, The centriolar satellite proteins Cep72 and Cep290 interact and are required for recruitment of BBS proteins to the cilium, Molecular Biology of the Cell 23 (17) (2012) 3322–3335, https://doi.org/10.1091/mbc.E12-02-0134. From NLM Medline).
[62] H. Pinto-Alphandary, A. Andremont, P. Couvreur, Targeted delivery of antibiotics using liposomes and nanoparticles: research and applications, International Journal of Antimicrobial Agents 13 (3) (2000) 155–168, https://doi.org/10.1016/s0924-8579(99)00121-1. From NLM Medline).
[63] G. Barratt, Colloidal drug carriers: achievements and perspectives, Cellular and Molecular Life Sciences 60 (1) (2003) 21–37, https://doi.org/10.1007/s000180300002. From NLM Medline).
[64] A. Sharma, R. Pandey, S. Sharma, G.K. Khuller, Chemotherapeutic efficacy of poly (DL-lactide-co-glycolide) nanoparticle encapsulated antitubercular drugs at sub-therapeutic dose against experimental tuberculosis, Article,

International Journal of Antimicrobial Agents 24 (6) (2004) 599–604, https://doi.org/10.1016/j.ijantimicag.2004.07.010. From NLM Medline).

[65] A. Sharma, S. Sharma, G.K. Khuller, Lectin-functionalized poly (lactide-co-glycolide) nanoparticles as oral/aerosolized antitubercular drug carriers for treatment of tuberculosis, Article, Journal of Antimicrobial Chemotherapy 54 (4) (2004) 761–766, https://doi.org/10.1093/jac/dkh411. From NLM Medline).

[66] J.M. Irache, I. Esparza, C. Gamazo, M. Agüeros, S. Espuelas, Nanomedicine: novel approaches in human and veterinary therapeutics, Veterinary Parasitology (2011), https://doi.org/10.1016/j.vetpar.2011.05.028. Articles.

[67] R.R. Jain, M.R. Mehta, A.R. Bannalikar, M.D. Menon, Alginate microparticles loaded with lipopolysaccharide subunit antigen for mucosal vaccination against *Klebsiella pneumoniae*, Biologicals 43 (3) (2015) 195–201, https://doi.org/10.1016/j.biologicals.2015.02.001. From NLM Medline).

[68] A. Farjah, P. Owlia, S.D. Siadat, S.F. Mousavi, M.S. Ardestani, H.K. Mohammadpour, Immunological evaluation of an alginate-based conjugate as a vaccine candidate against, Apmis 123 (2) (2015) 175–183, https://doi.org/10.1111/apm.12337.

[69] E. Cevher, S.K. Salomon, S. Somavarapu, S. Brocchini, H.O. Alpar, Development of chitosan-pullulan composite nanoparticles for nasal delivery of vaccines: in vivo studies, Journal of Microencapsulation 32 (8) (2015) 769–783, https://doi.org/10.3109/02652048.2015.1073393. From NLM Medline).

[70] T. Doavi, S.L. Mousavi, M. Kamali, J. Amani, M. Fasihi Ramandi, Chitosan-based intranasal vaccine against *Escherichia coli* O157:H7, Iranian Biomedical Journal 20 (2) (2016) 97–108, https://doi.org/10.7508/ibj.2016.02.005. From NLM Medline).

[71] Z. Cui, D. Han, X. Sun, M. Zhang, X. Feng, C. Sun, J. Gu, C. Tong, L. Lei, W. Han, Mannose-modified chitosan microspheres enhance OprF-OprI-mediated protection of mice against *Pseudomonas aeruginosa* infection via induction of mucosal immunity, Applied Microbiology and Biotechnology 99 (2) (2015) 667–680, https://doi.org/10.1007/s00253-014-6147-z. From NLM Medline).

[72] H.S. Oberoi, Y.M. Yorgensen, A. Morasse, J.T. Evans, D.J. Burkhart, PEG modified liposomes containing CRX-601 adjuvant in combination with methylglycol chitosan enhance the murine sublingual immune response to influenza vaccination, Journal of Controlled Release 223 (2016) 64–74, https://doi.org/10.1016/j.jconrel.2015.11.006. From NLM Medline).

[73] F. Lebre, G. Borchard, H. Faneca, M.C. Pedroso de Lima, O. Borges, Intranasal administration of novel chitosan nanoparticle/DNA complexes induces antibody response to hepatitis B surface antigen in mice, Molecular Pharmaceutics 13 (2) (2016) 472–482, https://doi.org/10.1021/acs.molpharmaceut.5b00707. From NLM Medline).

[74] B. Malathi, S. Mona, D. Thiyagarajan, P. Kaliraj, Immunopotentiating nano-chitosan as potent vaccine carter for efficacious prophylaxis of filarial antigens, International Journal of Biological Macromolecules 73 (2015) 131–137, https://doi.org/10.1016/j.ijbiomac.2014.11.014.

[75] T. Hunsawong, P. Sunintaboon, S. Warit, B. Thaisomboonsuk, R.G. Jarman, I.K. Yoon, S. Ubol, S. Fernandez, Immunogenic properties of a BCG adjuvanted chitosan nanoparticle-based dengue vaccine in human

dendritic cells, PLoS Neglected Tropical Diseases 9 (9) (2015) e0003958, https://doi.org/10.1371/journal.pntd.0003958. From NLM Medline).
[76] D.-P. Bai, X.-Y. Lin, Y.-F. Huang, X.-F. Zhang, Theranostics aspects of various nanoparticles in veterinary medicine, International Journal of Molecular Sciences (2018), https://doi.org/10.3390/ijms19113299. Articles.
[77] M.H. Xiong, Y.J. Li, Y. Bao, X.Z. Yang, B. Hu, J. Wang, Bacteria-responsive multifunctional nanogel for targeted antibiotic delivery, Advances in Materials 24 (46) (2012) 6175–6180, https://doi.org/10.1002/adma.201202847. From NLM Medline).
[78] M.H. Xiong, Y. Bao, X.Z. Yang, Y.C. Wang, B. Sun, J. Wang, Lipase-sensitive polymeric triple-layered nanogel for "on-demand" drug delivery, Journal of the American Chemical Society 134 (9) (2012) 4355–4362, https://doi.org/10.1021/ja211279u. From NLM Medline).
[79] M. Qindeel, M. Barani, A. Rahdar, R. Arshad, M. Cucchiarini, Nanomaterials for the diagnosis and treatment of urinary tract infections, Nanomaterials (2021), https://doi.org/10.22028/D291-33450. Articles.
[80] D. Campoccia, L. Montanaro, C.R. Arciola, The significance of infection related to orthopedic devices and issues of antibiotic resistance, Biomaterials 27 (11) (2006) 2331–2339, https://doi.org/10.1016/j.biomaterials.2005.11.044. From NLM Medline).
[81] D. Campoccia, L. Montanaro, C.R. Arciola, A review of the biomaterials technologies for infection-resistant surfaces, Biomaterials 34 (34) (2013) 8533–8554, https://doi.org/10.1016/j.biomaterials.2013.07.089. From NLM Medline).
[82] J. Han, A. Poma, Molecular targets for antibody-based anti-biofilm therapy in infective endocarditis, Polymers 14 (2022).
[83] D.P. Linklater, V.A. Baulin, S. Juodkazis, R.J. Crawford, P. Stoodley, E.P. Ivanova, Mechano-bactericidal actions of nanostructured surfaces, Nature Reviews Microbiology 19 (1) (2021) 8–22, https://doi.org/10.1038/s41579-020-0414-z.
[84] L. Wang, C. Hu, L. Shao, The antimicrobial activity of nanoparticles: present situation and prospects for the future, International Journal of Nanomedicine 12 (2017) 1227–1249, https://doi.org/10.2147/IJN.S121956. From NLM Medline).
[85] E. Cremonini, E. Zonaro, M. Donini, S. Lampis, M. Boaretti, S. Dusi, P. Melotti, M.M. Lleo, G. Vallini, Biogenic selenium nanoparticles: characterization, antimicrobial activity and effects on human dendritic cells and fibroblasts, Article, Microbial Biotechnology 9 (6) (2016) 758–771, https://doi.org/10.1111/1751-7915.12374. From NLM Medline).
[86] S. Sharmin, M.M. Rahaman, C. Sarkar, O. Atolani, M.T. Islam, O.S. Adeyemi, Nanoparticles as antimicrobial and antiviral agents: a literature-based perspective study, Heliyon 7 (3) (2021) e06456, https://doi.org/10.1016/j.heliyon.2021.e06456.
[87] Y. Abo-Zeid, G.R. Williams, The potential anti-infective applications of metal oxide nanoparticles: a systematic review, Wiley Interdisciplinary Reviews. Nanomedicine and Nanobiotechnology (2019), https://doi.org/10.1002/wnan.1592. Articles.
[88] H. Kumar, K. Bhardwaj, D.S. Dhanjal, E. Nepovimova, F. Sen, H. Regassa, R. Singh, R. Verma, V. Kumar, D. Kumar, et al., Fruit extract mediated green synthesis of metallic nanoparticles: a new avenue in pomology applications, International Journal of Molecular Sciences 21 (22) (2020), https://doi.org/10.3390/ijms21228458. From NLM Medline).

[89] E. Ghazy, A. Kumar, M. Barani, I. Kaur, A. Rahdar, T. Behl, Scrutinizing the therapeutic and diagnostic potential of nanotechnology in thyroid cancer: edifying drug targeting by nano-oncotherapeutics, Journal of Drug Delivery Science and Technology 61 (2021) 102221, https://doi.org/10.1016/j.jddst.2020.102221.
[90] M.R. Hajizadeh, H. Maleki, M. Barani, M.A. Fahmidehkar, M. Mahmoodi, M. Torkzadeh-Mahani, In vitro cytotoxicity assay of D-limonene niosomes: an efficient nano-carrier for enhancing solubility of plant-extracted agents, Research in Pharmaceutical Sciences 14 (5) (2019) 448–458, https://doi.org/10.4103/1735-5362.268206. From NLM PubMed-not-MEDLINE).
[91] P. Hasanein, A. Rahdar, M. Barani, F. Baino, S. Yari, Oil-in-water microemulsion encapsulation of antagonist drugs prevents renal ischemia-reperfusion injury in rats, Applied Science-Basel 11 (3) (2021) 1264, https://doi.org/10.3390/ap.11031264.
[92] M. Mukhtar, M. Bilal, A. Rahdar, M. Barani, R. Arshad, T. Behl, C. Brisc, F. Banica, S. Bungau, Nanomaterials for diagnosis and treatment of brain cancer: recent updates, Chemosensors 8 (4) (2020) 117, https://doi.org/10.3390/chemosensors8040117.
[93] S. Nikazar, M. Barani, A. Rahdar, M. Zoghi, G.Z. Kyzas, Photo- and magnetothermally responsive nanomaterials for therapy, controlled drug delivery and imaging applications, ChemistrySelect 5 (40) (2020) 12590–12609, https://doi.org/10.1002/slct.202002978.
[94] Y. Qin, Y.-H. Lao, H. Wang, J. Zhang, K. Yi, Z. Chen, J. Han, W. Song, Y. Tao, M. Li, Combatting *Helicobacter pylori* with oral nanomedicines, Journal of Materials Chemistry B (2021), https://doi.org/10.1039/d1tb02038b articles.
[95] S.V. Bhosale, P.S. Ekambe, S.V. Bhoraskar, V.L. Mathe, Effect of surface properties of NiFe2O4 nanoparticles synthesized by dc thermal plasma route on antimicrobial activity, Article, Applied Surface Science 441 (2018) 724–733, https://doi.org/10.1016/j.apsusc.2018.01.220. Scopus).
[96] O. Fabiyi, G. Olatunji, O. Atolani, O. Olawuyi, Preparation of bio-nematicidal nanoparticles of for the control of cyst nematode, Article, Journal of Animal and Plant Sciences 30 (5) (2020) 1172–1177, https://doi.org/10.36899/Japs.2020.5.0134. Scopus).
[97] S. Gurunathan, J.W. Han, A.A. Dayem, V. Eppakayala, J.H. Kim, Oxidative stress-mediated antibacterial activity of graphene oxide and reduced graphene oxide in *Pseudomonas aeruginosa*, International Journal of Nanomedicine 7 (2012) 5901–5914, https://doi.org/10.2147/IJN.S37397. From NLM Medline).
[98] M.A. Quinteros, V. Cano Aristizabal, P.R. Dalmasso, M.G. Paraje, P.L. Paez, Oxidative stress generation of silver nanoparticles in three bacterial genera and its relationship with the antimicrobial activity, Article, Toxicology in Vitro 36 (2016) 216–223, https://doi.org/10.1016/j.tiv.2016.08.007. From NLM Medline).
[99] A. Joe, S.H. Park, D.J. Kim, Y.J. Lee, K.H. Jhee, Y. Sohn, E.S. Jang, Antimicrobial activity of ZnO nanoplates and its Ag nanocomposites: insight into an ROS-mediated antibacterial mechanism under UV light, Article, Journal of Solid State Chemistry 267 (2018) 124–133, https://doi.org/10.1016/j.jssc.2018.08.003. Scopus).
[100] A. Nagy, A. Harrison, S. Sabbani, R.S. Munson Jr., P.K. Dutta, W.J. Waldman, Silver nanoparticles embedded in zeolite membranes: release of silver ions and mechanism of antibacterial action, Article,

International Journal of Nanomedicine 6 (2011) 1833–1852, https://doi.org/10.2147/IJN.S24019. From NLM Medline).

[101] B. Bagchi, S. Kar, S.K. Dey, S. Bhandary, D. Roy, T.K. Mukhopadhyay, S. Das, P. Nandy, In situ synthesis and antibacterial activity of copper nanoparticle loaded natural montmorillonite clay based on contact inhibition and ion release, Article, Colloids and Surfaces B: Biointerfaces 108 (2013) 358–365, https://doi.org/10.1016/j.colsurfb.2013.03.019. From NLM Medline).

[102] S. Panicker, I.M. Ahmady, C. Han, M. Chehimi, A.A. Mohamed, On demand release of ionic silver from gold-silver alloy nanoparticles: fundamental antibacterial mechanisms study, Materials Today Chemistry 16 (2020), https://doi.org/10.1016/j.mtchem.2019.100237. Article.

[103] N. Anic ic, M. Vukomanovic, T. Koklic, D. Suvorov, Fewer defects in the surface slows the hydrolysis rate, decreases the ROS generation potential, and improves the non-ROS antimicrobial activity of MgO, Article, Small 14 (26) (2018) e1800205, https://doi.org/10.1002/smll.201800205. From NLM Medline).

[104] K. Jun Sung, K. Eunye, Y. Kyeong Nam, K. Jong-Ho, K. Jong-Ho, K. Jong-Ho, P. Sungjin, P. Sung-Jin, P. Sungjin, L. Hu Jang, et al., Antimicrobial effects of silver nanoparticles, Nanomedicine: Nanotechnology, Biology and Medicine (2007), https://doi.org/10.1016/j.nano.2006.12.001.

[105] B. Le Ouay, F. Stellacci, Antibacterial activity of silver nanoparticles: a surface science insight, Nano Today 10 (3) (2015) 339–354, https://doi.org/10.1016/j.nantod.2015.04.002.

[106] D. Roe, B. Karandikar, N. Bonn-Savage, B. Gibbins, J.B. Roullet, Antimicrobial surface functionalization of plastic catheters by silver nanoparticles, Journal of Antimicrobial Chemotherapy 61 (4) (2008) 869–876, https://doi.org/10.1093/jac/dkn034. From NLM Medline).

[107] P. Kalfon, C. de Vaumas, D. Samba, E. Boulet, J.Y. Lefrant, D. Eyraud, T. Lherm, F. Santoli, W. Naija, B. Riou, Comparison of silver-impregnated with standard multi-lumen central venous catheters in critically ill patients, Critical Care Medicine 35 (4) (2007) 1032–1039, https://doi.org/10.1097/01.CCM.0000259378.53166.1B. From NLM Medline).

[108] K. Chaloupka, Y. Malam, A.M. Seifalian, Nanosilver as a new generation of nanoproduct in biomedical applications, Trends in Biotechnology 28 (11) (2010) 580–588, https://doi.org/10.1016/j.tibtech.2010.07.006. From NLM Medline).

[109] M. Rai, A. Yadav, A. Gade, Silver nanoparticles as a new generation of antimicrobials, Biotechnology Advance 27 (1) (2009) 76–83, https://doi.org/10.1016/j.biotechadv.2008.09.002. From NLM Medline).

[110] O. Choi, K.K. Deng, N.J. Kim, L. Ross Jr., R.Y. Surampalli, Z. Hu, The inhibitory effects of silver nanoparticles, silver ions, and silver chloride colloids on microbial growth, Water Research 42 (12) (2008) 3066–3074, https://doi.org/10.1016/j.watres.2008.02.021. From NLM Medline).

[111] C. Carlson, S.M. Hussain, A.M. Schrand, L.K. Braydich-Stolle, K.L. Hess, R.L. Jones, J.J. Schlager, Unique cellular interaction of silver nanoparticles: size-dependent generation of reactive oxygen species, Journal of Physical Chemistry B 112 (43) (2008) 13608–13619, https://doi.org/10.1021/jp712087m. From NLM Medline).

[112] H.J. Park, J.Y. Kim, J. Kim, J.H. Lee, J.S. Hahn, M.B. Gu, J. Yoon, Silver-ion-mediated reactive oxygen species generation affecting bactericidal

activity, Water Research 43 (4) (2009) 1027–1032, https://doi.org/10.1016/j.watres.2008.12.002. From NLM Medline).
[113] N.B. Ashley, S. Kathryn, A.S. Tova, L. Jiangrui, O.O. Sherine, E.S. Maria, Nanoparticles functionalized with ampicillin destroy multiple-antibiotic-resistant isolates of *Pseudomonas aeruginosa* and Enterobacter aerogenes and methicillin-resistant *Staphylococcus aureus*, Applied and Environmental Microbiology (2012), https://doi.org/10.1128/aem.06513-11.
[114] F. Ali, T. Shiva, N. Mahsa, Synthesis and characterization of core-shell bimetallic nanoparticles for synergistic antimicrobial effect studies in combination with doxycycline on burn specific pathogens, Journal of Photochemistry and Photobiology B-biology (2017), https://doi.org/10.1016/j.jphotobiol.2017.02.014.
[115] G. Hongwei, H. Pak-Leung, T. Edmond, W. Ling, X. Bing, Presenting vancomycin on nanoparticles to enhance antimicrobial activities, Nano Letters (2003), https://doi.org/10.1021/nl034396z.
[116] A. Rai, A. Prabhune, C.C. Perry, Antibiotic mediated synthesis of gold nanoparticles with potent antimicrobial activity and their application in antimicrobial coatings, Journal of Materials Chemistry 20 (32) (2010) 6789–6798.
[117] L. Ge, Q. Li, M. Wang, J. Ouyang, X. Li, M.M. Xing, Nanosilver particles in medical applications: synthesis, performance, and toxicity, International Journal of Nanomedicine 9 (2014) 2399–2407, https://doi.org/10.2147/IJN.S55015. From NLM Medline).
[118] H.L. Liu, S.A. Dai, K.Y. Fu, S.H. Hsu, Antibacterial properties of silver nanoparticles in three different sizes and their nanocomposites with a new waterborne polyurethane, International Journal of Nanomedicine 5 (2010) 1017–1028, https://doi.org/10.2147/Ijn.S14572.
[119] H. Derakhshankhah, S. Jafari, S. Sarvari, E. Barzegari, F. Moakedi, M. Ghorbani, B. Shiri Varnamkhasti, M. Jaymand, Z. Izadi, L. Tayebi, Biomedical applications of zeolitic nanoparticles, with an emphasis on medical interventions, International Journal of Nanomedicine 15 (2020), https://doi.org/10.2147/IJN.S234573 articles.
[120] C. Emerson Danguy, F. Luiz Francisco Poli de, F. Luiz Francisco Poli de, O. José Pinhata, S. Marcelo Martins, O. Roberto Angelo de, F. Fabiane Fantinelli, M. Valéria Spolon, Z. Valtencir, S.L. Anna, et al., Comparison of methods to detect the in vitro activity of silver nanoparticles (AgNP) against multidrug resistant bacteria, Journal of Nanobiotechnology (2015), https://doi.org/10.1186/s12951-015-0120-6.
[121] A. Baranwal, A. Srivastava, P. Kumar, V.K. Bajpai, P.K. Maurya, P. Chandra, Prospects of nanostructure materials and their composites as antimicrobial agents, Frontiers in Microbiology 9 (2018) 422, https://doi.org/10.3389/fmicb.2018.00422. From NLM PubMed-not-MEDLINE).
[122] F. Amanulla Mohammed, B. Kulandaivelu, G. Morukattu, M. Girilal, Y. Ruchi, Y. Ruchi, P.T. Kalaichelvan, K. Pudupalayam Thangavelu, V. Ramasamy, Biogenic synthesis of silver nanoparticles and their synergistic effect with antibiotics: a study against gram-positive and gram-negative bacteria, Nanomedicine: Nanotechnology, Biology and Medicine (2010), https://doi.org/10.1016/j.nano.2009.04.006.
[123] C. Arijit Kumar, C. Ruchira, B. Tarakdas, Mechanism of antibacterial activity of copper nanoparticles, Nanotechnology (2014), https://doi.org/10.1088/0957-4484/25/13/135101.

[124] S. Mehmood, M.A. Rehman, H. Ismail, B. Mirza, A.S. Bhatti, Significance of postgrowth processing of ZnO nanostructures on antibacterial activity against gram-positive and gram-negative bacteria, International Journal of Nanomedicine 10 (2015) 4521–4533, https://doi.org/10.2147/IJN.S83356. From NLM Medline).

[125] W. Liu, P. Su, A. Gonzales 3rd, S. Chen, N. Wang, J. Wang, H. Li, Z. Zhang, T.J. Webster, Optimizing stem cell functions and antibacterial properties of TiO2 nanotubes incorporated with ZnO nanoparticles: experiments and modeling, International Journal of Nanomedicine 10 (2015) 1997–2019, https://doi.org/10.2147/IJN.S74418. From NLM Medline).

[126] K.S. Babu, M. Anandkumar, T.Y. Tsai, T.H. Kao, B.S. Inbaraj, B.H. Chen, Cytotoxicity and antibacterial activity of gold-supported cerium oxide nanoparticles, International Journal of Nanomedicine 9 (2014) 5515–5531, https://doi.org/10.2147/IJN.S70087. From NLM Medline).

[127] K.K. Jain, Nanomedicine: application of nanobiotechnology in medical practice, Medical Principles and Practice: International Journal of the Kuwait University, Health Science Centre (2008), https://doi.org/10.1159/000112961. Articles.

[128] C. Sanjai, S. Kothan, P. Gonil, S. Saesoo, W. Sajomsang, Super-paramagnetic loaded nanoparticles based on biological macromolecules for in vivo targeted MR imaging, International Journal of Biological Macromolecules 86 (2016) 233–241, https://doi.org/10.1016/j.ijbiomac.2016.01.049. Scopus).

[129] Y. Kimura, T. Kurimoto, Y. Imai, H. Sugii, A. Toshimitsu, T. Matsuda, H. Imai, H. Yamada, T. Kondo, Novel biocompatible cobalt oxide nanoparticles for use in dual photoacoustic and magnetic resonance imaging, JSM Biotechnology Bioengineering 2 (2) (2014) (Scopus).

[130] N.F. Zadeh, Y. Sharifi, M. Gahremani, N.H. Jazani, Anti bacterial effects of nickel nano-particles on biofilm production amounts by B. Capacia ATCC 25416, Urmia University of Medical Sciences 28 (2017) 25–32 (Scopus).

[131] D.W. Hwang, H. Youn, D.S. Lee, Molecular imaging using PET/MRI particle, The Open Nuclear Medicine Journal 2 (2010) 186–191 (Scopus).

[132] M. Gogoi, K.S. Varadarajan, A.B. Patel, P. Deb, Facile development of iron-platinum nanoparticles to harness multifunctionality in single entity, Acta Metallurgica Sinica 29 (12) (2016) 1098–1106, https://doi.org/10.1007/s40195-016-0493-z. Scopus).

[133] J. Ma, K. Chen, Synthetic Ni3S2/Ni hybrid architectures as potential contrast agents in MRI, Materials Research Express 3 (4) (2016), https://doi.org/10.1088/2053-1591/3/4/045005. Scopus).

[134] N.V.S. Vallabani, S. Singh, A.S. Karakoti, Magnetic nanoparticles: current trends and future aspects in diagnostics and nanomedicine, Current Drug Metabolism (2019), https://doi.org/10.2174/1389200220666181122124458 articles.

[135] B. Ismail, M.N. Shafei, A. Harun, S. Ali, M. Omar, Z.Z. Deris, Predictors of polymyxin B treatment failure in Gram-negative healthcare-associated infections among critically ill patients, Journal of Microbiology, Immunology 51 (6) (2018) 763–769, https://doi.org/10.1016/j.jmii.2017.03.007.

[136] A.-J. Kuo, J.-C. Shu, T.-P. Liu, J.-J. Lu, M.-H. Lee, T.-S. Wu, L.-H. Su, T.-L. Wu, Vancomycin-resistant Enterococcus faecium at a university hospital in Taiwan, 2002–2015: fluctuation of genetic populations and emergence of a new structure type of the Tn1546-like element, Journal of Microbiology, Immunology, and Infection 51 (6) (2018) 821–828.

[137] S.W. Ting, C.H. Lee, J.W. Liu, Risk factors and outcomes for the acquisition of carbapenem-resistant Gram-negative bacillus bacteremia: a retrospective propensity-matched case control study, Journal of Microbiology, Immunology and Infection 51 (5) (2018) 621–628, https://doi.org/10.1016/j.jmii.2016.08.022. From NLM Medline).
[138] L.H. Tsao, C.Y. Hsin, H.Y. Liu, H.C. Chuang, L.Y. Chen, Y.J. Lee, Risk factors for healthcare-associated infection caused by carbapenem-resistant *Pseudomonas aeruginosa*, Journal of Microbiology, Immunology, and Infection 51 (3) (2018) 359–366, https://doi.org/10.1016/j.jmii.2017.08.015. From NLM Medline).
[139] N. Ismail, S.V. Omar, N.A. Ismail, R.P.H. Peters, Collated data of mutation frequencies and associated genetic variants of bedaquiline, clofazimine and linezolid resistance in *Mycobacterium tuberculosis*, Data in Brief 20 (2018) 1975–1983, https://doi.org/10.1016/j.dib.2018.09.057. From NLM PubMed-not-MEDLINE).
[140] P. Venkateswaran, S. Vasudevan, H. David, A. Shaktivel, K. Shanmugam, P. Neelakantan, A.P. Solomon, Revisiting ESKAPE Pathogens: virulence, resistance, and combating strategies focusing on quorum sensing, Frontiers in Cellular and Infection Microbiology 13 (2023) 1159798, https://doi.org/10.3389/fcimb.2023.1159798. From NLM Medline).
[141] J.J. Aguilera-Correa, J. Esteban, M. Vallet-Regi, Inorganic and polymeric nanoparticles for human viral and bacterial infections prevention and treatment, Nanomaterials 11 (1) (2021) articles, https://doi.org/10.3390/nano11010137. From NLM PubMed-not-MEDLINE).
[142] D.E. Bloom, D. Cadarette, Infectious disease threats in the twenty-first century: strengthening the global response, Frontiers in Immunology 10 (2019) 549, https://doi.org/10.3389/fimmu.2019.00549. From NLM Medline).
[143] S.L. Aitken, T.J. Dilworth, E.L. Heil, M.D. Nailor, Agricultural applications for antimicrobials. A danger to human health: an official position statement of the society of infectious diseases pharmacists, Articles, Pharmacotherapy: The Journal of Human Pharmacology and Drug Therapy 36 (4) (2016) 422–432, https://doi.org/10.1002/phar.1737. From NLM Medline).
[144] M.A. Alghamdi, A.N. Fallica, N. Virzi, P. Kesharwani, V. Pittala, K. Greish, The promise of nanotechnology in personalized medicine, Journal of Personalized Medicine 12 (5) (2022) articles, https://doi.org/10.3390/jpm12050673. From NLM PubMed-not-MEDLINE).
[145] H.T. Thuy, P. Nga le, T.T. Loan, Antibiotic contaminants in coastal wetlands from Vietnamese shrimp farming, Environmental Science and Pollution Research International 18 (6) (2011) 835–841, https://doi.org/10.1007/s11356-011-0475-7. From NLM Medline).
[146] P.K. Thornton, Livestock production: recent trends, future prospects, Philosophical Transactions of the Royal Society of London B Biological Sciences 365 (1554) (2010) 2853–2867, https://doi.org/10.1098/rstb.2010.0134. From NLM Medline).
[147] (FDA), F. a. D. A, 2018 Summary Report on Antimicrobials Sold or Distributed for Use in Food-Producing Animals, 2019.
[148] B.S. Lopez, Can infectious disease control Be achieved without antibiotics by exploiting mechanisms of disease tolerance?, Articles, Immunohorizons 6 (10) (2022) 730–740, https://doi.org/10.4049/immunohorizons.2200043. From NLM Medline).

[149] L. Taylor, B. Rodwell, Outbreak of foetal infection with bovine pestivirus in a central Queensland beef herd, Australian Veterinary Journal 79 (10) (2001) 682–685, https://doi.org/10.1111/j.1751-0813.2001.tb10670.x. From NLM Medline).

[150] K. Park, The beginning of the end of the nanomedicine hype, Journal of Controlled Release 305 (2019) 221–222, https://doi.org/10.1016/j.jconrel.2019.05.044. From NLM Medline).

[151] P. Grodzinski, NCI Centers of Cancer Nanotechnology Excellence (CCNEs) - a full story to set the record straight, Journal of Controlled Release 309 (2019) 341–342, https://doi.org/10.1016/j.jconrel.2019.08.016.

[152] J.P. Martins, J. das Neves, M. de la Fuente, C. Celia, H. Florindo, N. Gunday-Tureli, A. Popat, J.L. Santos, F. Sousa, R. Schmid, et al., The solid progress of nanomedicine, Drug Delivery and Translational Research 10 (3) (2020) 726–729, https://doi.org/10.1007/s13346-020-00743-2. From NLM Medline).

[153] M. Germain, F. Caputo, S. Metcalfe, G. Tosi, K. Spring, A.K.O. Åslund, A. Pottier, R. Schiffelers, A. Ceccaldi, R. Schmid, Delivering the power of nanomedicine to patients today, Journal of Controlled Release: Official Journal of the Controlled Release Society (2020), https://doi.org/10.1016/j.jconrel.2020.07.007. Articles.

[154] P. Boisseau, B. Loubaton, Nanomedicine, nanotechnology in medicine, Comptes Rendus Physique 12 (7) (2011) 620–636, https://doi.org/10.1016/j.crhy.2011.06.001. Articles.

[155] V.S. Chan, Nanomedicine: an unresolved regulatory issue, Articles, Regulatory Toxicology and Pharmacology 46 (3) (2006) 218–224, https://doi.org/10.1016/j.yrtph.2006.04.009. From NLM Medline).

[156] G. Oberdorster, A. Maynard, K. Donaldson, V. Castranova, J. Fitzpatrick, K. Ausman, J. Carter, B. Karn, W. Kreyling, D. Lai, et al., Principles for characterizing the potential human health effects from exposure to nanomaterials: elements of a screening strategy, Particle and Fibre Toxicology 2 (2005) 8, https://doi.org/10.1186/1743-8977-2-8. From NLM PubMed-not-MEDLINE).

[157] G. Oberdorster, E. Oberdorster, J. Oberdorster, Nanotoxicology: an emerging discipline evolving from studies of ultrafine particles, Environmental Health Perspectives 113 (7) (2005) 823–839, https://doi.org/10.1289/ehp.7339. From NLM Medline).

[158] Y. Muktar, T. Bikila, M. Keffale, Application of nanotechnology for animal health and production improvement: a review, World Applied Sciences Journal 33 (10) (2015) 1588–1596.

[159] A. Al-Qushawi, A. Rassouli, F. Atyabi, S.M. Peighambari, M. Esfandyari-Manesh, G.R. Shams, A. Yazdani, Preparation and characterization of three tilmicosin-loaded lipid nanoparticles: physicochemical properties and in-vitro antibacterial activities, Iranian Journal of Pharmaceutical Research 15 (4) (2016) 663–676 (From NLM PubMed-not-MEDLINE).

[160] M.Z. Troncarelli, H.d.M. Brandão, J.C. Gern, A.d.S. Guimarães, H. Langoni, Nanotechnology and Antimicrobials in Veterinary Medicine, 2013.

[161] S.K. Bhanja, A. Hotowy, M. Mehra, E. Sawosz, L. Pineda, K.P. Vadalasetty, N. Kurantowicz, A. Chwalibog, Ovo administration of silver nanoparticles and/or amino acids influence metabolism and immune gene expression in chicken embryos, International Journal of Molecular Sciences 16 (5) (2015) 9484–9503, https://doi.org/10.3390/ijms16059484. From NLM Medline).

[162] S. Bansod, M. Bawskar, M. Rai, In vitro effect of biogenic silver nanoparticles on sterilisation of tobacco leaf explants and for higher yield of protoplasts, IET Nanobiotechnology 9 (4) (2015) 239–245, https://doi.org/10.1049/iet-nbt.2014.0031. From NLM Medline).
[163] J. Lee, M. Jo, T.H. Kim, J.Y. Ahn, D.K. Lee, S. Kim, S. Hong, Aptamer sandwich-based carbon nanotube sensors for single-carbon-atomic-resolution detection of non-polar small molecular species, Lab on a Chip 11 (1) (2011) 52–56, https://doi.org/10.1039/c0lc00259c. From NLM Medline).
[164] C. Müller, A. Hohn, P.A. Schubiger, R. Schibli, Preclinical evaluation of novel organometallic 99m Tc-folate and 99m Tc-pteroate radiotracers for folate receptor-positive tumour targeting, European Journal of Nuclear Medicine and Molecular Imaging 33 (2006) 1007–1016.
[165] X. Pan, R.J. Lee, Tumour-selective drug delivery via folate receptor-targeted liposomes, Expert Opinion on Drug Delivery 1 (1) (2004) 7–17, https://doi.org/10.1517/17425247.1.1.7. From NLM Medline).
[166] Y. Lu, E. Sega, P.S. Low, Folate receptor-targeted immunotherapy: induction of humoral and cellular immunity against hapten-decorated cancer cells, International Journal of Cancer 116 (5) (2005) 710–719, https://doi.org/10.1002/ijc 21126. From NLM Medline).
[167] X.Y. Shi, S.H. Wang, S. Meshinchi, M.E. Van Antwerp, X.D. Bi, I.H. Lee, J.R. Baker, Dendrimer-entrapped gold nanoparticles as a platform for cancer-cell targeting and Imaging, Small 3 (7) (2007) 1245–1252, https://doi.org/10.1002/smll.200700054.
[168] O. Arome, O. Victoria, O. Comfort, A. Ogechukwu, U. Chimere, E. Affiong, U. Robert, O. Kingsley, Therapeutic Nanomedicine Surmounts the Limitations of Pharmacotherapy, 2017, https://doi.org/10.1515/med-2017-0041 articles.
[169] U.C. Oz, Z.B. Bolat, A. Poma, L. Guan, D. Telci, F. Sahin, G. Battaglia, A. Bozkır, Prostate cancer cell-specific BikDDA delivery by targeted polymersomes, Applied Nanoscience 10 (9) (2020) 3389–3401, https://doi.org/10.1007/s13204-020-01287-0.
[170] T.S. Bedwell, N. Anjum, Y. Ma, J. Czulak, A. Poma, E. Piletska, M.J. Whitcombe, S.A. Piletsky, New protocol for optimisation of polymer composition for imprinting of peptides and proteins, RSC Advances 9 (48) (2019) 27849–27855, https://doi.org/10.1039/C9RA05009D, 10.1039/C9RA05009D.
[171] E.-S. Kim, D. Kim, S. Nyberg, A. Poma, D. Cecchin, S.A. Jain, K.-A. Kim, Y.-J. Shin, E.-H. Kim, M. Kim. et al., LRP-1 functionalized polymersomes enhance the efficacy of carnosine in experimental stroke, Scientific Reports 10 (1) (2020) 699, https://doi.org/10.1038/s41598-020-57685-5.
[172] D. Radenkovic, S. Arjun, A. Poma, S. Nyberg, B. Battaglia, D.M. Yellon, S. Davidson, 162 polymersomes functionalized with HSP70 – novel, synthetic cardioprotective nanovesicles, Heart 102 (Suppl. 6) (2016), https://doi.org/10.1136/heartjnl-2016-309890.162. A115-A115.
[173] S. Hua, M.B.C. de Matos, J.M. Metselaar, G. Storm, Current trends and challenges in the clinical translation of nanoparticulate nanomedicines: pathways for translational development and commercialization, Frontiers in Pharmacology 9 (2018) 790, https://doi.org/10.3389/fphar.2018.00790. From NLM PubMed-not-MEDLINE).
[174] L.P. Wu, D. Wang, Z. Li, Grand challenges in nanomedicine, Materials Science & Engineering, C: Materials for Biological Applications 106 (2020) 110302, https://doi.org/10.1016/j.msec.2019.110302. From NLM Medline).

[175] Z. Lin, N.A. Monteiro-Riviere, J.E. Riviere, Pharmacokinetics of metallic nanoparticles, Wiley Interdisciplinary Reviews - Nanomedicine and Nanobiotechnology 7 (2) (2015) 189–217, https://doi.org/10.1002/wnan.1304. From NLM Medline).

[176] H. Zazo, C.I. Colino, J.M. Lanao, Current applications of nanoparticles in infectious diseases, Journal of Controlled Release 224 (2016) 86–102, https://doi.org/10.1016/j.jconrel.2016.01.008. From NLM Medline).

[177] C.A. Schutz, L. Juillerat-Jeanneret, H. Mueller, I. Lynch, M. Riediker, C. NanoImpactNet, Therapeutic nanoparticles in clinics and under clinical evaluation, Nanomedicine 8 (3) (2013) 449–467, https://doi.org/10.2217/nnm.13.8. From NLM Medline).

[178] S.S.A. Bala, K.R.B. Aamanchi, K.A.V. Phanindra, A. Amanchi, Novel Process of Preparing Nano Metal and the Products Thereof, Google Patents, 2015.

[179] C. Buzea, I.I. Pacheco, K. Robbie, Nanomaterials and nanoparticles: sources and toxicity, Biointerphases 2 (4) (2007) MR17–71, https://doi.org/10.1116/1.2815690 (From NLM PubMed-not-MEDLINE).

[180] V. Spampinato, G. Ceccone, S. Giordani, Surface analysis of zinc-porphyrin functionalized carbon nano-onions, Biointerphases 10 (1) (2015) 019006, https://doi.org/10.1116/1.4907726. From NLM Medline).

[181] X. Luo, A. Morrin, A.J. Killard, M.R. Smyth, Application of nanoparticles in electrochemical sensors and biosensors, Electroanalysis: An International Journal Devoted to Fundamental and Practical Aspects of Electroanalysis 18 (4) (2006) 319–326.

[182] Z. Feng, F. Ji-Quan, Research on catalytic properties of palladium catalyst prepared by biological reduction method, China Petroleum Processing and Petrochemical Technology 15 (2) (2013) 24.

[183] Y. Lee, M.A. Garcia, N.A.F. Huls, S. Sun, Synthetic tuning of the catalytic properties of Au-Fe 3 O 4 nanoparticles, Angewandte Chemie 7 (122) (2010) 1293–1296.

[184] M. Ananya Mandal, Properties of Nanoparticles, 2012. https://www.news-medical.net/life-sciences/Properties-of-Nanoparticles.aspx.

[185] B. Chen, R. Pan, D. Askhatova, P. Chen, Effective small interfering RNA delivery in vitro via a new stearylated cationic peptide, International Journal of Nanomedicine 10 (2015) 3303–3314, https://doi.org/10.2147/IJN.S79306. From NLM Medline).

[186] J. Estelrich, M.J. Sanchez-Martin, M.A. Busquets, Nanoparticles in magnetic resonance imaging: from simple to dual contrast agents, International Journal of Nanomedicine 10 (2015) 1727–1741, https://doi.org/10.2147/IJN.S76501. From NLM Medline).

[187] S.H. Hussein-Al-Ali, M.E. El Zowalaty, M.Z. Hussein, M. Ismail, D. Dorniani, T.J. Webster, Novel kojic acid-polymer-based magnetic nanocomposites for medical applications, International Journal of Nanomedicine 9 (2014) 351–362, https://doi.org/10.2147/IJN.S53847. From NLM Medline).

[188] J. Skopalik, K. Polakova, M. Havrdova, I. Justan, M. Magro, D. Milde, L. Knopfova, J. Smarda, H. Polakova, E. Gabrielova, et al., Mesenchymal stromal cell labeling by new uncoated superparamagnetic maghemite nanoparticles in comparison with commercial Resovist–an initial in vitro study, International Journal of Nanomedicine 9 (2014) 5355–5372, https://doi.org/10.2147/IJN.S66986. From NLM Medline).

[189] I. Gessner, Optimizing nanoparticle design and surface modification toward clinical translation, MRS Bulletin (2021), https://doi.org/10.1557/s43577-021-00132-1. Articles.

[190] A. Aghebati-Maleki, S. Dolati, M. Ahmadi, A. Baghbanzhadeh, M. Asadi, A. Fotouhi, M. Yousefi, L. Aghebati-Maleki, Nanoparticles and cancer therapy: perspectives for application of nanoparticles in the treatment of cancers, Journal of Cellular Physiology 235 (3) (2020) 1962–1972, https://doi.org/10.1002/jcp.29126. From NLM Medline).
[191] M.R. Miller, J.B. Raftis, J.P. Langrish, S.G. McLean, P. Samutrtai, S.P. Connell, S. Wilson, A.T. Vesey, P.H. Fokkens, A.J.F. Boere, Inhaled nanoparticles accumulate at sites of vascular disease, ACS Nano 11 (5) (2017) 4542–4552.
[192] L.J.F. Peters, A. Jans, M. Bartneck, E.P.C. van der Vorst, Immunomodulatory nanomedicine for the treatment of atherosclerosis, Journal of Clinical Medicine (2021), https://doi.org/10.3390/jcm10143185. Articles.
[193] M.A. Munger, P. Radwanski, G.C. Hadlock, G. Stoddard, A. Shaaban, J. Falconer, D.W. Grainger, C.E. Deering-Rice, In vivo human time-exposure study of orally dosed commercial silver nanoparticles, Nanomedicine 10 (1) (2014) 1–9, https://doi.org/10.1016/j.nano.2013.06.010. From NLM Medline).
[194] X. Zhang, Gold nanoparticles: recent advances in the biomedical applications, Cell Biochemistry and Biophysics 72 (3) (2015) 771–775, https://doi.org/10.1007/s12013-015-0529-4. From NLM Medline).
[195] X.D. Zhang, D. Wu, X. Shen, P.X. Liu, N. Yang, B. Zhao, H. Zhang, Y.M. Sun, L.A. Zhang, F.Y. Fan, Size-dependent in vivo toxicity of PEG-coated gold nanoparticles, International Journal of Nanomedicine 6 (2011) 2071–2081, https://doi.org/10.2147/IJN.S21657. From NLM Medline).
[196] Z. Zdrojewicz, M. Waracki, B. Bugaj, D. Pypno, K. Cabała, Medical applications of nanotechnology, Postepy Higieny i Medycyny Doświadczalnej (2015) (articles).
[197] J. Alper, National cancer Institute alliance for nanotechnology in cancer: shining a light on cancer research, Jan/Feb issue, in: Azo Nanotechnology Article: Nanomedicine-How Nanotechnology Can Be Used in the Healthcare/drug Markets for Humans and Animals, 2005.
[198] C.W. Lam, J.T. James, R. McCluskey, R.L. Hunter, Pulmonary toxicity of single-wall carbon nanotubes in mice 7 and 90 days after intratracheal instillation, Toxicological Sciences 77 (1) (2004) 126–134, https://doi.org/10.1093/toxsci/kfg243. From NLM Medline).
[199] D.B. Warheit, B.R. Laurence, K.L. Reed, D.H. Roach, G.A. Reynolds, T.R. Webb, Comparative pulmonary toxicity assessment of single-wall carbon nanotubes in rats, Toxicological Sciences 77 (1) (2004) 117–125, https://doi.org/10.1093/toxsci/kfg228. From NLM Medline).
[200] V. Labhasetwar, C. Song, W. Humphrey, R. Shebuski, R.J. Levy, Arterial uptake of biodegradable nanoparticles: effect of surface modifications, Journal of Pharmaceutical Sciences 87 (10) (1998) 1229–1234, https://doi.org/10.1021/js980021f. From NLM Medline).
[201] K. Donaldson, V. Stone, C. Tran, W. Kreyling, P.J. Borm, Nanotoxicology, BMJ Publishing Group Ltd 61 (2004) 727–728.
[202] D.M. Brown, M.R. Wilson, W. MacNee, V. Stone, K. Donaldson, Size-dependent proinflammatory effects of ultrafine polystyrene particles: a role for surface area and oxidative stress in the enhanced activity of ultrafines, Toxicology and Applied Pharmacology 175 (3) (2001) 191–199, https://doi.org/10.1006/taap.2001.9240. From NLM Medline).

[203] P.G. Barlow, K. Donaldson, J. MacCallum, A. Clouter, V. Stone, Serum exposed to nanoparticle carbon black displays increased potential to induce macrophage migration, Toxicology Letters 155 (3) (2005) 397–401, https://doi.org/10.1016/j.toxlet.2004.11.006. From NLM Medline).
[204] E. Baranowska-Wójcik, Factors conditioning the potential effects TiO2 NPs exposure on human microbiota: a mini-review, Biological Trace Element Research (2021), https://doi.org/10.1007/s12011-021-02578-5. Articles.
[205] M. Trop, M. Novak, S. Rodl, B. Hellbom, W. Kroell, W. Goessler, Silver-coated dressing acticoat caused raised liver enzymes and argyria-like symptoms in burn patient, Journal of Trauma and Acute Care Surgery 60 (3) (2006) 648–652.
[206] H.J. Johnston, G. Hutchison, F.M. Christensen, S. Peters, S. Hankin, V. Stone, A review of the in vivo and in vitro toxicity of silver and gold particulates: particle attributes and biological mechanisms responsible for the observed toxicity, Critical Reviews in Toxicology 40 (4) (2010) 328–346, https://doi.org/10.3109/10408440903453074. From NLM Medline).
[207] I. Chopra, The increasing use of silver-based products as antimicrobial agents: a useful development or a cause for concern? Journal of antimicrobial Chemotherapy 59 (4) (2007) 587–590.
[208] J. Singh, T. Dutta, K.H. Kim, M. Rawat, P. Samddar, P. Kumar, Green' synthesis of metals and their oxide nanoparticles: applications for environmental remediation, Journal of Nanobiotechnology 16 (1) (2018) 84, https://doi.org/10.1186/s12951-018-0408-4. From NLM Medline).
[209] R. Arshad, M.F. Sohail, H.S. Sarwar, H. Saeed, I. Ali, S. Akhtar, S.Z. Hussain, I. Afzal, S. Jahan, R. Anees Ur, et al., ZnO-NPs embedded biodegradable thiolated bandage for postoperative surgical site infection: in vitro and in vivo evaluation, PLoS One 14 (6) (2019) e0217079, https://doi.org/10.1371/journal.pone.0217079. From NLM Medline).
[210] I. Khan, K. Saeed, I. Khan, Nanoparticles: properties, applications and toxicities, Arabian Journal of Chemistry 12 (7) (2019) 908–931, https://doi.org/10.1016/j.arabjc.2017.05.011.
[211] D. Ashish, et al., Future Effect of Nano-Medicine on Human Generation, 2015 (articles).
[212] E. Fasoli, Protein corona: dr. Jekyll and mr. Hyde of nanomedicine, Biotechnology and Applied Biochemistry (2020), https://doi.org/10.1002/bab.2035. Articles.
[213] S. Naahidi, M. Jafari, F. Edalat, K. Raymond, A. Khademhosseini, P. Chen, Biocompatibility of engineered nanoparticles for drug delivery, Journal of Controlled Release 166 (2) (2013) 182–194, https://doi.org/10.1016/j.jconrel.2012.12.013. From NLM Medline).
[214] C.Z. Bueno, A.C. Apolinário, A. Duro-Castano, A. Poma, A. Pessoa, C.O. Rangel-Yagui, G. Battaglia, l-Asparaginase encapsulation into asymmetric permeable polymersomes, ACS Macro Letters 9 (10) (2020) 1471–1477, https://doi.org/10.1021/acsmacrolett.0c00619.
[215] X. Ma, J.C. Knowles, A. Poma, Biodegradable and sustainable synthetic antibodies—a perspective, in: Pharmaceutics, vol 15, 2023.
[216] K.K. Jain, The Handbook of Nanomedicine, Humana, Totowa, NJ, 2008, https://doi.org/10.1007/978-1-60327-319-0.
[217] A. Kuzmov, T. Minko, Nanotechnology approaches for inhalation treatment of lung diseases, Journal of Controlled Release 219 (2015)

500–518, https://doi.org/10.1016/j.jconrel.2015.07.024. From NLM Medline).
[218] M. Doroudian, R. MacLoughlin, F. Poynton, A. Prina-Mello, S.C. Donnelly, Nanotechnology based therapeutics for lung disease, Thorax (2019), https://doi.org/10.1136/thoraxjnl-2019-213037. Articles.
[219] C.M. Goodman, C.D. McCusker, T. Yilmaz, V.M. Rotello, Toxicity of gold nanoparticles functionalized with cationic and anionic side chains, Bioconjugate Chemistry 15 (4) (2004) 897–900, https://doi.org/10.1021/bc049951i. From NLM).
[220] V. Kattumuri, K. Katti, S. Bhaskaran, E.J. Boote, S.W. Casteel, G.M. Fent, D.J. Robertson, M. Chandrasekhar, R. Kannan, K.V. Katti, Gum Arabic as a phytochemical construct for the stabilization of gold nanoparticles: in vivo pharmacokinetics and X-ray-contrast-imaging studies, Small 3 (2) (2007) 333–341, https://doi.org/10.1002/smll.200600427. From NLM).
[221] V. Kandi, S. Kandi, Antimicrobial properties of nanomolecules: potential candidates as antibiotics in the era of multi-drug resistance, Epidemiol Health 37 (2015) e2015020, https://doi.org/10.4178/epih/e2015020. From NLM).
[222] D.B. Warheit, Nanoparticles: health impacts?, Review, Materials Today 7 (2) (2004) 32–35, https://doi.org/10.1016/S1369-7021(04)00081-1. Scopus).
[223] C.A. Dos Santos, M.M. Seckler, A.P. Ingle, I. Gupta, S. Galdiero, M. Galdiero, A. Gade, M. Rai, Silver nanoparticles: therapeutical uses, toxicity, and safety issues, Journal of Pharmaceutical Sciences 103 (7) (2014) 1931–1944, https://doi.org/10.1002/jps.24001. From NLM).
[224] W.I. Hagens, A.G. Oomen, W.H. de Jong, F.R. Cassee, A.J. Sips, What do we (need to) know about the kinetic properties of nanoparticles in the body? Regulatory Toxicology and Pharmacology 49 (3) (2007) 217–229, https://doi.org/10.1016/j.yrtph.2007.07.006. From NLM).
[225] S.E. Leucuta, Systemic and biophase bioavailability and pharmacokinetics of nanoparticulate drug delivery systems, Current Drug Delivery 10 (2) (2013) 208–240, https://doi.org/10.2174/1567201811310020007. From NLM).
[226] J. Sengupta, S. Ghosh, P. Datta, A. Gomes, A. Gomes, Physiologically important metal nanoparticles and their toxicity, Journal of Nanoscience and Nanotechnology 14 (1) (2014) 990–1006, https://doi.org/10.1166/jnn.2014.9078. From NLM).
[227] L. Wei, J. Lu, H. Xu, A. Patel, Z.S. Chen, G. Chen, Silver nanoparticles: synthesis, properties, and therapeutic applications, Drug Discovery Today 20 (5) (2015) 595–601, https://doi.org/10.1016/j.drudis.2014.11.014. From NLM).
[228] R. Duncan, R. Gaspar, Nanomedicine(s) under the microscope, Molecular Pharmaceutics 8 (6) (2011) 2101–2141, https://doi.org/10.1021/mp200394t. From NLM).
[229] R.R. Arvizo, S. Bhattacharyya, R.A. Kudgus, K. Giri, R. Bhattacharya, P. Mukherjee, Intrinsic therapeutic applications of noble metal nanoparticles: past, present and future, Chemical Society Reviews 41 (7) (2012) 2943–2970, https://doi.org/10.1039/c2cs15355f. From NLM).
[230] Safety, H. a.; Executive, Using Nanomaterials at Work, Health and Safety Executive, 2013.
[231] S. Ghosh, S. Patil, M. Ahire, R. Kitture, D.D. Gurav, A.M. Jabgunde, S. Kale, K. Pardesi, V. Shinde, J. Bellare, et al., Gnidia glauca flower extract mediated synthesis of gold nanoparticles and evaluation of its

chemocatalytic potential, Journal of Nanobiotechnology 10 (2012), https://doi.org/10.1186/1477-3155-10-17. Scopus).
[232] P. Daisy, K. Saipriya, Biochemical analysis of Cassia fistula aqueous extract and phytochemically synthesized gold nanoparticles as hypoglycemic treatment for diabetes mellitus, International Journal of Nanomedicine 7 (2012) 1189–1202, https://doi.org/10.2147/IJN.S26650. Scopus).
[233] I.R. Bell, G.E. Schwartz, N.N. Boyer, M. Koithan, A.J. Brooks, Advances in integrative nanomedicine for improving infectious disease treatment in public health, European journal of integrative medicine (2013), https://doi.org/10.1016/j.eujim.2012.11.002. Articles.
[234] W. Luther, R. Nass, F. Schuster, M. Kallio, P. Lintunen, et al., Industrial Application of Nanomaterials - Changes and Risks, 2004.
[235] L. Milane, M. Amiji, Clinical approval of nanotechnology-based SARS-CoV-2 mRNA vaccines: impact on translational nanomedicine, Drug Delivery and Translational Research (2021), https://doi.org/10.1007/s13346-021-00911-y. Articles.
[236] J.,R.A. Freitas, Current status of nanomedicine and medical nanorobotics, Journal of Computational and Theoretical Nanoscience 2 (1) (2005) 1–25 (Review. Scopus).
[237] A. Hafner, J. Lovrić, G.P. Lakŏ, I. Pepić, Nanotherapeutics in the EU: an overview on current state and future directions, International Journal of Nanomedicine 9 (1) (2014) 1005–1023, https://doi.org/10.2147/IJN.S55359. Scopus).
[238] A.S. Rathore, H. Winkle, Quality by design for biopharmaceuticals, Nature Biotechnology 27 (1) (2009) 26–34, https://doi.org/10.1038/nbt0109-26. Scopus).
[239] T. Bastogne, Quality-by-design of nanopharmaceuticals - a state of the art, Nanomedicine: Nanotechnology, Biology and Medicine (2017), https://doi.org/10.1016/j.nano.2017.05.014. Articles.
[240] K.M. Tyner, P. Zou, X. Yang, H. Zhang, C.N. Cruz, S.L. Lee, Product quality for nanomaterials: current U.S. experience and perspective, Article, Wiley Interdisciplinary Reviews - Nanomedicine and Nanobiotechnology 7 (5) (2015) 640–654, https://doi.org/10.1002/wnan.1338. From NLM Medline).
[241] S. Mignani, X. Shi, J. Rodrigues, R. Roy, Á. Muñoz-Fernández, V. Ceña, J.-P. Majoral, Dendrimers toward translational nanotherapeutics: concise key step analysis, Bioconjugate Chemistry (2020), https://doi.org/10.1021/acs.bioconjchem.0c00395. Articles.
[242] B. Flühmann, I. Ntai, G. Borchard, S. Simoens, S. Mühlebach, Nanomedicines: the magic bullets reaching their target? European Journal of Pharmaceutical Sciences 128 (2019) 73–80, https://doi.org/10.1016/j.ejps.2018.11.019. From NLM).
[243] Y.H. Choi, H.-K. Han, Nanomedicines: current status and future perspectives in aspect of drug delivery and pharmacokinetics, Journal of pharmaceutical investigation 48 (1) (2018) 43–60.
[244] FDA, A. CDER, Drug Products, Including Biological Products, that Contain Nanomaterials-Guidance for Industry, 2017.
[245] D. Bobo, K.J. Robinson, J. Islam, K.J. Thurecht, S.R. Corrie, Nanoparticle-based medicines: a review of FDA-approved materials and clinical trials to date, Pharmaceutical Research 33 (10) (2016) 2373–2387, https://doi.org/10.1007/s11095-016-1958-5. From NLM Medline).

[246] A.D. Jones, G. Mi, T.J. Webster, A status report on FDA approval of medical devices containing nanostructured materials, Trends in Biotechnology 37 (2) (2019) 117–120, https://doi.org/10.1016/j.tibtech.2018.06.003. From NLM Medline).
[247] S. Mignani, J. Rodrigues, R. Roy, X. Shi, V. Ceña, S. El Kazzouli, J.P. Majoral, Exploration of biomedical dendrimer space based on in-vivo physicochemical parameters: key factor analysis (Part 2), Drug Discovery Today 24 (5) (2019) 1184–1192, https://doi.org/10.1016/j.drudis.2019.03.001. From NLM).
[248] D.A. Tomalia, L.S. Nixon, D.M. Hedstrand, The role of branch cell symmetry and other critical nanoscale design parameters in the determination of dendrimer encapsulation properties, Biomolecules 10 (4) (2020), https://doi.org/10.3390/biom10040642. From NLM).
[249] N.P. Suh, The Principles of Design, 1990 *(No Title)*.
[250] P. Satalkar, B.S. Elger, P. Hunziker, D. Shaw, Challenges of clinical translation in nanomedicine: a qualitative study, Nanomedicine 12 (4) (2016) 893–900, https://doi.org/10.1016/j.nano.2015.12.376. From NLM).
[251] Nanotechnology Task Force Report 2007, Deputy Commissioner for Policy Associate Commissioner for Science, 2007. https://www.fda.gov/science-research/nanotechnology-programs-fda/nanotechnology-task-force-report-2007.
[252] P. Bhatia, S. Vasaikar, A. Wali, A landscape of nanomedicine innovations in India, Nanotechnology Reviews 7 (2) (2018) 131–148, https://doi.org/10.1515/ntrev-2017-0196. (Accessed 6 January 2024).
[253] R.M. Kannan, E. Nance, S. Kannan, D.A. Tomalia, Emerging concepts in dendrimer-based nanomedicine: from design principles to clinical applications, Journal of Internal Medicine 276 (6) (2014) 579–617, https://doi.org/10.1111/joim.12280. From NLM Medline).
[254] S. Mignani, J. Rodrigues, H. Tomas, R. Roy, X. Shi, J.P. Majoral, Bench-to-bedside translation of dendrimers: reality or utopia? A concise analysis, Advanced Drug Delivery Reviews 136–137 (2018) 73–81, https://doi.org/10.1016/j.addr.2017.11.007. From NLM Medline).
[255] T. Stylianopoulos, R.K. Jain, Design considerations for nanotherapeutics in oncology, Nanomedicine 11 (8) (2015) 1893–1907, https://doi.org/10.1016/j.nano.2015.07.015. From NLM).
[256] J. Yue, T.J. Feliciano, W. Li, A. Lee, T.W. Odom, Gold nanoparticle size and shape effects on cellular uptake and intracellular distribution of siRNA nanoconstructs, Bioconjugate Chemistry 28 (6) (2017) 1791–1800, https://doi.org/10.1021/acs.bioconjchem.7b00252. From NLM).
[257] E. Morgan, D. Wupperfeld, D. Morales, N. Reich, Shape matters: gold nanoparticle shape impacts the biological activity of siRNA delivery, Bioconjugate Chemistry 30 (3) (2019) 853–860, https://doi.org/10.1021/acs.bioconjchem.9b00004. From NLM).
[258] D. Papahadjopoulos, T.M. Allen, A. Gabizon, E. Mayhew, K. Matthay, S.K. Huang, K.D. Lee, M.C. Woodle, D.D. Lasic, C. Redemann, et al., Sterically stabilized liposomes: improvements in pharmacokinetics and antitumor therapeutic efficacy, Proceedings of the National Academy of Sciences of the U S A 88 (24) (1991) 11460–11464, https://doi.org/10.1073/pnas.88.24.11460. From NLM).
[259] A. Poma, M. Whitcombe, S. Piletsky, Plastic antibodies, in: S.A. Piletsky, M.J. Whitcombe (Eds.), Designing Receptors for the Next Generation of Biosensors, Springer Berlin Heidelberg, 2013, pp. 105–129.

[260] A. Poma, A.P.F. Turner, S.A. Piletsky, Advances in the manufacture of MIP nanoparticles, Trends in Biotechnology 28 (12) (2010) 629–637, https://doi.org/10.1016/j.tibtech.2010.08.006.
[261] A. Poma, H. Brahmbhatt, H.M. Pendergraff, J.K. Watts, N.W. Turner, Generation of novel hybrid aptamer-molecularly imprinted polymeric nanoparticles, Advanced Materials 27 (4) (2015) 750–758, https://doi.org/10.1002/adma.201404235. From NLM).
[262] D.C. Thang, Z. Wang, X. Lu, B. Xing, Precise cell behaviors manipulation through light-responsive nano-regulators: recent advance and perspective, Theranostics (2019), https://doi.org/10.7150/thno.33888 articles.
[263] R.O. Hynes, Integrins: bidirectional, allosteric signaling machines, Cell 110 (6) (2002) 673–687, https://doi.org/10.1016/s0092-8674(02)00971-6. From NLM).
[264] K.T. Nguyen, Y. Zhao, Engineered hybrid nanoparticles for on-demand diagnostics and therapeutics, Accounts of Chemical Research (2015), https://doi.org/10.1021/acs.accounts.5b00316. Articles.
[265] Authorizations of Emergency Use of Two Biological Products during the COVID-19 Pandemic; Availability, Department of Health and Human Services, F. a. D. A., 2021.
[266] Nanomedicine and the COVID-19 vaccines, Nature Nanotechnology 15 (12) (2020) 963, https://doi.org/10.1038/s41565-020-00820-0. From NLM Medline).
[267] M.C. Roco, National Nanotechnology Initiative at 20 years: enabling new horizons, Journal of Nanoparticle Research 25 (10) (2023) 197, https://doi.org/10.1007/s11051-023-05829-9.
[268] Nanomedicine Market Size, Share & Trends Analysis Report by Application (Drug Delivery), by Indication (Clinical Oncology, Infectious Diseases), by Molecule Type, by Region, and Segment Forecasts, 2023 - 2030, 2023. https://www.grandviewresearch.com/industry-analysis/nanomedicine-market.
[269] X. Shan, X. Gong, J. Li, J. Wen, Y. Li, Z. Zhang, Current approaches of nanomedicines in the market and various stage of clinical translation, Acta Pharmaceutica Sinica B 12 (7) (2022) 3028–3048, https://doi.org/10.1016/j.apsb.2022.02.025 (From NLM PubMed-not-MEDLINE).
[270] R.K. Thapa, J.O. Kim, Nanomedicine-based commercial formulations: current developments and future prospects, Journal of Pharmaceutical Investigation 53 (1) (2023) 19–33, https://doi.org/10.1007/s40005-022-00607-6. From NLM PubMed-not-MEDLINE).
[271] S. Marchal, A. El Hor, M. Millard, V. Gillon, L. Bezdetnaya, Anticancer drug delivery: an update on clinically applied nanotherapeutics, Drugs 75 (14) (2015) 1601–1611, https://doi.org/10.1007/s40265-015-0453-3. From NLM Medline).
[272] Y. Barenholz, Doxil(R)–the first FDA-approved nano-drug: lessons learned, Journal of Controlled Release 160 (2) (2012) 117–134, https://doi.org/10.1016/j.jconrel.2012.03.020. From NLM Medline).
[273] C. Kleinstreuer, S.V. Chari, S. Vachhani, Potential use of multifunctional nanoparticles for the treatment of cardiovascular diseases, Journal of Cardiology and Cardiovascular Sciences 2 (3) (2018).
[274] C.L. Ventola, Progress in nanomedicine: approved and investigational nanodrugs, P and T 42 (12) (2017) 742–755 (From NLM PubMed-not-MEDLINE).

[275] Y.X. Wang, Current status of superparamagnetic iron oxide contrast agents for liver magnetic resonance imaging, World Journal of Gastroenterology 21 (47) (2015) 13400–13402, https://doi.org/10.3748/wjg.v21.i47.13400. From NLM Medline).
[276] A.C. Anselmo, S. Mitragotri, Nanoparticles in the clinic: an update, Bioengineering & Translational Medicine 4 (3) (2019) e10143, https://doi.org/10.1002/btm2.10143. From NLM PubMed-not-MEDLINE).
[277] J.K. Patra, G. Das, L.F. Fraceto, E.V.R. Campos, M.D.P. Rodriguez-Torres, L.S. Acosta-Torres, L.A. Diaz-Torres, R. Grillo, M.K. Swamy, S. Sharma, et al., Nano based drug delivery systems: recent developments and future prospects, Journal of Nanobiotechnology 16 (1) (2018) 71, https://doi.org/10.1186/s12951-018-0392-8. From NLM Medline).
[278] N.A. Mohamed, I. Marei, S. Crovella, H. Abou-Saleh, Recent developments in nanomaterials-based drug delivery and upgrading treatment of cardiovascular diseases, International Journal of Molecular Sciences (2022), https://doi.org/10.3390/ijms23031404. Articles.
[279] W.W.Y. Wong, A commuting-vector-field approach to some dispersive estimates, Archiv der Mathematik 110 (3) (2018) 273–289, https://doi.org/10.1007/s00013-017-1114-4. Scopus).
[280] J.M. Caster, A.N. Patel, T. Zhang, A. Wang, Investigational nanomedicines in 2016: a review of nanotherapeutics currently undergoing clinical trials, Wiley Interdiscip Rev Nanomed Nanobiotechnol 9 (1) (2017) e1416, https://doi.org/10.1002/wnan.1416. From NLM Medline).
[281] D. Lebeaux, A. Chauhan, O. Rendueles, C. Beloin, From in vitro to in vivo models of bacterial biofilm-related infections, Pathogens 2 (2) (2013) 288–356, https://doi.org/10.3390/pathogens2020288. From NLM PubMed-not-MEDLINE).
[282] D.B. Barbosa, A.M. Agostinho Hunt, A. Berretta, E. Rodrigues de Camargo, L.F. Gorup, D.R. Monteiro, G.L. Fernandes, R.A. Fernandes, K.R. Kirker, The importance of preventing and controlling biofilm in wounds, in: M.S. Ågren (Ed.), Wound Healing Biomaterials, Woodhead Publishing, 2016, pp. 79–105.
[283] T. Bjarnsholt, M. Alhede, M. Alhede, S.R. Eickhardt-Sorensen, C. Moser, M. Kuhl, P.O. Jensen, N. Hoiby, The in vivo biofilm, Trends in Microbiology 21 (9) (2013) 466–474, https://doi.org/10.1016/j.tim.2013.06.002. From NLM Medline).
[284] F. Andrade, D. Rafael, M. Videira, D. Ferreira, A. Sosnik, B. Sarmento, Nanotechnology and pulmonary delivery to overcome resistance in infectious diseases, Advanced Drug Delivery Reviews 65 (13–14) (2013) 1816–1827, https://doi.org/10.1016/j.addr.2013.07.020. From NLM Medline).
[285] Health, U. N. I. o. ClinicalTrials. gov, On Demand Antiretroviral Preexposure Prophylaxis for HIV Infection in Men Who Have Sex with Men (IPERGAY), 2015, 2015.
[286] E. Beltrán-Gracia, A. López-Camacho, I. Higuera-Ciapara, J.B. Velázquez-Fernández, A.A. Vallejo-Cardona, Nanomedicine review: clinical developments in liposomal applications, Cancer Nanotechnology 10 (1) (2019) 1–40.
[287] P. Ma, R.J. Mumper, Paclitaxel nano-delivery systems: a comprehensive review, Journal of Nanomedicine & Nanotechnology 4 (2) (2013) 1000164, https://doi.org/10.4172/2157-7439.1000164 (From NLM PubMed-not-MEDLINE).

[288] B. Li, X. Zhang, Y. Dong, Nanoscale platforms for messenger RNA delivery, Wiley Interdisciplinary Reviews - Nanomedicine and Nanobiotechnology 11 (2) (2019) e1530, https://doi.org/10.1002/wnan.1530. From NLM Medline).

[289] A. Akinc, M.A. Maier, M. Manoharan, K. Fitzgerald, M. Jayaraman, S. Barros, S. Ansell, X. Du, M.J. Hope, T.D. Madden, et al., The Onpattro story and the clinical translation of nanomedicines containing nucleic acid-based drugs, Nature Nanotechnology 14 (12) (2019) 1084–1087, https://doi.org/10.1038/s41565-019-0591-y. From NLM Medline).

[290] Y. Xin, M. Huang, W.W. Guo, Q. Huang, L.Z. Zhang, G. Jiang, Nano-based delivery of RNAi in cancer therapy, Molecular Cancer 16 (1) (2017) 134, https://doi.org/10.1186/s12943-017-0683-y. From NLM Medline).

[291] Study to Evaluate Arikace™ in CF Patients with Chronic Infection Due to Pseudomonas Aeruginosa, US National Library of Medicine, 2018. https://clinicaltrials.gov/study/NCT01315691#more-information.

[292] K. Bush, Alarming beta-lactamase-mediated resistance in multidrug-resistant Enterobacteriaceae, Current Opinion in Microbiology 13 (5) (2010) 558–564, https://doi.org/10.1016/j.mib.2010.09.006. From NLM Medline).

[293] J.M. Sallovitz, M.I.Z. Menghini, C.E. Lanusse, Impact of liposomes as delivery systems in veterinary medicine, Veterinary Research 29 (5) (1998) 409–430.

[294] C.E. Swenson, W.R. Perkins, P. Roberts, I. Ahmad, R. Stevens, D.A. Stevens, A.S. Janoff, In vitro and in vivo antifungal activity of amphotericin B lipid complex: are phospholipases important? Antimicrobial Agents and Chemotherapy 42 (4) (1998) 767–771, https://doi.org/10.1128/AAC.42.4.767. From NLM Medline).

[295] P. Meers, M. Neville, V. Malinin, A.W. Scotto, G. Sardaryan, R. Kurumunda, C. Mackinson, G. James, S. Fisher, W.R. Perkins, Biofilm penetration, triggered release and in vivo activity of inhaled liposomal amikacin in chronic *Pseudomonas aeruginosa* lung infections, Journal of Antimicrobial Chemotherapy 61 (4) (2008) 859–868, https://doi.org/10.1093/jac/dkn059 (From NLM Medline). (Accessed 1 May 2024).

[296] Z. Ehsan, J.P. Clancy, Management of *Pseudomonas aeruginosa* infection in cystic fibrosis patients using inhaled antibiotics with a focus on nebulized liposomal amikacin, Future Microbiology 10 (12) (2015) 1901–1912, https://doi.org/10.2217/fmb.15.117. From NLM Medline).

[297] V. Waters, F. Ratjen, Inhaled liposomal amikacin, Expert Review of Respiratory Medicine 8 (4) (2014) 401–409, https://doi.org/10.1586/17476348.2014.918507. From NLM Medline).

[298] J. Costa-Gouveia, E. Pancani, S. Jouny, A. Machelart, V. Delorme, G. Salzano, R. Iantomasi, C. Piveteau, C.J. Queval, O.R. Song, et al., Combination therapy for tuberculosis treatment: pulmonary administration of ethionamide and booster co-loaded nanoparticles, Scientific Reports 7 (1) (2017) 5390, https://doi.org/10.1038/s41598-017-05453-3. From NLM Medline).

[299] J. Zhang, F. Leifer, S. Rose, D.Y. Chun, J. Thaisz, T. Herr, M. Nashed, J. Joseph, W.R. Perkins, K. DiPetrillo, Amikacin liposome inhalation suspension (ALIS) penetrates non-tuberculous mycobacterial biofilms and enhances amikacin uptake into macrophages, Frontiers in Microbiology 9 (2018) 915.

[300] D. Caimmi, N. Martocq, D. Trioleyre, C. Guinet, S. Godreuil, T. Daniel, R. Chiron, Positive effect of liposomal amikacin for inhalation on

Mycobacterium abcessus in cystic fibrosis patients, in: Open Forum Infectious Diseases, vol 5, Oxford University Press US, 2018, p. ofy034.
[301] K.N. Olivier, D.E. Griffith, G. Eagle, J.P. McGinnis 2nd, L. Micioni, K. Liu, C.L. Daley, K.L. Winthrop, S. Ruoss, D.J. Addrizzo-Harris, et al., Randomized trial of liposomal amikacin for inhalation in nontuberculous mycobacterial lung disease, American Journal of Respiratory and Critical Care Medicine 195 (6) (2017) 814–823, https://doi.org/10.1164/rccm.201604-0700OC. From NLM Medline).
[302] O.O. Okusanya, S.M. Bhavnani, J. Hammel, P. Minic, L.J. Dupont, A. Forrest, G.J. Mulder, C. Mackinson, P.G. Ambrose, R. Gupta, Pharmacokinetic and pharmacodynamic evaluation of liposomal amikacin for inhalation in cystic fibrosis patients with chronic pseudomonal infection, Antimicrobial Agents and Chemotherapy 53 (9) (2009) 3847–3854, https://doi.org/10.1128/AAC.00872-08. From NLM Medline).
[303] M.-X. Luo, S. Hua, Q.-Y. Shang, Application of nanotechnology in drug delivery systems for respiratory diseases (Review), Molecular Medicine Reports (2021), https://doi.org/10.3892/mmr.2021.11964. Articles.
[304] M. Shirley, Amikacin liposome inhalation suspension: a review in *Mycobacterium avium* complex lung disease, Drugs 79 (2019) 555–562.
[305] D. Bilton, T. Pressler, I. Fajac, J.P. Clancy, D. Sands, P. Minic, M. Cipolli, I. Galeva, A. Sole, A.L. Quittner, et al., Amikacin liposome inhalation suspension for chronic *Pseudomonas aeruginosa* infection in cystic fibrosis, Journal of Cystic Fibrosis 19 (2) (2020) 284–291, https://doi.org/10.1016/j.jcf.2019.08.001. From NLM Medline).
[306] J. Adler-Moore, R.E. Lewis, R.J.M. Bruggemann, B.J.A. Rijnders, A.H. Groll, T.J. Walsh, Preclinical safety, tolerability, pharmacokinetics, pharmacodynamics, and antifungal activity of liposomal amphotericin B, Clinical Infectious Diseases 68 (Suppl. 4) (2019) S244–S259, https://doi.org/10.1093/cid/ciz064. From NLM Medline).
[307] D.J. Serisier, D. Bilton, A. De Soyza, P.J. Thompson, J. Kolbe, H.W. Greville, D. Cipolla, P. Bruinenberg, I. Gonda, O.-. investigators, Inhaled, dual release liposomal ciprofloxacin in non-cystic fibrosis bronchiectasis (ORBIT-2): a randomised, double-blind, placebo-controlled trial, Thorax 68 (9) (2013) 812–817, https://doi.org/10.1136/thoraxjnl-2013-203207. From NLM Medline).
[308] M. Doroudian, R. MacLoughlin, F. Poynton, A. Prina-Mello, S.C. Donnelly, Nanotechnology based therapeutics for lung disease, Thorax 74 (10) (2019) 965–976, https://doi.org/10.1136/thoraxjnl-2019-213037. From NLM Medline).
[309] K.A. Hamblin, J.P. Wong, J.D. Blanchard, H.S. Atkins, The potential of liposome–encapsulated ciprofloxacin as a tularemia therapy, Frontiers in Cellular and Infection Microbiology 4 (2014) 79.
[310] J.P. Wong, H. Yang, K.L. Blasetti, G. Schnell, J. Conley, L.N. Schofield, Liposome delivery of ciprofloxacin against intracellular Francisella tularensis infection, Journal of Controlled Release 92 (3) (2003) 265–273, https://doi.org/10.1016/s0168-3659(03)00358-4. From NLM Medline).
[311] C. Haworth, A. Wanner, J. Froehlich, T. O'Neal, A. Davis, I. Gonda, A. O'Donnell, Inhaled liposomal ciprofloxacin in patients with bronchiectasis and chronic *Pseudomonas aeruginosa* infection: results from two parallel phase III trials (ORBIT-3 and-4), in: B14. Clinical Trials across Pulmonary Disease, American Thoracic Society, 2017. A7604-A7604.

[312] D.L. MacLeod, J.F. Prescott, The use of liposomally-entrapped gentamicin in the treatment of bovine *Staphylococcus aureus* mastitis, Canadian Journal of Veterinary Research 52 (4) (1988) 445–450 (From NLM Medline).
[313] C. Beaulac, S. Sachetelli, J. Lagace, In-vitro bactericidal efficacy of sub-MIC concentrations of liposome-encapsulated antibiotic against gram-negative and gram-positive bacteria, Journal of Antimicrobial Chemotherapy 41 (1) (1998) 35–41, https://doi.org/10.1093/jac/41.1.35. From NLM Medline).
[314] S. Sachetelli, H. Khalil, T. Chen, C. Beaulac, S. Sénéchal, J. Lagacé, Demonstration of a fusion mechanism between a fluid bactericidal liposomal formulation and bacterial cells, Biochimica et Biophysica Acta (BBA) - Biomembranes 1463 (2) (2000) 254–266.
[315] P. Dissaya, Z. Li, I.Z. Li, Z. Li, Z. Li, O. Sage, A. Santosh, O. Marygorret, S.V. Kenneth, H. Chun-Ming, et al., Bacterial toxin-triggered drug release from gold nanoparticle-stabilized liposomes for the treatment of bacterial infection, Journal of the American Chemical Society (2011), https://doi.org/10.1021/ja111110e.
[316] V.V. Mody, R. Siwale, A. Singh, H.R. Mody, Introduction to metallic nanoparticles, Journal of Pharmacy and BioAllied Sciences 2 (4) (2010) 282–289, https://doi.org/10.4103/0975-7406.72127 (From NLM PubMed-not-MEDLINE).
[317] S. Stankic, S. Suman, F. Haque, J. Vidic, Pure and multi metal oxide nanoparticles: synthesis, antibacterial and cytotoxic properties, Journal of Nanobiotechnology 14 (1) (2016) 73, https://doi.org/10.1186/s12951-016-0225-6. From NLM Medline).
[318] P.K. Jain, M.A. El-Sayed, Universal scaling of plasmon coupling in metal nanostructures: extension from particle pairs to nanoshells, Nano Letters 7 (9) (2007) 2854–2858, https://doi.org/10.1021/nl071496m. From NLM Medline).
[319] S. Gurunathan, J.W. Han, D.N. Kwon, J.H. Kim, Enhanced antibacterial and anti-biofilm activities of silver nanoparticles against Gram-negative and Gram-positive bacteria, Nanoscale Research Letters 9 (1) (2014) 373, https://doi.org/10.1186/1556-276X-9-373. From NLM PubMed-not-MEDLINE).
[320] S. Gurunathan, J.W. Han, J.H. Park, E. Kim, Y.J. Choi, D.N. Kwon, J.H. Kim, Reduced graphene oxide-silver nanoparticle nanocomposite: a potential anticancer nanotherapy, International Journal of Nanomedicine 10 (2015) 6257–6276, https://doi.org/10.2147/IJN.S92449. From NLM Medline).
[321] X. Wang, D. Wang, H. Lu, X. Wang, X. Wang, J. Su, G. Xia, Strategies to promote the journey of nanoparticles against biofilm-associated infections, Small (2024) e2305988, https://doi.org/10.1002/smll.202305988. From NLM Publisher).
[322] M. Antonelli, G. De Pascale, V.M. Ranieri, P. Pelaia, R. Tufano, O. Piazza, A. Zangrillo, A. Ferrario, A. De Gaetano, E. Guaglianone, et al., Comparison of triple-lumen central venous catheters impregnated with silver nanoparticles (AgTive(R)) vs conventional catheters in intensive care unit patients, Journal of Hospital Infection 82 (2) (2012) 101–107, https://doi.org/10.1016/j.jhin.2012.07.010. From NLM Medline).
[323] J. Li, D. Guo, X. Wang, H. Wang, H. Jiang, B. Chen, The photodynamic effect of different size ZnO nanoparticles on cancer cell proliferation

in vitro, Nanoscale Research Letters 5 (6) (2010) 1063–1071, https://doi.org/10.1007/s11671-010-9603-4. From NLM PubMed-not-MEDLINE).
[324] W. He, H.K. Kim, W.G. Warner, D. Melka, J.H. Callahan, J.J. Yin, Photogenerated charge carriers and reactive oxygen species in ZnO/Au hybrid nanostructures with enhanced photocatalytic and antibacterial activity, Journal of the American Chemical Society 136 (2) (2014) 750–757, https://doi.org/10.1021/ja410800y. From NLM Medline).
[325] H. Xiang, Y. Chen, Energy-converting nanomedicine, Small (2019), https://doi.org/10.1002/smll.201805339 articles.
[326] Y. Liu, J. He, K. Yang, C. Yi, Y. Liu, L. Nie, N.M. Khashab, X. Chen, Z. Nie, Folding up of gold nanoparticle strings into plasmonic vesicles for enhanced photoacoustic imaging, Angewandte Chemie International Edition in English 54 (52) (2015) 15809–15812, https://doi.org/10.1002/anie.201508616. From NLM Medline).
[327] A.C. Anselmo, S. Mitragotri, A review of clinical translation of inorganic nanoparticles, The AAPS Journal 17 (5) (2015) 1041–1054, https://doi.org/10.1208/s12248-015-9780-2. From NLM Medline).
[328] A.C. Anselmo, S. Mitragotri, Nanoparticles in the clinic, Bioengineering & Translational Medicine 1 (1) (2016) 10–29, https://doi.org/10.1002/btm2.10003 (From NLM PubMed-not-MEDLINE).
[329] B.S. Spinowitz, M.H. Schwenk, P.M. Jacobs, W.K. Bolton, M.R. Kaplan, C. Charytan, M. Galler, The safety and efficacy of ferumoxytol therapy in anemic chronic kidney disease patients, Kidney International 68 (4) (2005) 1801–1807, https://doi.org/10.1111/j.1523-1755.2005.00598.x. From NLM Medline).
[330] B.S. Spinowitz, A.T. Kausz, J. Baptista, S.D. Noble, R. Sothinathan, M.V. Bernardo, L. Brenner, B.J. Pereira, Ferumoxytol for treating iron deficiency anemia in CKD, Journal of the American Society of Nephrology 19 (8) (2008) 1599–1605, https://doi.org/10.1681/ASN.2007101156. From NLM Medline).
[331] D. Pantarotto, C.D. Partidos, J. Hoebeke, F. Brown, E. Kramer, J.P. Briand, S. Muller, M. Prato, A. Bianco, Immunization with peptide-functionalized carbon nanotubes enhances virus-specific neutralizing antibody responses, Chemical Biology 10 (10) (2003) 961–966, https://doi.org/10.1016/j.chembiol.2003.09.011. From NLM Medline).
[332] B. Fadeel, A.E. Garcia-Bennett, Better safe than sorry: understanding the toxicological properties of inorganic nanoparticles manufactured for biomedical applications, Advanced Drug Delivery Reviews 62 (3) (2010) 362–374, https://doi.org/10.1016/j.addr.2009.11.008. From NLM Medline).
[333] C. Lamprecht, I. Liashkovich, V. Neves, J. Danzberger, E. Heister, M. Rangl, H.M. Coley, J. McFadden, E. Flahaut, H.J. Gruber, et al., AFM imaging of functionalized carbon nanotubes on biological membranes, Nanotechnology 20 (43) (2009) 434001, https://doi.org/10.1088/0957-4484/20/43/434001. From NLM Medline).
[334] A. Surendiran, S. Sandhiya, S.C. Pradhan, C. Adithan, Novel applications of nanotechnology in medicine, Indian Journal of Medical Research 130 (6) (2009) 689–701 (From NLM Medline).
[335] J.J. Richardson, F. Caruso, Nanomedicine toward 2040, Article, Nano Letters 20 (3) (2020) 1481–1482, https://doi.org/10.1021/acs.nanolett.0c00620. From NLM Medline).
[336] Jop de Vrieze, Suspicions grow that nanoparticles in Pfizer's COVID-19 vaccine trigger rare allergic reactions, Science 10 (10.1126) (2020).

[337] A. Diaz, Boston Health Care Worker Who Experienced Reaction to Moderna Coronavirus Vaccine Has History of Allergies, CNN health, 2020. https://edition.cnn.com/2020/12/25/health/boston-health-care-worker-allergic-reaction-moderna-coronavirus-vaccine/index.html.

[338] A.V. Singh, P. Laux, A. Luch, C. Sudrik, S. Wiehr, A.M. Wild, G. Santomauro, J. Bill, M. Sitti, Review of emerging concepts in nanotoxicology: opportunities and challenges for safer nanomaterial design, Toxicology Mechanisms and Methods 29 (5) (2019) 378–387, https://doi.org/10.1080/15376516.2019.1566425. From NLM Medline).

[339] H. Langauer-Lewowicka, K. Pawlas, Nanoparticles, nanotechnology—potential environmental and occupational hazards, Medycyna Srodowiskowa 17 (2) (2014) 7–14.

[340] Y. Zhao, X. Jiang, Multiple strategies to activate gold nanoparticles as antibiotics, Nanoscale 5 (18) (2013) 8340–8350, https://doi.org/10.1039/c3nr01990j. From NLM Medline).

[341] P.J. Finley, R. Norton, C. Austin, A. Mitchell, S. Zank, P. Durham, Unprecedented silver resistance in clinically isolated enterobacteriaceae: major implications for burn and wound management, Antimicrobial Agents and Chemotherapy 59 (8) (2015) 4734–4741, https://doi.org/10.1128/AAC.00026-15. From NLM Medline).

[342] C.H.N. Barros, S. Fulaz, D. Stanisic, L. Tasic, Biogenic nanosilver against multidrug-resistant bacteria (MDRB), Antibiotics 7 (3) (2018), https://doi.org/10.3390/antibiotics7030069. From NLM PubMed-not-MEDLINE).

[343] J.L. Graves Jr., M. Tajkarimi, Q. Cunningham, A. Campbell, H. Nonga, S.H. Harrison, J.E. Barrick, Rapid evolution of silver nanoparticle resistance in *Escherichia coli*, Frontiers in Genetics 6 (2015) 42, https://doi.org/10.3389/fgene.2015.00042. From NLM PubMed-not-MEDLINE).

[344] A. Panacek, L. Kvitek, M. Smekalova, R. Vecerova, M. Kolar, M. Roderova, F. Dycka, M. Sebela, R. Prucek, O. Tomanec, et al., Bacterial resistance to silver nanoparticles and how to overcome it, Nature Nanotechnology 13 (1) (2018) 65–71, https://doi.org/10.1038/s41565-017-0013-y. From NLM Medline).

[345] M.G. Bianchetti, G.D. Simonetti, A. Bettinelli, Body fluids and salt metabolism - Part I, Italian Journal of Pediatrics 35 (1) (2009) 36, https://doi.org/10.1186/1824-7288-35-36. From NLM PubMed-not-MEDLINE).

[346] J.J. Aguilera-Correa, A. Conde, M.A. Arenas, J.J. de-Damborenea, M. Marin, A.L. Doadrio, J. Esteban, Bactericidal activity of the Ti-13Nb-13Zr alloy against different species of bacteria related with implant infection, Biomedical Materials 12 (4) (2017) 045022, https://doi.org/10.1088/1748-605X/aa770c. From NLM Medline).

[347] L. Ding, Z. Liu, M.O. Aggrey, C. Li, J. Chen, L. Tong, Nanotoxicity: the toxicity research progress of metal and metal-containing nanoparticles, Mini Reviews in Medicinal Chemistry 15 (7) (2015) 529–542, https://doi.org/10.2174/1389557515071504241043334. From NLM Medline).

[348] D.M. Tobin, Modelling infectious disease to support human health, Disease Models & Mechanisms (2022), https://doi.org/10.1242/dmm.049824 articles.

[349] D.M. Musher, R.J. Arasaratnam, Contributions of animal studies to the understanding of infectious diseases, Clinical Infectious Diseases: An Official Publication of the Infectious Diseases Society of America (2022), https://doi.org/10.1093/cid/ciab844. Articles.

[350] I.A. Bakker-Woudenberg, A.F. Lokerse, M.T. ten Kate, J.W. Mouton, M.C. Woodle, G. Storm, Liposomes with prolonged blood circulation and selective localization in Klebsiella pneumoniae-infected lung tissue, The Journal of Infectious Diseases 168 (1) (1993) 164–171, https://doi.org/10.1093/infdis/168.1.164. From NLM Medline).
[351] S.E. Blutt, M.K. Estes, Organoid models for infectious disease, Annual Review of Medicine (2021), https://doi.org/10.1146/annurev-med-042320-023055. Articles.
[352] M.A. Tutty, G. Vella, A. Prina-Mello, Pre-clinical 2D and 3D toxicity response to a panel of nanomaterials; comparative assessment of NBM-induced liver toxicity, Drug delivery and translational research (2022), https://doi.org/10.1007/s13346-022-01170-1. Articles.
[353] S.L. Mitchell, E.E. Carlson, Tiny things with enormous impact: nanotechnology in the fight against infectious disease, ACS Infectious Diseases 4 (10) (2018) 1432–1435, https://doi.org/10.1021/acsinfecdis.8b00138. From NLM Medline).
[354] P.E. Williams, H.M. Crauwels, E.D. Basstanie, Formulation and pharmacology of long-acting rilpivirine, Current Opinion in HIV and AIDS 10 (4) (2015) 233–238, https://doi.org/10.1097/COH.0000000000000164. From NLM Medline).
[355] J. McMillan, A. Szlachetka, L. Slack, B. Sillman, B. Lamberty, B. Morsey, S. Callen, N. Gautam, Y. Alnouti, B. Edagwa, et al., Pharmacokinetics of a long-acting nanoformulated dolutegravir prodrug in rhesus macaques, Antimicrobial Agents and Chemotherapy 62 (1) (2018), https://doi.org/10.1128/AAC.01316-17. From NLM Medline).
[356] E. Wistrand-Yuen, M. Knopp, K. Hjort, S. Koskiniemi, O.G. Berg, D.I. Andersson, Evolution of high-level resistance during low-level antibiotic exposure, Nature Communications 9 (1) (2018) 1599, https://doi.org/10.1038/s41467-018-04059-1. From NLM Medline).
[357] K. Bruynesteyn, V. Gant, C. McKenzie, T. Pagliuca, C. Poynton, R.N. Kumar, J.P. Jansen, A cost-effectiveness analysis of caspofungin vs. liposomal amphotericin B for treatment of suspected fungal infections in the UK, Article, European Journal of Haematology 78 (6) (2007) 532–539, https://doi.org/10.1111/j.1600-0609.2007.00850.x. From NLM Medline).
[358] D. Al-Badriyeh, D. Liew, K. Stewart, D.C. Kong, Economic impact of caspofungin as compared with liposomal amphotericin B for empirical therapy in febrile neutropenia in Australia, Article, Journal of Antimicrobial Chemotherapy 63 (6) (2009) 1276–1285, https://doi.org/10.1093/jac/dkp119. From NLM Medline).
[359] S. Naik, J. Lundberg, R. Kumar, J. Sjolin, J.P. Jansen, Economic evaluation of caspofungin versus liposomal amphotericin B for empirical antifungal therapy in patients with persistent fever and neutropenia in Sweden, Article, Scandinavian Journal of Infectious Diseases 43 (6–7) (2011) 504–514, https://doi.org/10.3109/00365548.2011.556145. From NLM Medline).
[360] G. Bozzuto, A. Molinari, Liposomes as nanomedical devices, International Journal of Nanomedicine 10 (2015) 975–999, https://doi.org/10.2147/IJN.S68861. From NLM Medline).
[361] D. Mishra, N. Jain, V. Rajoriya, A.K. Jain, Glycyrrhizin conjugated chitosan nanoparticles for hepatocyte-targeted delivery of lamivudine, Article, Journal of Pharmacy and Pharmacology 66 (8) (2014) 1082–1093, https://doi.org/10.1111/jphp.12235. From NLM Medline).

[362] R. Bosetti, W. Marneffe, L. Vereeck, Assessing the need for quality-adjusted cost-effectiveness studies of nanotechnological cancer therapies, Article, Nanomedicine 8 (3) (2013) 487–497, https://doi.org/10.2217/nnm.13.15. From NLM Medline).
[363] J.A. Jackman, J. Lee, N.-J. Cho, Nanomedicine for infectious disease applications: innovation towards broad-spectrum treatment of viral infections, Small (2015), https://doi.org/10.1002/smll.201500854 articles.

Index

'*Note:* Page numbers followed by "f" indicate figures and "t" indicate tables.'

Printed and bound by CPI Group (UK) Ltd, Croydon, CR0 4YY
05/09/2024
01032133-0002